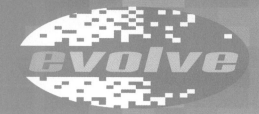

The Latest *Evolution* in Learning.

Evolve provides online access to free learning resources and activities designed specifically for the textbook you are using in your class. The resources will provide you with information that enhances the material covered in the book and much more.

Visit the Web address listed below to start your learning evolution today!

▶▶ **LOGIN:** *http://evolve.elsevier.com/Buck/certification/*

Evolve Student Learning Resources for Buck: *The Certification Step: 2004 Physician Coding Exam Review Guide* offers the following features:

- **Study Tips**
  Thoughts and advice from the author to help medical coding students.

- **Medical Coding in the News**
  The latest developments in the world of coding, updated quarterly.

- **WebLinks**
  Links to places of interest on the web specific to your classroom needs.

- **Links to Related Products**
  See what else Elsevier has to offer in your specific field of interest.

Think outside the book... evolve.

copy

P. 226

(p. 247)
248
249
⋆ 250

Combination Code
Uncertain Cond,
impending or Threatened

The
Certification Step

2004 Physician Coding Exam
Review Guide

The Certification Step

2004 Physician Coding Exam
Review Guide

Carol J. Buck, MS, CPC

Program Director, Retired
Medical Secretary Programs
Northwest Technical College
East Grand Forks, Minnesota

with 45 illustrations

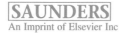
SAUNDERS
An Imprint of Elsevier Inc

SAUNDERS
An Imprint of Elsevier Inc

11830 Westline Industrial Drive
St. Louis, Missouri 63146

The Certification Step: 2004 Physician Coding Exam Review Guide   ISBN 0-7216-0209-6

NOTICE

Medical Coding is an ever-changing field. Standard safety precautions must be followed, but as new research and clinical experience broaden our knowledge, changes in treatment and drug therapy may become necessary or appropriate. Readers are advised to check the most current product information provided by the manufacturer of each drug to be administered to verify the recommended dose, the method and duration of administration, and contraindications. It is the responsibility of the licensed prescriber, relying on experience and knowledge of the patient, to determine dosages and the best treatment for each individual patient. Neither the publisher nor the author assumes any liability for any injury and/or damage to persons or property arising from this publication.

Library of Congress Cataloging-in-Publication Data

Buck, Carol J.
    The certification step : 2004 physician coding exam review guide / Carol J. Buck
    p. ; cm.
    Includes index.
    ISBN 0-7216-0209-6 (alk paper)
    1. Nosology—Code numbers—Examinations, questions, etc.   I. Title.
[DNLM: 1. Classification—Examination Questions.   2. Terminology—Examination Questions. WB 18.2 B922c 2004]
RB115.B824 2004
616'.001'2—dc22   2003058660

Acquisitions Editor: Susan Cole
Developmental Editor: Beth LoGiudice
Publishing Services Manager: Pat Joiner
Project Manager: Rachel E. Dowell
Senior Designer: Mark A. Oberkrom

Printed in the United States of America
Last digit is the print number: 9 8 7 6 5 4 3 2 1

Dedication

To coding instructors, who each day strive to enhance the lives of their students and provide the next generation of knowledgeable medical coders.

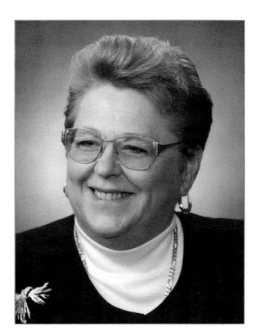

Carol J. Buck

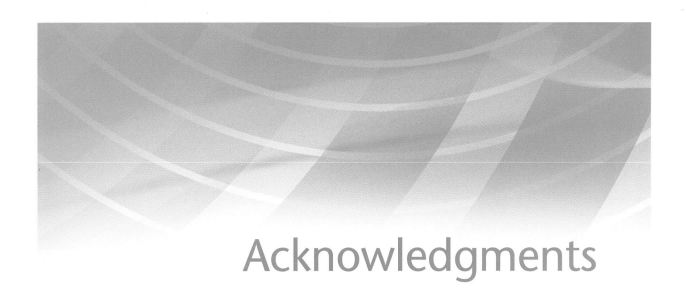

Acknowledgments

There are so many, many that participated in the development of this text and only through the effort of all the team members has it been possible to publish this text. **Jackie Grass,** who lent her technical coding knowledge and enthusiasm to this project. **Jody Klitz,** who spent endless hours ensuring this material was correct. **Marilyn Rasmussen,** who provided her coding skills to this task with great determination. **Mary Lazareus** and **Betty Nelson,** both provided technical support by reviewing the examinations. **Loraine Barge** and **Carol Enz,** who both spent endless hours keying in the material. **Sue Moe,** whose exceptional knowledge of medical terminology improved the terminology material.

    Sally Schrefer, Executive Vice President, Nursing and Health Professions, who possesses great listening skills and the ability to ensure the publication of high-quality educational materials. **Andrew Allen,** Publishing Director, Health Professions, who sees the bigger picture and shares the vision. **Adrianne Cochran,** Executive Editor, who is always ready and willing to venture into uncharted territories with the greatest of enthusiasm. **Susan Cole,** Acquisitions Editor, who guided this project to completion with her steady hand. **Beth LoGiudice,** Developmental Editor, who has performed minor miracles daily during the development of this text. **Rachel Dowell,** Project Manager, who ensured that we all completed our work on time. The employees of Elsevier have participated in the publication of this text and demonstrated the highest levels of professionalism and competence.

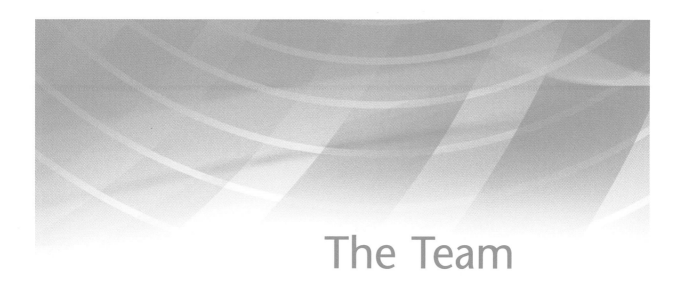

The Team

Data Entry Specialist, **Loraine Barge**
Data Entry Specialist, **Carol Ensz**
Coding Specialist, **Jody Klitz**
Coding Specialist, **Mary Lazareus**
Coding Specialist, **Betty Nelson**
Coding Specialist, **Marilyn Rasmussen**
Terminology Specialist, **Sue Moe**
Student Coder, **Barb Maslack**

Technical Collaborator
Jacqueline Grass, MA, CPC
Reimbursement and Coding
Altru Clinic
Grand Forks, North Dakota

About the CD-ROM

The companion CD-ROM included in the back of this review guide contains valuable software to assist you with your preparation for the physician coding certification examination. It includes a timed and scored 150-question practice exam, modeled after the actual certification exams, that contains three major sections of 50 questions. The exam is designed to be taken twice—once as a pre-exam and once as a post-exam. The Pre-Exam must be completed at the start of your study, and the Post-Exam should be taken after your study is complete. By comparing the results of both exam modes, you can see your improvement after using the review guide.

SUMMARY SCREEN

When using the program, the Summary screen serves as home base. Here you can find information relating to your progress and performance in different exam sections and subject areas. From this screen, you can choose an exam mode, submit an exam section, check your progress, or review your results.

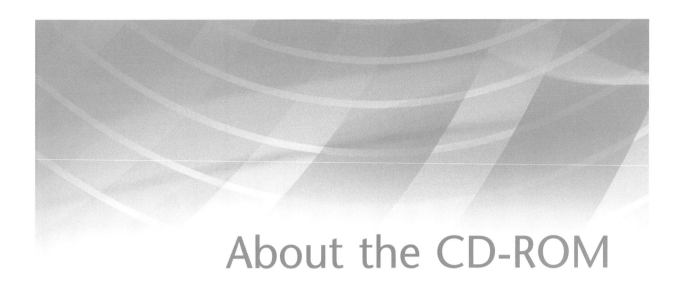

Summary Screen

In addition to displaying your scores for completed sections and tracking the total elapsed time, this screen also shows the answered, unanswered, and flagged questions in each subsection. You can return to the Summary screen at any point while taking or reviewing an exam, and all information related to your answers and position is saved.

TAKING THE EXAM

While taking the exam, click on the letter of your answer choice, and the answer will be highlighted in red. You can also use the corresponding letter keys and arrows on the keyboard to answer and navigate. The exam screen displays the current question number, which doubles a pull-down menu that allows you to jump to any question in the current section. Additionally, the Flag button at the bottom of the screen allows you to mark questions for later reference.

REVIEWING YOUR RESULTS

Once you have taken both exam modes, you have the option to review all the exam questions with rationales, even the ones you answered correctly. The correct answer is shown for each question, and a rationale is given for each answer option. You can also compare your results on the Pre- and Post-Exams by viewing the bar graph or printing out a score sheet.

TUTORIAL MODE

For extra practice a Tutorial mode is available after you have completed and submitted the Pre-Exam. You can create short, customizable quizzes by choosing a small number of questions in different subject areas. The quizzes are not scored, but rationales are given for each answer choice to help you study.

Additional instructions and help files are included on the CD-ROM to assist you in using the software.

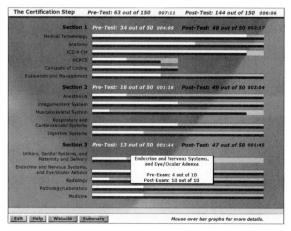

Review Graph

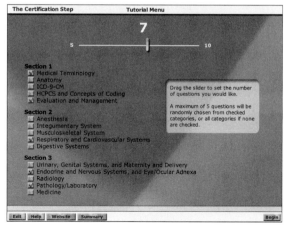

Tutorial Menu

Contents

The
Certification Step

2004 Physician Coding Exam
Review Guide

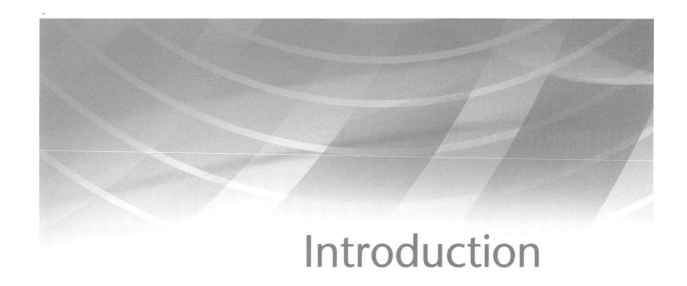

Introduction

This review was developed to help you as you prepare for your certification examination. First, congratulations on your initiative. Preparing for a certification examination can seem like a daunting and formidable task. You have already taken the first and hardest step: you have made a commitment. Your steely determination and organizational skills are your best tools as you organize to complete this exciting journey successfully.

This text has been developed to serve as a tool in your preparation for the outpatient (physician-based) certification examination. There are two outpatient, physician-based coding certifications: **CCS-P** (Certified Coding Specialist—Physician-based) and **CPC** (Certified Professional Coder). The American Health Information Management Association (AHIMA) offers the CCS-P, and the American Academy of Professional Coders offers the CPC. Although the formats of the examinations are different, the commonality is that both assess your medical coding ability. Regardless of which examination you take, you will have to know how to assign medical codes to patient services and diagnoses. This textbook is focused on providing you with that coding practice as well as anatomy, terminology, reimbursement, and coding concepts in preparation for the CPC.

This text is divided into:
- Success Strategies
- Unit I Anatomy and Terminology
- Unit II Reimbursement Issues
- Unit III Overview of CPT, ICD-9-CM, and HCPCS Coding
- Unit IV Examinations
- Appendix A, Official Guidelines for Coding and Reporting
- Appendix B, Medical Terminology
- Appendix C, Combining Forms
- Appendix D, Prefixes
- Appendix E, Suffixes

- Appendix F, Abbreviations
- Appendix G, Further Text References

Appendices B-F are combined lists of Medical Terminology, Combining Forms, Prefixes, and Suffixes used within Unit I, Anatomy and Terminology.

The material in this review features the following:

- Comprehensive guide in outline format
- Photos and drawings to illustrate key points
- Practice Examination (CD)—150 questions
- Final Examination (text)—150 questions

My personal best wishes to you as prepare for your certification. You can do this!

Our goals can only be reached through a vehicle of a plan, in which we must fervently believe, and upon which we must vigorously act. There is no other route to success.

Stephen A. Brennen

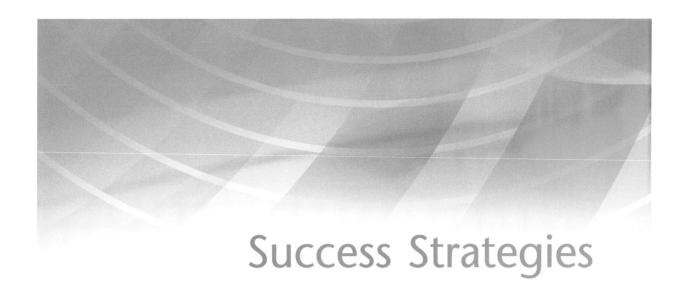

Success Strategies

How do you prepare for a certification examination? The answers to that question are as varied as the persons preparing for it. Each person comes to the preparation with different educational, coding, and personal experiences. Therefore, each must develop a plan that meets his or her individual needs and preferences. Success Strategies will help you to develop your individual plan.

CERTIFICATION EXAMINATIONS

- The CCS-P certification examination consists of Part I (60 multiple-choice questions) and Part II (21 medical records cases). The 60-multiple choice questions cover documentation, CPT, ICD-9-CM, HCPCS, reimbursement, and data quality. The examination is administered over 5 hours.
- The CPC certification examination consists of Section 1, 2, and 3 covering medical terminology, anatomy, CPT, ICD-9-CM, HCPCS, and coding concepts. The examination is administered over 5 hours.

Date and Location

Although every journey begins with the first step, you have to know where you are going to make a plan to get there.

- Choose the **date and location** for taking the certification examination. The certifying organizations' web sites contain detailed information about the examination sites and dates.
- The American Academy of Professional Coders has an Examination Packet that can be downloaded from their website at www.aapc.com or sent for by contacting:
  American Academy of Professional Coders
  309 West 700 South
  Salt Lake City, UT 84101
  Telephone: 800-626-2633

- The AAPC Candidate Handbook can be downloaded from the their website at www.ahima.org or send for by contacting:
  American Health Information Management Association
  Attn: CCS/CCS-P Examination
  233 North Michigan Avenue, Suite 2150
  Chicago, IL 60601-5800
  Telephone: 312-233-1100
- After you have obtained the examination materials, read all the information carefully. Review all competencies outlined in the material to ensure that your study plan contains strategies to address each of these competencies.
- The questions within this textbook are not the same questions that are in the certification examinations, but the skill and knowledge that you gain through analysis, coding, and recall will increase your ability to be successful on examination day.
- The certification organization's handbook will indicate the coding specifics. For example, the levels of the evaluation and management key components (history, examination, and medical decision making complexity) are stated in the certification questions so you will not be required to assign the levels.

MANAGING YOUR TIME

Role strain! That is what you get when you have so many different roles in your life and you cannot find time for all of them! Know that feeling? Are you a daughter/son, mother/father, wife/husband, student, friend, worker, volunteer, hobbyist—the list is endless. Each takes time from your schedule, and somehow you now need to fit into the role of successful learner. Because you have only 24 hours in your day, being a successful learner requires a time-balancing act. Maybe you will have to be satisfied with dust bunnies under your bed, dishes in your kitchen sink, or fewer visits with your friends. Whatever you have to do to juggle the time around to give yourself ample time to devote to this important task of examination preparation, you must do and make a plan for in advance; otherwise, life just takes over and you find you do not have adequate study time.

If you are planning a big event in your life—moving, a trip, and so on, think about postponing it until after the examination. Your focus right now has to be on yourself. Make your motto **"It's All About Me!"** Sounds self-centered, I know, and most likely very different from who you are, but just this once, you need to carve out the time you need to accomplish this important goal. This time is for yourself. Make it happen for yourself. Move everything you can out of the way, focus on this preparation, and give this preparation your best effort.

SCHEDULE

Each person has an individual learning style. The coding profession seems to attract those most influenced by logic and facts. The best way for a logical and factual person to learn is to problem-solve and apply the information. Hands-on practice is how you will build your skill and confidence for the examination.

- Choose a location to be your Study Central.
- Gather into Study Central the following study resources
  - Certification packet or handbook from the certifying organization
  - CPT, current edition
  - ICD-9-CM, current edition
  - HCPCS, current edition

- Official Guidelines for Coding and Reporting (Appendix A)
- Medical dictionary
- Coding textbooks, professional journals, and magazines
- Terminology, anatomy, or pathology text, as needed
- See Appendix G for Further Text References

Make Study Central your special place where you can get away from all other responsibilities. Make it a quiet, calm get away, even if it is a corner of your bedroom. In this quiet place have a comfortable chair, adequate lighting, supplies, and sufficient desktop surface to use all your coding books. This is your place to focus all your attention on preparation for the examination, without distractions.

- Plan your **schedule** from now until the certification examination using a calendar. Make weekly goals so that you have definite tasks to accomplish each week and you can check the tasks off—a great feeling of accomplishment comes from being able to check off a task. In this way, you can see your progress on your countdown to success.

- Choose a specific **time** each day or several times a week when you are going to study and mark them on your calendar. Make this commitment in writing. After each study session, you should check off that date on the calendar as a visual reminder that you are sticking to your plan and are one step closer to your goal.

- You should plan your study time in advance, know what you are going to be studying the next session, and **be prepared** for that upcoming study session. This will greatly increase the amount of material you are able to cover during the session. At the end of each session, decide what you are going to study next session and ensure that you have all the material and references you will need readily available. At the end of each session, you should be ready for the next study session.

- Your plan should include those areas where you know you will need improvement. For example, when is the last time you read, not referenced or reviewed, but really read, the CPT Anesthesia Guidelines? You probably do not code anesthesia services often, if ever, and as such are not familiar with the information in these guidelines. That is an area of improvement, and your plan should include a thorough reading of all the CPT section guidelines.

- **DO THIS BEFORE YOU BEGIN YOUR STUDY: Assess** your strengths and weaknesses. By making this assessment, you will know where to concentrate your efforts and where to focus your study schedule. You know those areas where you already have strong skills and knowledge and will not need to spend as much time preparing in these areas. The **Practice Examination** is a 150-question examination that you can use as a tool to assess your current skill level. This examination should be taken before you begin your study and then again immediately after you have completed your entire study schedule. Do not analyze the questions by reviewing the rationales provided in the Practice Examination; rather, wait until after you have completed your studies and have taken this same examination a second time. If you review the rationales after the first time you take the examination, you will know the answers too well to provide a valid comparison between examinations. See Unit IV of this textbook for further directions on the Practice Examination.

- After you have completed your course of study, take the Practice Examination again. You should plan to cover the examination in the same amount of time as will be given for the certification examination you are going to take. Compare your scores to those from the first time you took this examination. Note the areas where you did not demonstrate sufficient skills and knowledge.

- Develop a **second plan** to improve the specific areas where you believe you need further study.

- You are now ready to take the **Final Examination** that is located in this text. Take the examination in the same amount of time that will be allocated for the certification examination. It is best if you do this final in one sitting, thereby mimicking the actual examination. If your schedule does not allow for taking the examination in one sitting, plan to take it in several sessions, but always keep track of the time used to ensure that you take the examination in the same amount time allowed for the official examination. Learning to work within the time allocated is part of the skill you are developing. Remember the certification examinations assess not only your coding knowledge but also your efficiency in completing the test within the allocated time.

USING THIS TEXT

- **Unit I** is a review of the anatomy and terminology by organ systems designed to provide you with a quick review of that organ system. In addition, there is a list of combining forms, prefixes, suffixes, and abbreviations that are often used in that organ system. At the end of each organ system, there is a quiz that will give you an opportunity to assess your knowledge.
- **Unit II** is a review of reimbursement issues and terminology. A quiz is located at the end of the unit to assess your knowledge.
- **Unit III** is a review of CPT, HCPCS, and ICD-9-CM. The CPT and ICD-9-CM material follows the order of the manuals. There is no quiz at the end of this unit because you will be applying this material in the Practice Examination and in the Final Examination.
- **Unit IV** contains the examinations. The Practice Examination is a 150-question examination located on the **CD** and is to be taken twice—once before you begin your study and the second time after you have completed your study. You should allow 5 hours (300 minutes) to complete the Practice Examination because this is the amount of time you will have for the certification review. The CD stores your score from your Practice Examination and compares the results from the first and second time you took the examination; so you can see not only your score on each section but also the improvement from the first to the second examination. The Final Examination is also a 150-question, paper and pencil examination that is located in the text, and you should allow 5 hours (300 minutes) to complete the examination. Both examinations are divided into the following sections:
  - **Section 1—50 questions**
    - Medical Terminology (10)
    - Anatomy (10)
    - ICD-9-CM (10)
    - HCPCS (5)
    - Concepts of Coding (5)
    - Evaluation and Management (10)
  - **Section 2—50 questions**
    - Anesthesia (10)
    - Integumentary System (10)
    - Musculoskeletal System (10)
    - Respiratory and Cardiovascular Systems (10)
    - Digestive System (10)
  - **Section 3—50 questions**
    - Urinary, Male Genital, Female Genital Systems, and Maternity Care and Delivery (10)

  ▪ Endocrine and Nervous Systems, and Eye/Ocular Adnexa (10)
  ▪ Radiology (10)
  ▪ Pathology/Laboratory (10)
  ▪ Medicine (10)

There are many ways you could use this text. However you decide to prepare, you should take the examination before you begin your study to ensure that you develop a study plan that includes time and activities that will increase your knowledge in those areas where your test scores indicate areas of weakness. You could then take the units in the order they are presented, or you may want to review the anatomy and terminology for a body system and then review the CPT material for that body system. There is no one set way to approach the use of this text because each individual will have a personal learning style and preferences that will direct how the material is used. Your skills may be very strong in one or more coding or knowledge areas, and you will want to delete those areas from your individual study plan.

   This text is not meant to be the only study source, but only one tool of many that you will use. For example, if your terminology skills need a complete overhaul, this brief overview in this text may not meet your needs. You may want to supplement this text with a terminology text and an in-depth study of terminology.

- **Appendices** are a resource for you as you prepare your study plan.
  ○ **Appendix A,** Official Guidelines for Coding and Reporting, is the rules for use of ICD-9-CM codes and will be referenced in Unit III when reviewing the use of ICD-9-CM codes.
  ○ **Appendix B,** Medical Terminology, is a complete alphabetic list of all the medical terms listed in the Medical Terminology portion of the organ system reviews used in Unit I.
  ○ **Appendix C,** Combining Forms, is a complete alphabetic list of the combining forms used in Unit I.
  ○ **Appendix D,** Prefixes, is a complete alphabetic list of the prefixes used in Unit I.
  ○ **Appendix E,** Suffixes, is a complete alphabetic list of the suffixes used in Unit I.
  ○ **Appendix F,** Abbreviations, is a complete list of the abbreviations referenced in Unit I.
  ○ **Appendix G,** Further Text References, is a list of texts that you may want to obtain to supplement your study plan.

DAY BEFORE THE EXAMINATION

- No cramming! Your study time is now over, and cramming the day before the test is not a good idea because it just increases your anxiety level. This day is your day to prepare yourself. Do some things you enjoy this day. Take your mind off the examination. Pamper yourself: you deserve it.
- Prepare pencils (no. 2), erasers, picture identification, CPT, ICD-9-CM, HCPCS code books if necessary for your specific examination, and examination admission card.
- You cannot have excessive writing, sticky notes, labels, etc. in your code books. Check the examination packet to ensure that your books meet the specifications identified by the testing organization.
- If allowed, take bottled water and snacks because the day is long.
- Review the certification packet information one last time to ensure that you have all the required material.

- Listen to the weather and traffic reports. Plan your route to the examination site. If it is in a new location, drive to the location before the big day.
- Eat a light supper and get to bed early. Set the alarm in plenty of time to arrive at the site early. It is a good idea to have a friend or family member give you an early wake-up call to ensure that you do not oversleep.

DAY OF THE EXAMINATION

- Wear comfortable clothes and be prepared for any room temperature. A short-sleeved shirt with a sweater is a good plan. Dress in layers so you can ensure that you will be comfortable in any environment.
- Take a watch with you.
- Eat a good breakfast. Avoid caffeine because it initially stimulates you, but in the long run will decrease your concentration.
- Arrive early. The doors are locked to those who arrive late. This is a day to be early.
- Ensure that you have the correct room for your examination. Often there are several examinations being administered at one time, so be certain you are in the correct room for your examination.

THE CERTIFICATION EXAMINATION

You are ready for this! You have planned your work and have worked your plan. Now it is time to reap the rewards for all that hard work.

- Choose a good location in which to sit. Choose a location that will not get a lot of traffic from those leaving the room.
- Place all your supplies on the table.
- Someone will distribute the examination after the general directions have been given to the group.
- Take several deep breaths before you begin to help relax you.
- Quickly review the entire examination. Note the location of the halfway mark. This will help you to keep on schedule.
- Some prefer to take the parts of the examination out of order, taking those questions they are most confident of first. Others prefer to start at the beginning and work through all questions in order. The approach that you use will depend on your individual test-taking style.
- When you come to a question for which you are unsure of the answer, you may wish to skip over and come back to all those ones you were unsure of at the end of the examination, depending on the time available. Or you may want to attempt each question and mark those you are unsure of to return to when you have finished the entire examination. Again, the approach you will use depends on your individual style. If you mark questions to return to and are using a scan sheet on which to enter your answers, be certain that you return and remove the erasure marks because these tests are machine-scanned and those stray pencil marks can give inaccurate responses. You will receive your score back only, not the test or the answer sheet; so if your stray pencil marks give inaccurate responses, you will have no way to fix those mistakes.
- Read the directions. This may sound too simple, but many persons do not completely read the directions, only to find that the directions gave specific directions about what or what not to code on a certain case (for example, "code only this certain portion of the procedure"). Yet the choices for answers included the full coding of the case as a selection; if you did not read all the directions, you would choose the response with codes for all the items listed in the report. For

example, the question may have directed you to code the service only, not the diagnosis, and yet one of the choices would be the correct service and diagnosis codes, which of course would be an incorrect answer based on the directions. So read all of the directions.

- Your speed and accuracy are being tested. You do not have time to labor over each question for a long time if you intend to complete all the questions. Read the directions, read the question, put down your best assessment of the answer, and then move on to the next question. Place a light mark by the question about which you have doubts.
- Words such as *always, every, never,* and *all* generally indicate broad terms that, with true/false questions, usually indicate a false question.
- If you do not know the answer to the question, try eliminating those that you know are incorrect first and then select that answer that seems more likely to be correct.
- Judge the time as you are moving through the examination. Keep assessing whether you are making sufficient progress or whether you can slow down or need to speed up.
- Answer all questions. Even if you have to guess quickly, at least fill in an answer. The best situation is that you answer all questions and have time left over to go back over the questions about which you are in doubt.
- Erase all stray pencil marks on your test. Be neat with your work; neatness makes a difference when the machine scores your test.
- Be certain to carefully complete the information sheet that accompanies the examination. This sheet will include your name, address, and other information that ensures that your test results are accurately recorded.
- Use every minute of the test time, but it is not a good idea to begin second-guessing yourself. Do not return to those questions for which you did not have serious doubts about the correct answer. Usually, your first answer is the best.
- When the time is finished, hand in your examination, and pat yourself on the back! You have done an excellent job. Now it is time to go get a good supper and a good night's sleep.

DAYS AFTER THE EXAMINATION

- You will miss the preparation! Okay, maybe not miss it exactly, but your life will be different now without that constant preparation.
- Relax and await the results in confidence. You have done your best. That is always good enough!
- Be proud of yourself; this was no small undertaking, and you did it.

UNIT I

Anatomy and Terminology

INTEGUMENTARY SYSTEM

The skin and accessory organs (nails, hair, and glands)

Layers (Figure 1-1)

Epidermis: outermost layer

Basal layer deepest region of epidermis (stratum germinativum)

Stratum corneum is the outermost layer of epidermis

Dermis: middle layer, also known as corium, meaning true skin

Two layers of stratum

Subcutaneous Tissue or Hypodermis: innermost layer contains fat tissue

Nails

- Keratin plates covering the dorsal surface of each finger and toe
- Lunula—semilunar or half-moon, white area at base of nail plate
- Cuticle, narrow band of epidermis at base and sides of nail
- Paronychia, soft tissue around nail border

Glands

- Sebaceous glands located in dermal layer
  Secrete sebum, which lubricates skin and hair
- Sweat glands (sudoriferous) originate in dermis and extend up through epidermis
  Openings are pores

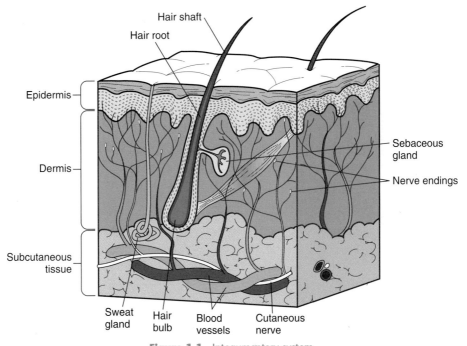

Figure 1-1 Integumentary system.

COMBINING FORMS

1.	aden/o	gland
2.	albin/o	white
3.	adip/o	fat
4.	aut/o	self
5.	bi/o	life
6.	cauter/o	burn
7.	crypt/o	hidden
8.	cutane/o	skin
9.	cyan/o	blue
10.	derm/o	skin
11.	eosin/o	rosy
12.	erythem/o	red
13.	erythr/o	red
14.	heter/o	different
15.	hidr/o	sweat
16.	ichthy/o	dry/scaly
17.	jaund/o	yellow
18.	kerat/o	hard
19.	lip/o	fat
20.	lute/o	yellow
21.	melan/o	black
22.	myc/o	fungus
23.	necr/o	death
24.	onych/o	nail
25.	pachy/o	thick
26.	pil/o	hair
27.	poli/o	gray
28.	rhytid/o	wrinkle
29.	rube/o	red
30.	seb/o	sebum/oil
31.	staphyl/o	clusters
32.	steat/o	fat
33.	strept/o	twisted chain
34.	trich/o	hair
35.	ungu/o	nail

36. xanth/o   yellow

37. xer/o   dry

PREFIXES

1. epi-   on/upon
2. hyper-   over
3. hypo-   under
4. intra-   within
5. para-   beside
6. per-   through
7. sub-   under

SUFFIXES

1. -coccus   spherical bacterium
2. -ectomy   removal
3. -ia   condition
4. -malacia   softening
5. -opsy   view of
6. -plasty   surgical repair
7. -rrhea   discharge
8. -tome   an instrument to cut
9. -tomy   to cut

MEDICAL ABBREVIATIONS

1. bx   biopsy
2. ca   cancer
3. derm   dermatology
4. I&D   incision and drainage
5. subcu, subq   subcutaneous

MEDICAL TERMS

Adipose   Fatty

Albinism   Lack of color pigment

Allograft   Homograft, same species graft

Alopecia   Condition in which hair falls out

Anhidrosis   Deficiency of sweat

Autograft   From patient's own body

Biopsy   Removal of a small piece of living tissue for diagnostic purposes

Causalgia	Burning pain
Collagen	Protein substance of skin
Debridement	Cleansing of or removal of dead tissue from a wound
Delayed flap	Pedicle of skin with blood supply that is separated from origin over time
Dermabrasion	Planing of the skin by means of sander, brush, or sandpaper
Dermatologist	Physician who treats conditions of the skin
Dermatoplasty	Surgical repair of skin
Electrocautery	Cauterization by means of heated instrument
Epidermolysis	Loosening of the epidermis
Epidermomycosis	Superficial fungal infection
Epithelium	Surface covering of internal and external organs of the body
Erythema	Redness of skin
Escharotomy	Surgical incision into necrotic (dead) tissue
Fissure	Cleft or groove
Free full-thickness graft	Graft of epidermis and dermis that is completely removed from donor area
Furuncle	Nodule in the skin caused by staphylococci entering through hair follicle
Homograft	Allograft, same species graft
Ichthyosis	Skin disorder characterized by scaling
Incise	To cut into
Island pedicle flap	Contains a single artery and vein that remains attached to origin temporarily or permanently
Leukoderma	Depigmentation of skin
Leukoplakia	White patch on mucous membrane
Lipocyte	Fat cell
Lipoma	Fatty tumor
Melanin	Dark pigment of skin
Melanoma	Tumor of epidermis, malignant and black in color
Mohs surgery or Mohs micrographic surgery	Removal of skin cancer in layers by a surgeon who also acts as a pathologist during surgery
Muscle flap	Transfer of muscle from origin to recipient site
Neurovascular flap	Contains artery, vein, and nerve
Pedicle	Tumor on a stem
Pilosebaceous	Pertains to hair follicles and sebaceous glands
Sebaceous gland	Secretes sebum
Seborrhea	Excess sebum secretion
Sebum	Oily substance
Split-thickness graft	All epidermis and some of dermis

Steatoma	Fat mass in sebaceous gland
Stratified	Layered
Stratum (strata)	Layer
Subungual	Beneath the nail
Xanthoma	Tumor composed of cells containing lipid material, yellow in color
Xenograft	Different species graft
Xeroderma	Dry, discolored, scaly skin

INTEGUMENTARY SYSTEM QUIZ

1. This is the outermost layer of the skin:
    a. basal
    b. dermis
    c. epidermis
    d. subcutaneous

2. Which of the following is NOT a part of the skin or accessory organs:
    a. hair
    b. sebaceous gland
    c. nail
    d. haversian

3. This prefix means beside:
    a. para-
    b. intra-
    c. per-
    d. epi-

4. This combining form means hair:
    a. xanth/o
    b. trich/o
    c. ichthy/o
    d. kerat/o

5. The lunula is the:
    a. narrow band of epidermis at the base of the nail
    b. opening of the pores
    c. outermost layer of epidermis
    d. white area at the base of the nail plate

6. The subcutaneous tissue is also known as:
    a. dermal
    b. adipose
    c. hypodermis
    d. stratum corneum

7. Which of the follow combining forms does not refer to a color:
    a. cyan/o
    b. jaund/o
    c. eosin/o
    d. pachy/o

8. This medical term mean the surgical incision into dead tissue:
    a. onychomycosis
    b. escharotomy
    c. keratotomy
    d. curettage

9. This suffix means surgical repair:
   a. -opsy
   b. -rrhea
   c. -plasty
   d. -tome

10. The soft tissue around the nail border is the:
    a. cuticle
    b. lunula
    c. paronychium
    d. corium

MUSCULOSKELETAL SYSTEM

Skeletal System

- Comprises 206 bones, cartilage, and ligaments
- Provides organ protection, movement, framework, stores calcium, hematopoiesis (formation of blood cells)

Classification of Bones

Long bones (tubular)

- Length exceeds width of bone
- Broad at ends, such as the thigh, lower leg, upper arm, and lower arm

Short bones (cuboidal)

- Larger ends on short bones, such as the wrist and ankle

Flat

- Thin
- Cover body parts, such as the skull

Irregular

- Varied shapes, such as zygoma of face or vertebrae

Sesamoid

- Rounded
- Found near joint, such as the kneecap

Structure

Long Bones (Figure 1-2)

Diaphysis: shaft
Epiphysis: ends
- Articular cartilage covers epiphyses and serves as a cushion
Epiphyseal line or plate: growth plate that disappears when fully grown
Metaphysis: flared portion of bone near epiphyseal plate
Periosteum: outer covering
Cortical or compact bone: hard bone beneath periosteum mainly found in shaft
- Medullary cavity contains yellow marrow (fatty bone marrow)
Cancellous bones: spongy or trabecular
- Contains red bone marrow (blood cell development)

Two Skeletal Divisions

Axial

Appendicular

Axial Skeleton, 80

Skull (Figure 1-3)
Cranial
- Frontal (forehead)
- Parietal (sides and top)

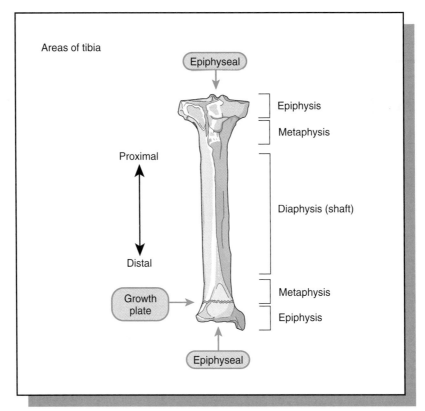

Figure 1-2 Structure of bones.

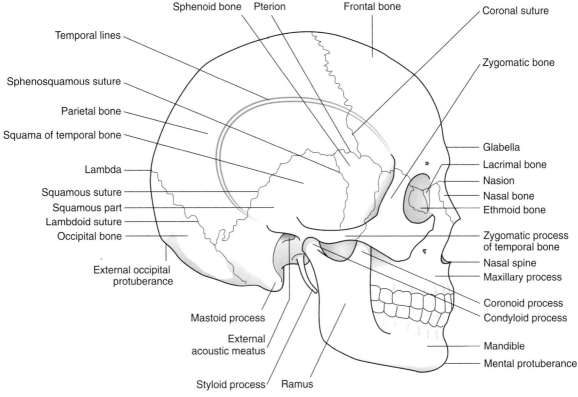

Figure 1-3 Lateral view of the skull.

- Temporal (lower sides)
- Occipital (posterior of cranium)
- Sphenoid (floor of cranium)
- Ethmoid (area between orbits and nasal cavity)
- Styloid process (below ear)
- Zygomatic process (cheek)

Ear bones (Figure 1-4)

- Malleus
- Incus
- Stapes

Face (Figure 1-5)

- Nasal (bridge of nose)
- Maxilla (upper jaw)
- Zygomatic (arch of cheekbone)
- Mandible (lower jawbone)
- Lacrimal (near orbits)
- Palate (separates oral and nasal cavities)
- Vomer (base, nasal septum)

Hyoid

- Supports tongue
- U shaped
- Attached by ligaments and muscles to larynx and skull

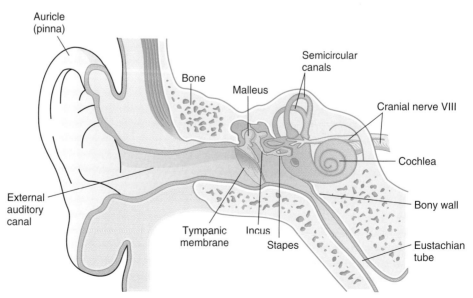

Figure 1-4   Structure of the ear and the three divisions of external, middle, and inner ear.

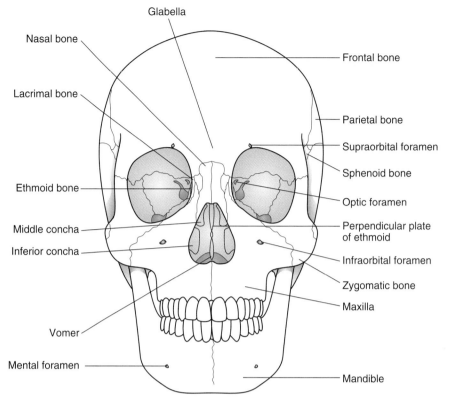

Glabella

Nasal bone

Frontal bone

Lacrimal bone

Parietal bone

Supraorbital foramen

Sphenoid bone

Ethmoid bone

Optic foramen

Middle concha

Perpendicular plate of ethmoid

Inferior concha

Infraorbital foramen

Zygomatic bone

Maxilla

Vomer

Mental foramen

Mandible

Figure 1-5   Frontal view of the skull.

Spine (Figure 1-6)

Cervical vertebra

C1-7

1st atlas (C1)

2nd axis (C2)

Thoracic vertebra (T1-12)

Lumbar vertebra (L1-5)

Sacrum

Coccyx

Thorax (Figure 1-7)

Ribs, 12 pairs

True ribs, 1-7

False ribs, 8-10

Floating ribs, 11 and 12

Sternum

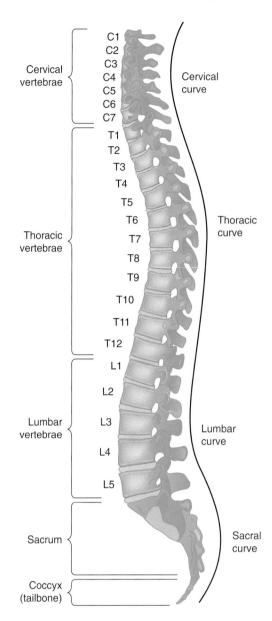

Figure 1-6 Anterior view of the vertebral column.

Cervical vertebrae

C1
C2
C3
C4
C5
C6
C7

Cervical curve

Thoracic vertebrae

T1
T2
T3
T4
T5
T6
T7
T8
T9
T10
T11
T12

Thoracic curve

Lumbar vertebrae

L1
L2
L3
L4
L5

Lumbar curve

Sacrum

Sacral curve

Coccyx (tailbone)

Appendicular Skeleton, 126 (Figure 1-8)

Lower extremities

Pelvis

Ilium (uppermost part) wing shaped
• Acetabulum, depression on lateral hip surface into which head of femur fits

Ischium (posterior part)

Pubis (anterior part)

Pubis symphysis (cartilage between pubic bones)

Femur (thighbone)

Trochanter (processes at neck of femur)

Head fits into the acetabulum

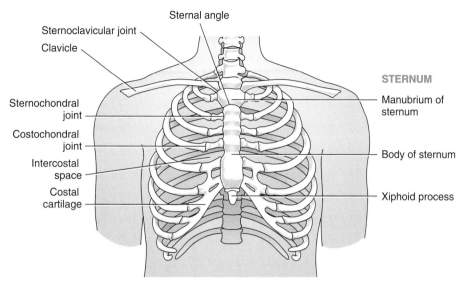

Figure 1-7   The thoracic cage.

Patella (kneecap)

Tibia (shinbone)

Fibula (smaller bone in lower leg)

Tarsal (ankle bone)

Calcaneus (heel bone)

Metatarsal (foot instep)

Phalanges (toes)

Lateral malleolus (lower part of fibula)

Medial malleolus (lower part of tibia)

Upper extremities

Clavicle (collarbone)

Scapula (shoulder bone)

Humerus (upper arm)

Radius (forearm, thumb side)

Ulna (forearm, little finger side)

Carpals (wrist)

Metacarpals (hand)

Phalanges (finger)

Olecranon (tip of elbow)

Joints (Reticulations)

Condyle, rounded ends of bones

Classified by degree of movement

Synarthroses (immovable)

Example: joint between cranial bones

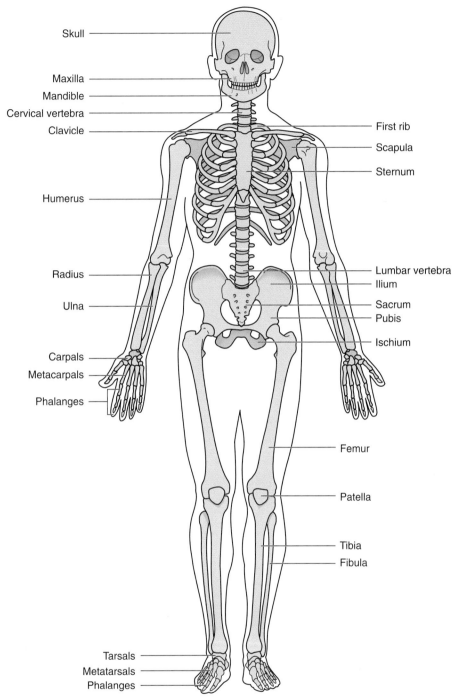

Skull

Maxilla

Mandible

Cervical vertebra

Clavicle

First rib

Scapula

Sternum

Humerus

Radius

Lumbar vertebra

Ilium

Ulna

Sacrum

Pubis

Ischium

Carpals

Metacarpals

Phalanges

Femur

Patella

Tibia

Fibula

Tarsals

Metatarsals

Phalanges

Figure 1-8 Skeletal system.

Amphiarthroses (slightly movable)

Example: intervertebral the joint between bodies of the vertebra

Diarthroses (considerably movable)

Types, hinge or ball and socket

Example: elbow

Bursa, sacs of synovial fluid located near joints

Muscular System

Functions

- Heat production
- Movement
- Posture
- Protection
- Shape

Muscle Tissue Types

Skeletal

Striated (cross stripes) (Figures 1-9 and 1-10)

Move body

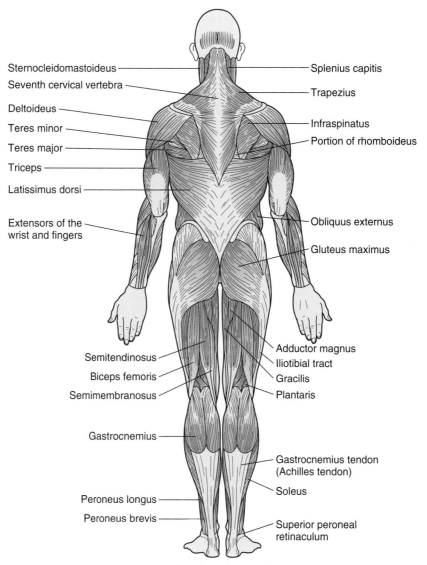

Sternocleidomastoideus

Seventh cervical vertebra

Deltoideus

Teres minor

Teres major

Triceps

Latissimus dorsi

Extensors of the
wrist and fingers

Splenius capitis

Trapezius

Infraspinatus

Portion of rhomboideus

Obliquus externus

Gluteus maximus

Semitendinosus

Biceps femoris

Semimembranosus

Adductor magnus

Iliotibial tract

Gracilis

Plantaris

Gastrocnemius

Gastrocnemius tendon
(Achilles tendon)

Soleus

Peroneus longus

Peroneus brevis

Superior peroneal
retinaculum

Figure 1-9   Muscular system, posterior view.

Voluntary

Attaches to bones
  - Most attach to two bones with a joint in between
  - Origin, point where muscle attaches to stationary bone
  - Insertion, where muscle attaches to movable bone
  - Body of muscle, main part of muscle

Cardiac/Heart Muscle

Striated

Involuntary

Moves blood by means of contractions

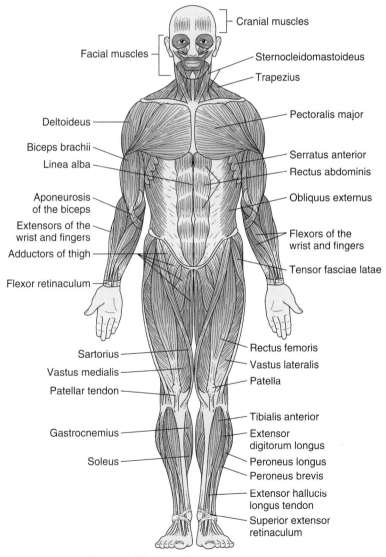

Figure 1-10 Muscular system, anterior view.

Smooth/Visceral

- Linings such as bowel, urethra, blood vessels
- Nonstriated
- Involuntary

Tendons Anchor Muscle to Bone

Ligaments anchor bones to bones

Muscle Action

Muscle Capabilities

- Stretch
- Contract
- Receive and respond to stimulus
- Returns to original shape and length

Muscle Movement

- Prime mover, responsible for movement
- Synergist, assist prime mover
- Antagonist, relaxes as prime mover and synergists contract, resulting in movement

Terms of Movement

- Flexion (bend)
- Extension (straighten)
- Abduction (away)
- Adduction (toward)
- Rotation (turn on axis)
- Circumduction (circular)
- Supination (upward)
- Pronation (downward)
- Hyperextension (overextension)
- Inversion (inward)
- Eversion (outward)

Names of Bones

Head and Neck

Facial
- Orbicularis oris (opens mouth)
- Zygomaticus (elevates corners of mouth)
- Orbicularis oculi (opens and closes eyelid)

Mastication (chewing)
- Masseter (used to chew)
- Temporal (closes jaw)

Sternocleidomastoid (rotates head and neck)

Trapezius (extends head)

Upper Extremities

Biceps (flexes elbow)

Triceps brachii (extends elbow)

Deltoid (abducts upper arm)

Latissimus dorsi (extends upper arm)

Pectoralis major (flexes upper arm)

Trunk

Abdominal

External oblique (compresses abdomen)

Internal oblique (compresses abdomen)

Transversus abdominis (compresses abdomen)

Rectus abdominis (flexes trunk)

Respiratory

Diaphragm (separates thorax from abdomen)

Intercostal (between ribs)

Lower Extremities

Thigh

Gluteus maximus (abducts thigh)

Abductor brevis (abducts thigh)

Iliopsoas (flexes thigh)

Hamstring (flexes lower leg)

Quadriceps (extends lower leg)

Sartorius (flexes and rotates leg)

Tibialis anterior (dorsiflexes foot)

Peroneus longus (everts foot)

Gastrocnemius (calf, with soleus flexes foot, also flexes knee)

Soleus (calf, flexes foot)

Achilles tendon (largest tendon)

COMBINING FORMS

1.	acetabul/o	hip socket
2.	ankyl/o	bent
3.	aponeur/o	tendon type
4.	arthr/o	joint
5.	burs/o	fluid-filled sac in a joint
6.	calc/o, calci/o	calcium
7.	carp/o	carpals (wrist bones)

8. chondr/o   cartilage
9. clavic/o, clavicul/o clavicle (collar bone)
10. cost/o: rib
11. crani/o   cranium (skull)
12. disk/o   intervertebral disk
13. femor/o   thighbone
14. fibul/o   fibula
15. humer/o   humerus (upper arm bone)
16. ili/o   ilium (upper pelvic bone)
17. isch/o   ischium (posterior pelvic bone)
18. kinesi/o   movement
19. kyph/o   hump
20. lamin/o   lamina
21. lord/o   curve
22. lumb/o   lower back
23. mandibul/o   mandible (lower jawbone)
24. maxill/o   maxilla (upper jawbone)
25. menisci/o   meniscus
26. metacarp/o   metacarpals (hand)
27. metatars/o   metatarsals (foot)
28. menisc/o   meniscus
29. myel/o   bone marrow
30. my/o, myos/o   muscle
31. olecran/o   olecranon (elbow)
32. orth/o   straight
33. oste/o   bone
34. patell/o   patella (kneecap)
35. pelv/i   pelvis (hip)
36. petr/o   stone
37. phalang/o   phalanges (finger or toe)
38. pub/o   pubis
39. rachi/o   spine
40. radi/o   radius (lower arm)
41. sacr/o   sacrum
42. scapul/o   scapular (shoulder)
43. scoli/o   bent
44. spondyl/o   vertebra

45.	stern/o	sternum (breast bone)
46.	synovi/o	synovial membrane
47.	tars/o	tarsal (ankle)
48.	ten/o	tendon
49.	tend/o	tendon (connective tissue)
50.	tendin/o	tendon (connective tissue)
51.	tibi/o	shin bone
52.	uln/o	ulna (lower arm bone)
53.	vertebr/o	vertebra

PREFIXES

1.	inter-	between
2.	supra-	above
3.	sym-	together
4.	syn-	together

SUFFIXES

1.	-asthenia	weakness
2.	-blast	embryonic
3.	-clast, -clasia, -clasis	break
4.	-desis	fusion
5.	-listhesis	slipping
6.	-malacia	softening
7.	-physis	to grow
8.	-porosis	passage
9.	-schisis	split
10.	-tome	instrument that cuts
11.	-tomy	incision

MEDICAL ABBREVIATIONS

1.	ACL	anterior cruciate ligament
2.	AKA	above-knee amputation
3.	BKA	below-knee amputation
4.	C1-C7	cervical vertebrae
5.	CTS	carpal tunnel syndrome
6.	fx	fracture
7.	L1-L5	lumbar vertebrae
8.	OA	osteoarthritis

9. RA	rheumatoid arthritis
10. T1-T12	thoracic vertebrae
11. TMJ	temporomandibular joint

MEDICAL TERMS

Articular	Pertains to a joint
Arthrocentesis	Injection and/or aspiration of joint
Arthrodesis	Surgical immobilization of a joint
Arthrography	Radiography of joint
Arthroplasty	Reshaping or reconstruction of a joint
Arthroscopy	Use of scope to view inside joint
Arthrotomy	Incision into a joint
Aspiration	Use of a needle and a syringe to withdraw fluid
Atrophy	Wasting away
Bunion	Hallux valgus, abnormal increase in size of metatarsal head that results in displacement of the great toe
Bursitis	Inflammation of bursa
Chondral	Referring to the cartilage
Closed fracture repair	Not surgically opened with/without manipulation and with/without traction
Closed treatment	Fracture site that is not surgically opened and visualized
Colles' fracture	Fracture at lower end of radius that displaces the bone posteriorly
Dislocation	Placement in a location other than the original location
Endoscopy	Inspection of body organs or cavities using a lighted scope that may be inserted through an existing opening or through a small incision
Fasciectomy	Removal of the band of fibrous tissue
Fissure	Groove
Fracture	Break in a bone
Ganglion	Knot
Internal/external fixation	Application of pins, wires, screws, placed externally or internally to immobilize a body part
Kyphosis	Humpback
Lamina	Flat plate
Ligament	Fibrous band of tissue that connects cartilage or bones
Lordosis	Anterior curve of spine
Lumbodynia	Pain in the lumbar area
Lysis	Releasing
Manipulation or reduction	Alignment of a fracture or joint dislocation to normal position

Open fracture repair	Surgical opening over or remotely opening of a fracture site
Osteoarthritis	Degenerative condition of articular cartilage
Osteoclast	Absorption or removal of bone
Osteotomy	Cutting into bone
Percutaneous	Through the skin
Percutaneous fracture repair	Repair of a fracture by means of pins and wires inserted through the fracture site
Percutaneous skeletal fixation	Considered neither open nor closed; the fracture is not visualized, but fixation is placed across the fracture site under x-ray imaging
Reduction	Replace to normal position
Scoliosis	Lateral curve of the spine
Skeletal traction	Application of pressure to bone by means of pins and/or wires inserted into the bone
Skin traction	Application of pressure to bone by means of tape applied to the skin
Spondylitis	Inflammation of vertebrae
Subluxation	Partial dislocation
Supination	Supine position
Synchondrosis	Union between two bones (connected by cartilage)
Tendon	Attaches a muscle to a bone
Tenodesis	Suturing of a tendon to a bone
Tenorrhaphy	Suture repair of tendon
Traction	Application of force to a limb
Trocar needle	Needle with a tube on the end; used to puncture and withdraw fluid from a cavity

MUSCULOSKELETAL SYSTEM QUIZ

1. Tubular is another name for these bones:
   a. short
   b. long
   c. flat
   d. irregular

2. These bones are found near joints:
   a. irregular
   b. flat
   c. sesamoid
   d. broad

3. The zygoma is an example of this type of bone:
   a. irregular
   b. flat
   c. sesamoid
   d. broad

4. The diaphysis is this part of the bone:
   a. end
   b. surface
   c. shaft
   d. marrow

5. Which is NOT a part of the cranium:
   a. condyle
   b. sphenoid
   c. ethmoid
   d. parietal

6. This is NOT an ear bone:
   a. malleus
   b. stapes
   c. incus
   d. styloid

7. This term describes the growth plate:
   a. endosteum
   b. epiphyseal
   c. metaphysis
   d. periosteum

8. This is a depression on the lateral hip surface into which the head of the femur fits:
   a. ilium
   b. ischium
   c. patella
   d. acetabulum

9. The tip of the elbow is the:
   a. olecranon
   b. trapezium
   c. humerus
   d. tarsal

10. This term describes an immovable joint:
    a. amphiarthroses
    b. diarthroses
    c. synarthroses
    d. ischium

RESPIRATORY SYSTEM

Supplies oxygen to body and helps clean body of waste
Two tracts (Figure 1-11)

Upper respiratory tract (nose, sinuses, pharynx, and larynx)

Lower respiratory tract (trachea, bronchial tree, and lungs)

Lined with specialized membranes
- Purifies air by trapping irritants
- Covered with cilia that move mucus upward

Upper Respiratory Tract (URT)

Nose

Sense of smell (olfactory)

Moistens and warms air

Nasal septum divides interior

Sinuses

Frontal

Ethmoid

Maxillary

Sphenoidal

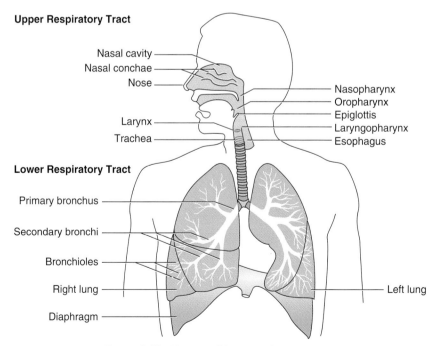

Figure 1-11 Upper and lower respiratory system.

Pharynx (Throat)

Passageway for both food and air

Nasopharynx contains adenoids

Oropharynx contains tonsils

Laryngopharynx leads to larynx

Larynx (Voice Box)

Contains vocal cords

Lower Respiratory Tract (LRT)

Trachea (Windpipe)

Mucus-lined tube with C-shaped cartilage rings to hold windpipe open

Air passageway

Bronchi

Trachea divides into branches—right branch and left branch

Branches divide into smaller bronchioles that are tipped with alveoli (air sacs that exchange gases)

Lungs

Covered by pleura

Cone-shaped organs

Base rests on diaphragm

Left lung contains two lobes

Right lung contains three lobes

Respiration

Inspiration—oxygen moves in

Expiration—carbon dioxide moves out

COMBINING FORMS

1. adenoid/o   adenoid
2. alveol/o   alveolus
3. atel/o   incomplete
4. bronch/o   bronchus
5. bronchi/o   bronchus
6. bronchiol/o   bronchiole
7. coni/o   dust
8. diaphragmat/o diaphragm

9.	epiglott/o	epiglottis
10.	laryng/o	larynx
11.	lob/o	lobe
12.	muc/o	mucus
13.	nas/o	nose
14.	rhin/o	nose
15.	orth/o	straight
16.	ox/i	oxygen
17.	oxy/o	oxygen
18.	pharyng/o	pharynx
19.	pleur/o	pleura
20.	pneum/o	lung/air
21.	pneumat/o	air
22.	pneumon/o	lung/air
23.	pulmon/o	lung
24.	py/o	pus
25.	sept/o	septum
26.	sinus/o	sinus
27.	spir/o	breath
28.	thorac/o	thorax
29.	tonsill/o	tonsil
30.	trache/o	trachea

PREFIXES

1.	a-	not
2.	an-	not
3.	endo-	within
4.	eu-	good
5.	pan-	all
6.	poly-	many

SUFFIXES

1.	-algia	pain
2.	-ar	pertaining to
3.	-ary	pertaining to
4.	-capnia	carbon dioxide
5.	-centesis	puncture to remove

6.	-dynia	pain
7.	-eal	pertaining to
8.	-ectasis	stretching
9.	-emia	blood
10.	-gram	record
11.	-graph	recording instrument
12.	-graphy	recording process
13.	-itis	inflammation
14.	-meter	measure
15.	-metry	measurement of
16.	-oxia	oxygen
17.	-pexy	fixation
18.	-phonia	sound
19.	-pnea	breathing
20.	-rrhgia	bursting of blood
21.	-scopy	to examine
22.	-spasm	contraction of muscle
23.	-stenosis	blockage, narrowing
24.	-stomy	opening
25.	-thorax	chest
26.	-tomy	cutting, incision

MEDICAL ABBREVIATIONS

1.	ABG	arterial blood gas
2.	AFB	acid-fast bacillus
3.	ARDS	adult respiratory distress syndrome
4.	BiPAP	bi-level positive airway pressure
5.	COPD	chronic obstructive pulmonary disease
6.	CPAP	continuous positive airway pressure
7.	DLCO	diffuse capacity of lungs for carbon monoxide
8.	FEF	forced expiratory flow
9.	FEV_1	forced expiratory volume in one second
10.	FEV_1:FVC	ratio of forced expiratory volume in one second to forced vital capacity ratio
11.	FRC	functional residual capacity
12.	FVC	forced vital capacity
13.	HHN	hand-held nebulizer

14.	IPAP	inspiratory positive airway pressure
15.	IRDS	idiopathic respiratory distress syndrome
16.	MDI	metered dose inhaler
17.	MVV	maximum voluntary ventilation
18.	PAWP	pulmonary artery wedge pressure
19.	PCWP	pulmonary capillary wedge pressure
20.	PEAP	positive end-airway pressure
21.	PEEP	positive end-expiratory pressure
22.	PFT	pulmonary function test
23.	PND	paroxysmal nocturnal dyspnea
24.	RDS	respiratory distress syndrome
25.	RV	respiratory volume
26.	RV:TLC	respiratory volume to total lung capacity ratio
27.	TLC	total lung capacity
28.	TLV	total lung volume
29.	URI	upper respiratory infection
30.	V/Q	ventilation/perfusion scan

MEDICAL TERMS

Ablation	Removal by cutting
Adenoidectomy	Removal of adenoids
Apnea	Stop breathing
Asphyxia	Lack of oxygen
Asthma	Shortage of breath caused by contraction of bronchi
Atelectasis	Incomplete expansion of lung, collapse
Auscultation	Listening to sounds, such as to lung sounds
Bacilli	Plural of bacillus, a rod-shaped bacteria
Bilobectomy	Surgical removal of two lobes of a lung
Bronchiole	Smaller division of bronchial tree
Bronchoplasty	Surgical repair of the bronchi
Bronchoscopy	Inspection of the bronchial tree using a bronchoscope
Catheter	Tube placed into the body to put fluid in or take fluid out
Cauterization	Destruction of tissue by the use of cautery
Cordectomy	Surgical removal of the vocal cord(s)
Crackle	Abnormal sound when breathing
Cyanosis	Bluish
Drainage	Free flow or withdrawal of fluids from a wound or cavity

Dysphonia	Speech impairment
Dyspnea	Shortage of breath
Emphysema	Air accumulated in organ or tissue
Epiglottidectomy	Excision of the covering of the larynx
Epistaxis	Nose bleed
Glottis	True vocal cords
Hemoptysis	Bloody sputum
Intramural	Within the organ wall
Intubation	Insertion of a tube
Laryngeal web	Congenital abnormality of connective tissue between the vocal cords
Laryngectomy	Surgical removal of the larynx
Laryngoplasty	Surgical repair of the larynx
Laryngoscope	Fiberoptic scope used to view the inside of the larynx
Laryngoscopy	Direct visualization and examination of the interior of larynx with a laryngoscope
Laryngotomy	Incision into the larynx
Lavage	Washing out of an organ
Lobectomy	Surgical excision of a lobe of the lung
Nasal button	Synthetic circular disk used to cover a hole in the nasal septum
Orthopnea	Difficulty in breathing, needing to be upright to breathe
Percussion	Tapping with sharp blows as a diagnostic technique
Pharyngolaryngectomy	Surgical removal of the pharynx and larynx
Pleura	Covers the lungs and lines the thoracic cavity
Pleurectomy	Surgical excision of the pleura
Pleuritis	Inflammation of the pleura
Pneumonocentesis	Surgical puncturing of a lung to withdraw fluid
Pneumonolysis	Surgical separation of the lung from the chest wall to allow the lung to collapse
Pneumonotomy	Incision of the lung
Rales	Coarse sound on inspiration, also known as crackle
Rhinoplasty	Surgical repair of nose
Rhinorrhea	Nasal mucous discharge
Segmentectomy	Surgical removal of a portion of a lung
Septoplasty	Surgical repair of the nasal septum
Sinusotomy	Surgical incision into a sinus
Spirometry	Measuring breathing capacity
Tachypnea	Quick, shallow breathing

Thoracentesis	Surgical puncture of the thoracic cavity, usually using a needle, to remove fluids
Thoracoplasty	Surgical procedure that removes rib(s) and thereby allows the collapse of a lung
Thoracoscopy	Use of a lighted endoscope to view the pleural spaces and thoracic cavity or to perform surgical procedures
Thoracostomy	Surgical incision into the chest wall and insertion of a chest tube
Thoracotomy	Surgical incision into the chest wall
Total pneumonectomy	Surgical removal of an entire lung
Tracheostomy	Creation of an opening into the trachea
Tracheotomy	Incision into the trachea
Transtracheal	Across the trachea

RESPIRATORY SYSTEM QUIZ

1. This is NOT a part of the lower respiratory tract:
   a. trachea
   b. larynx
   c. bronchi
   d. lungs

2. Another name for the voice box is:
   a. oropharynx
   b. pharynx
   c. laryngopharynx
   d. larynx

3. This is the windpipe:
   a. pharynx
   b. larynx
   c. trachea
   d. sphenoid

4. The interior of the nose is divided by the:
   a. septum
   b. sphenoid
   c. oropharynx
   d. apical

5. This combining form means incomplete:
   a. atel/o
   b. alveol/o
   c. ox/i
   d. pneumat/o

6. This prefix means breathe:
   a. py/o
   b. lob/o
   c. spir/o
   d. pleur/o

7. This prefix means all:
   a. a-
   b. an-
   c. pan-
   d. poly-

8. This abbreviation refers to a syndrome that involves difficulty in breathing:
   a. ABG
   b. ARDS
   c. BiPAP
   d. FEF

9. This abbreviation refers to the amount of air the patient can expel from the lungs in one second:
   a. PFT
   b. PND
   c. RDS
   d. FEV_1

10. This suffix means breathing:
   a. -stenosis
   b. -spasm
   c. -pexy
   d. -pnea

CARDIOVASCULAR SYSTEM

Consists of blood, blood vessels, and heart

Blood

Carries

Oxygen and nutrients to cells

Waste and carbon dioxide to kidneys, liver, and lungs

Hormones from endocrine system

Regulates

Temperature by circulating blood

Protection

White cells produce antibodies

Composed of Two Parts:

Liquid part (extracellular): plasma

Water 91%

Protein 1%, albumin, globulins, fibrinogen

Or 2%, ions, nutrients, waste products, gases, regulating substances

Formed part

Leukocytes (WBC)

Neutrophils

Lymphocytes

Monocytes

Eosinophils

Basophils

Erythrocytes (RBC)

Platelets/thrombocytes

Vessels

Function

To carry nutrients and oxygen (blood)

Types

Arteries (Figure 1-12)

Inner layer, endothelium

Lead away from heart

Branches are arterioles

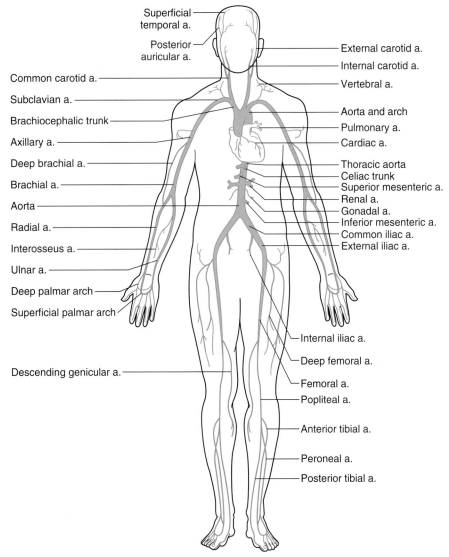

Figure 1-12   Arteries of the circulatory system.

Capillaries

Carries blood from arterioles to venules

Exchange vessels

Veins (Figure 1-13)

Carries blood to heart

Venules are small branches

Heart

Circulates blood

Four Chambers (Figure 1-14)

Two upper: right and left atria (singular atrium) receive blood

Two lower: right and left ventricles, discharge blood (pump)

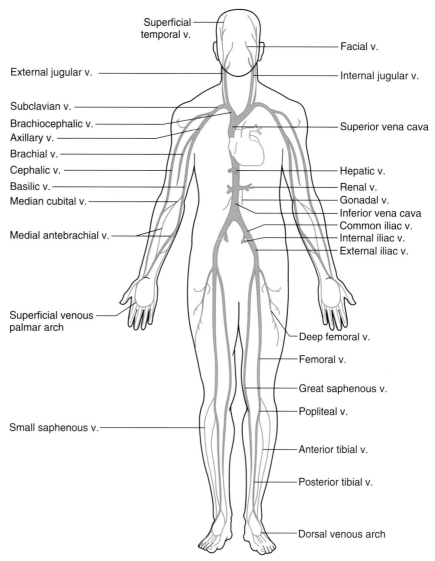

Figure 1-13 Veins of the circulatory system.

Chamber Walls

Composed of three layers

Endocardium: smooth inner layer
Myocardium: middle muscular layer
Epicardium: outer layer

Septa (Singular Septum)

Divides chambers

Interatrial septum: separates two upper chambers
Interventricular: separates two lower chambers

Pericardium

Sac that covers heart in two layers

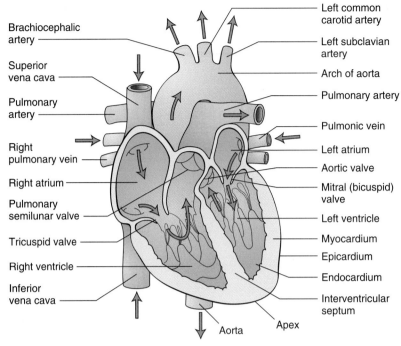

Figure 1-14   Internal view of the heart.

Parietal pericardium: outermost covering
Visceral pericardium: innermost (epicardium)
Pericardial cavity: contains fluid

Valves

Tricuspid: right atrium to left ventricle
Pulmonary: at entrance of pulmonary artery
Aortic: at entrance of aorta
Bicuspid (mitral): left atrium to left ventricle

Conduction System (Figure 1-15)

Sinoatrial node: SA node, nature's pacemaker sends impulses to atrioventricular node
Atrioventricular node: AV node, located on interatrial septum and sends impulses to bundle of His
Bundle of His: divides into right and left bundle branches in septum
Purkinje fibers: in walls of ventricles

Heartbeat

Two Phases

Diastole: relaxation
Systole: contraction

COMBINING FORMS

1. angi/o   vessel

2. aort/o   aorta

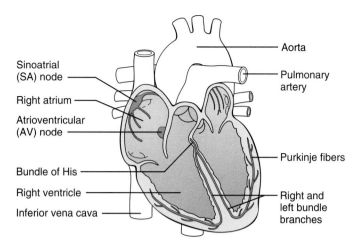

Sinoatrial (SA) node
Right atrium
Atrioventricular (AV) node
Bundle of His
Right ventricle
Inferior vena cava
Aorta
Pulmonary artery
Purkinje fibers
Right and left bundle branches

Figure 1-15   Electrical system of the heart.

3.	ar/o	plaque
4.	arter/o	artery
5.	arteri/o	artery
6.	atri/o	atrium
7.	brachi/o	arm
8.	cardi/o	heart
9.	cholester/o	cholesterol
10.	coron/o	heart
11.	cyano/cyan/o	blue
12.	myo/myx/o/muscul/o	muscle
13.	ox/o	oxygen
14.	pericardi/o	pericardium
15.	phleb/o	vein
16.	sphygm/o	pulse
17.	steth/o	chest
18.	thromb/o	clot
19.	valvul/o	valve
20.	valv/o	valve
21.	vascul/o	vessel
22.	vas/o	vessel
23.	ven/o	vein
24.	ventriculo/ventrcul/o	ventricle

PREFIXES

1.	a-	not
2.	an-	not

3.	bi-	two
4.	brady-	slow
5.	de-	lack of
6.	dys-	bad
7.	endo-	in
8.	hyper-	over
9.	hypo-	under
10.	inter-	between
11.	intra-	within
12.	meta-	change
13.	peri-	surrounding
14.	tachy-	fast
15.	tetra-	four
16.	tri-	three

SUFFIXES

1.	-dilation	widening, expanding
2.	-emia	blood
3.	-graphy	recording process
4.	-lysis	separation
5.	-megaly	enlargement
6.	-oma	tumor
7.	-osis	condition
8.	-plasty	repair
9.	-sclerosis	hardening
10.	-stenosis	blockage, narrowing
11.	-tomy	cutting into

MEDICAL ABBREVIATIONS

1.	ASCVD	arteriosclerotic cardiovascular disease
2.	ASD	atrial septal defect
3.	ASHD	arteriosclerotic heart disease
4.	AV	atrioventricular
5.	CABG	coronary artery bypass graft
6.	CHF	congestive heart failure
7.	CK	creatine kinase
8.	CPK	creatine phosphokinase
9.	CVI	cerebrovascular insufficiency

10.	DSE	dobutamine stress echocardiography
11.	HCVD	hypertensive cardiovascular disease
12.	LBBB	left bundle branch block
13.	LVH	left ventricular hypertrophy
14.	MAT	multifocal atrial tachycardia
15.	MI	myocardial infarction
16.	NSR	normal sinus rhythm
17.	PAC	premature atrial contraction
18.	PAT	paroxysmal atrial tachycardia
19.	PST/PSVT	paroxysmal supraventricular tachycardia
20.	PTCA	percutaneous transluminal coronary angioplasty
21.	PVC	premature ventricular contraction
22.	RBBB	right bundle branch block
23.	RSR	regular sinus rhythm
24.	RVH	right ventricular hypertrophy
25.	SVT	supraventricular tachycardia
26.	TEE	transesophageal echocardiography
27.	TST	treadmill stress test

MEDICAL TERMS

Anastomosis	Connection of two vessels
Aneurysm	Sac formed outside the vessel, artery, or heart
Angina	Sudden pain
Angiography	Radiography of the blood vessels
Angioplasty	Procedure in a vessel to dilate the vessel opening
Atherectomy	Removal of plaque by percutaneous method
Auscultation	Listening for sounds within the body
Bundle of His	Muscular cardiac fibers that provide the heart rhythm to the ventricles
Bypass	To go around
Cardiopulmonary	Refers to the heart and lungs
Cardiopulmonary bypass	Blood bypasses the heart through a heart-lung machine
Cardioverter-defibrillator	Surgically placed device that directs an electric current shock to the heart to restore rhythm
Circumflex	A coronary artery that circles the heart
Cutdown	Incision into a vessel for placement of a catheter
Edema	Swelling due to abnormal fluid collection in the tissue spaces
Electrode	Lead attached to a generator that carries the electric current from the generator to the atria or ventricles

Electrophysiology	Study of the electrical system of the heart, including study of arrhythmias
Embolectomy	Removal of blockage (embolism) from vessels
Endarterectomy	Incision into an artery to remove inner lining
Epicardial	Over the heart
False aneurysm	Sac of clotted blood that has completely destroyed the vessel and is being contained by the tissue that surrounds the vessel
Fistula	Abnormal opening from one area to another area or to the outside of the body
Hematoma	Mass of blood that forms outside the vessel
Hemolytic	Breakdown of red blood cells
Hypoxemia	Low level of oxygen in the blood
Hypoxia	Low level of oxygen in the tissue
Intracardiac	Inside the heart
Invasive	Entering the body, breaking skin
Noninvasive	Not entering the body, not breaking skin
Nuclear cardiology	Diagnostic specialty that uses radiologic procedures to aid in diagnosis of cardiologic conditions
Order	Shows subordination of one to another
Pericardiocentesis	Procedure in which a surgeon withdraws fluid from the pericardial space by means of a needle inserted percutaneously
Pericardium	Membranous sac enclosing heart and ends of great vessels
Swan Ganz catheter	A catheter that measures pressure in heart
Thoracostomy	Incision into the chest wall and insertion of a chest tube
Thromboendarterectomy	Procedure to remove plaque or clot formations from an artery by percutaneous method
Transvenous	Through a vein

CARDIOVASCULAR SYSTEM QUIZ

1. Carry blood to the heart:
   a. capillaries
   b. arteries
   c. arterioles
   d. veins

2. The relaxation phase of the heartbeat:
   a. diastole
   b. systole

3. Nature's pacemaker is this node:
   a. atrioventricular
   b. Bundle of His
   c. sinoatrial
   d. mitral

4. Node located on the interatrial septum:
   a. atrioventricular
   b. Bundle of His
   c. sinoatrial
   d. Purkinje

5. Which of the following is NOT one of the three layers of the chamber walls of the heart:
   a. endocardium
   b. myocardium
   c. epicardium
   d. pericardium

6. Divides the upper two chambers of the heart:
   a. intraventricular
   b. interatrial
   c. tricuspid
   d. myocardium

7. This is the valve between the right atrium and left ventricle:
   a. pulmonary
   b. aortic
   c. bicuspid
   d. tricuspid

8. The outer two-layer covering of the heart:
   a. pericardium
   b. parietal pericardium
   c. myocardium
   d. epicardium

9. These are the chambers that receive blood:
    a. right and left ventricle
    b. left ventricle and right atrium
    c. right atrium and right ventricle
    d. right and left atria

10. This combining form means plaque:
    a. atri/o
    b. brachi/o
    c. cyan/o
    d. ather/o

FEMALE GENITAL SYSTEM AND PREGNANCY

Terminology

Ovaries (pair): produce ovum (single female gamete), ova: plural; ovum: singular (Figure 1-16)

Fallopian Tubes: (uterine tubes or oviducts): ducts from ovary to uterus

Uterus (womb): muscular organ that holds embryo

Three layers:

Endometrium: inner mucosa
Myometrium: middle layer/muscle
Perimetrium/Uterine serosa: outer layer
    Cervix: lower narrow portion of uterus
    Fundus: the upper rounded part of the uterus

Vagina: tube from uterus to outside of body

Vulva: external genitalia
    Clitoris: erectile tissue
    Labia majora: outer lips of vagina
    Labia minor: inner lips of vagina
    Bartholin gland: glands on either side of vagina
    Hymen: membrane that covers entrance to vagina

Perineum: area between anus and vaginal orifice

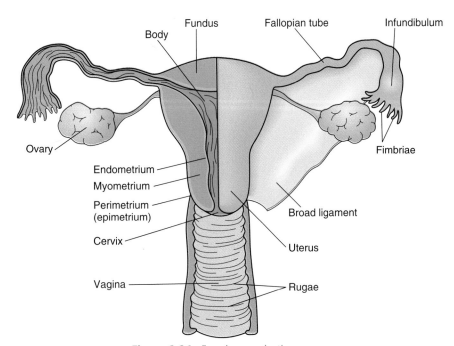

Figure 1-16 Female reproductive organs.

Accessory Organs (Figure 1-17)

Breasts: mammary glands

Composed of glandular tissue containing milk glands/lactiferous

In response to hormones, develop milk by means of lactiferous or milk ducts

Sinus cavities transfer milk to nipple

Nipple, surrounded by areola

Menstruation and Pregnancy

Proliferation Phase

Menstruation (Days 1-5): discharge of blood fluid containing endometrial cells, blood cells, and glandular secretions from endometrium

Endometrium repair (Days 6-12): begins by means of estrogen (hormone) and during which endometrium thickens and the ovum (egg) matures in graafian follicles

Secretory Phase

Ovulation (Days 13-14): occurs when the graafian follicles rupture and ovum travels down fallopian tube

Premenstruation (Days 15-28): a period of time in which graafian follicles fill with corpus luteum and secrete estrogen and progesterone to stimulate build up of uterine lining. If after 5 days no fertilization occurs, cycle repeats

Pregnancy

- Prenatal stage of development from fertilization to birth (39 weeks)
- Fertilized ovum or zygote develops in a double cavity: yolk sac (produces blood cells) and amniotic cavity (contains amniotic fluid)
- Embryo, fertilized ovum
- Fetus, unborn offspring, 9 weeks until birth

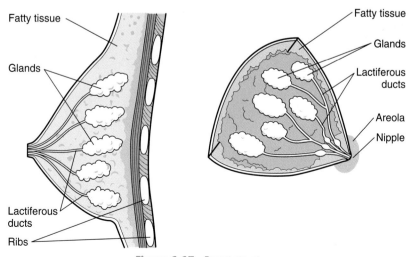

Figure 1-17 Breast structure.

Placenta Forms Within Uterine Wall and Produces Hormone Human Chorionic Gonadotropin (HCG)

- HCG stimulates corpus luteum to produce estrogen and progesterone for several months
- Placenta then produces hormones
- Expelled after delivery (afterbirth)

Gestation, Approximately 266 Days

- 280 days used when calculating Estimated Date of Delivery (EDD) or that time from last menstrual period (LMP)
- Three trimesters

First	LMP-12 weeks
Second	13-27 weeks
Third	28 weeks-EDD

COMBINING FORMS

1.	amni/o	amnion
2.	arche/o	first
3.	cephal/o	head
4.	cervic/o	cervix
5.	chori/o	chorion
6.	colp/o	vagina
7.	crypt/o	hidden
8.	culd/o	cul-de-sac
9.	episi/o	vulva
10.	fet/o	fetus
11.	galact/o	milk
12.	gynec/o	female
13.	gyn/o	female
14.	hymen/o	hymen
15.	hyster/o	uterus
16.	lact/o	milk
17.	lapar/o	abdominal wall
18.	mamm/o	breast
19.	mast/o	breast
20.	men/o	menstruation, month
21.	metr/o	uterus, measure
22.	metri/o	uterus
23.	my/o	muscle
24.	nat/a	birth

25. nati/i	birth
26. olig/o	few
27. oo/o	egg
28. oopho/o	ovary
29. ov/o	egg
30. ovari/o	ovary
31. ovul/o	ovulation
32. perine/o	perineum
33. peritone/o	peritoneum
34. salping/o	uterine tube
35. top/o	place
36. uter/o	uterus
37. vagin/o	vagina
38. vulv/o	vulva

PREFIXES

1. ante-	before
2. dys-	painful
3. ecto-	outside
4. endo-	within
5. extra-	outside
6. in-	in
7. intra-	within
8. multi-	many
9. neo-	new
10. nulli-	none
11. nulti-	none
12. post-	after
13. primi-	first
14. pseudo-	false
15. retro-	backwards
16. uni-	one

SUFFIXES

1. -arche	beginning
2. -cyesis	pregnancy
3. -gravida	pregnancy
4. -o/rrhexis	rupture

5. -para   woman who has given birth
6. -parous   to bear
7. -rrhea   discharge
8. -tocia   labor
9. -version   turning

MEDICAL ABBREVIATIONS

1. AFI   amniotic fluid index
2. AGA   appropriate for gestational age
3. ARM   artificial rupture of membrane
4. BPD   biparietal diameter
5. BPP   biophysical profile
6. BV   bacterial vaginosis
7. CHL   crown to heel length
8. CNM   certified nurse midwife
9. CPD   cephalopelvic disproportion
10. CPP   chronic pelvic pain
11. D&C   dilation and curettage
12. D&E   dilation and evacuation
13. DUB   dysfunctional uterine bleeding
14. ECC   endocervical curettage
15. EDC   estimated date of confinement
16. EDD   estimated date of delivery
17. EFM   electronic fetal monitoring
18. EFW   estimated fetal weight
19. EGA   estimated gestational age
20. EMC   endometrial curettage
21. ERT   estrogen replacement therapy
22. FAS   fetal alcohol syndrome
23. FHR   fetal heart rate
24. FSH   follicle-stimulating hormone
25. HPV   human papillomavirus
26. HSG   hysterosalpingogram
27. HSV   herpes simplex virus
28. IVF   in vitro fertilization
29. LEEP   loop electrosurgical excision procedure
30. LGA   large for gestational age

31. PID   pelvic inflammatory disease

32. PROM   premature rupture of membranes

33. SHG   sonohysterogram

34. SROM   spontaneous rupture of membrane

35. SUI   stress urinary incontinence

36. TAH   total abdominal hysterectomy

37. VBAC   vaginal birth after cesarean

MEDICAL TERMS

Abortion	Termination of pregnancy
Amniocentesis	Percutaneous aspiration of amniotic fluid
Amniotic sac	Fluid containing the fetus and amniotic fluid
Antepartum	Before childbirth
Cesarean	Surgical opening through abdominal wall for delivery
Chorionic villus sampling (CVS)	Biopsy of the outermost part of the placenta
Cordocentesis	Procedure to obtain a fetal blood sample; also called a percutaneous umbilical blood sampling
Curettage	Scraping of a cavity using a spoon-shaped instrument
Cystocele	Herniation of the bladder into the vagina
Delivery	Childbirth
Dilation	Expansion (of the cervix)
Ectopic	Pregnancy outside the uterus (i.e., in the fallopian tube)
Hysterectomy	Surgical removal of the uterus
Hysterorrhaphy	Suturing of the uterus
Hysteroscopy	Visualization of the canal and cavity of the uterus using a scope placed through the vagina
Introitus	Opening or entrance to the vagina from the uterus
Ligation	Binding or tying off, as in constricting the blood flow of a vessel or binding fallopian tubes for sterilization
Oophorectomy	Surgical removal of the ovary(ies)
Perineum	Area between the vulva and anus; also known as the pelvic floor
Placenta	An organism that connects the fetus and mother during pregnancy
Postpartum	After childbirth
Salpingectomy	Surgical removal of the uterine tube
Salpingostomy	Creation of a fistula into the uterine tube
Tocolysis	Repression of uterine contractions
Vesicovaginal fistula	Creation of a tube between the vagina and the bladder

FEMALE GENITAL SYSTEM AND PREGNANCY QUIZ

1. This is NOT one of the three layers of the uterus:
   a. perimetrium
   b. endometrium
   c. myometrium
   d. epimetrium

2. The lower portion of the uterus is the:
   a. cervix
   b. vagina
   c. perineum
   d. labia majora

3. The approximate gestation of a human fetus is:
   a. 266 days
   b. 276 days
   c. 290 days
   d. 292 days

4. The LMP is the:
   a. later maternity phase
   b. last menstrual period
   c. low metabolic pregnancy
   d. late menstruation phase

5. Name of the stage that describes the development of the fetus from fertilization to birth is the:
   a. postpartum
   b. antepartum
   c. prenatal
   d. natal

6. Which of the following correctly identifies the three trimesters of gestation:
   a. LMP-12 weeks, 13-27 weeks, 28-EDD
   b. LMP-14 weeks, 15-27 weeks, 28-EDD
   c. LMP-14 weeks, 15-28 weeks, 29-EDD
   d. LMP-11 weeks, 12-26 weeks, 27-EDD

7. Combining form means few:
   a. oopho/o
   b. olig/o
   c. nati/i
   d. top/o

8. Combining form means hidden:
   a. amni/o
   b. crypt/o
   c. chori/o
   d. fet/o

9. Suffix means the beginning:
   a. -cyesis
   b. -rrhea
   c. -arche
   d. -orrhexis

10. Prefix meaning within:
    a. ante-
    b. dys-
    c. ecto-
    d. endo-

MALE GENITAL SYSTEM

- Function, reproduction
- Structure, essential organs, and accessory organs (Figure 1-18)

Essential Organs

Testes (Gonads)

Produces sperm (male gamete)

Covered by tunica albuginea, located in scrotum

Produces testosterone

Vas Deferens

Is a tube

End of epididymis

Accessory Organs

- Ducts (carry sperm from testes to exterior), sex glands (produce solutions that mix with sperm), and external genitalia
- Seminal vesicles produce most seminal fluid
- Prostate gland produces some seminal fluid and activates sperm
- Bulbourethral gland (Cowper's glands) secretes a very small amount of seminal fluid
- External genitalia: penis and scrotum
    Penis contains three columns of erectile tissue: two corpora cavernosa and one spongiosum
    Scrotum encloses testes

COMBINING FORMS

1. andr/o   male
2. balan/o   glans penis

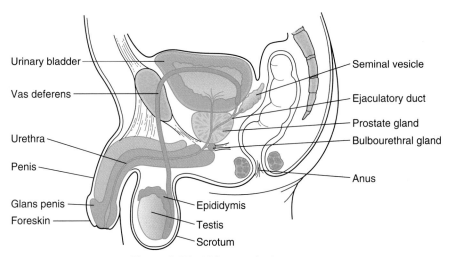

Figure 1-18   Male reproductive organs.

3.	epididym/o	epididymis
4.	orch/i	testicle
5.	orch/o	testicle
6.	orchi/o	testicle
7.	orchid/o	testicle
8.	prostat/o	prostate gland
9.	semin/i	semen
10.	sperm/o	sperm
11.	spermat/o	sperm
12.	test/o	testicle
13.	vas/o	vessel, vas deferens
14.	vesicul/o	seminal vesicles

SUFFIXES

1.	-one	hormone
2.	-pexy	fixation

MEDICAL ABBREVIATIONS

1.	BPH	benign prostatic hypertrophy
2.	PSA	prostate-specific antigen
3.	TURBT	transurethral resection of bladder tumor
4.	TURP	transurethral resection of prostate

MEDICAL TERMS

Cavernosa	Creation of a connection between the cavity of the penis and a vein
Cavernosography	Radiographic recording of a cavity, e.g., the pulmonary cavity or the main part of the penis
Cavernosometry	Measurement of the pressure in a cavity, e.g., the penis
Chordee	Condition resulting in the penis' being bent downward
Corpora cavernosa	The two cavities of the penis
Epididymectomy	Surgical removal of the epididymis
Epididymis	Tube located at the top of the testes that stores sperm
Epididymovasostomy	Creation of a new connection between the vas deferens and epididymis
Meatotomy	Surgical enlargement of the opening of the urinary meatus
Orchiectomy	Castration, removal of the testes
Orchiopexy	Surgical procedure to release undescended testis and fixate within the scrotum

Penoscrotal	Referring to the penis and scrotum
Plethysmography	Determining the changes in volume of an organ part or body
Priapism	Painful condition in which the penis is constantly erect
Prostatotomy	Incision into the prostate
Transurethral resection, prostate	Procedure performed through the urethra by means of a cystoscopy to remove part or all of the prostate
Tumescence	State of being swollen
Tunica vaginalis	Covering of testes
Varicocele	Swelling of a scrotal vein
Vas deferens	Tube that carries sperm from the epididymis to the urethra
Vasogram	Recording flow in vas deferens
Vasotomy	Creation of an opening in vas deferens
Vasovasorrhaphy	Suturing of vas deferens
Vasovasostomy	Reversal of vasectomy
Vesiculectomy	Excision of the seminal vesicle
Vesiculotomy	Incision into the seminal vesicle

MALE GENITAL SYSTEM QUIZ

1. This gland activates the sperm and produces some seminal fluid:
   a. seminal vesicles
   b. bulbourethral
   c. prostate gland
   d. scrotum

2. Carries the sperm from the testes to the exterior:
   a. duct
   b. sex gland
   c. tunica
   d. seminal

3. The penis contains these erectile tissues:
   a. one corpora cavernosa and two spongiosa
   b. two corpora cavernosa and two spongiosa
   c. one corpora cavernosa and one spongiosum
   d. two corpora cavernosa and one spongiosum

4. Also known as the Cowper's gland:
   a. seminal vesicles
   b. bulbourethral
   c. prostate gland
   d. scrotum

5. Which of the following is NOT an accessory organ:
   a. gonads
   b. seminal vesicles
   c. prostate
   d. penis

6. Combining form meaning male:
   a. andr/o
   b. balan/o
   c. orchi/o
   d. test/o

7. Combining form meaning glans penis:
   a. balan/o
   b. vas/o
   c. vesicul/o
   d. orch/o

8. The testes are covered by the:
   a. seminal vesicles
   b. androgen
   c. chancre
   d. tunica albuginea

9. This abbreviation describes a surgical resection of the prostate that is accomplished by means of an endoscope inserted into the urethra:
    a. TURBT
    b. BPH
    c. UPJ
    d. TURP

10. This abbreviation describes a condition of the prostate in which there is an enlargement that is benign:
    a. TURBT
    b. BPH
    c. UPJ
    d. TURP

URINARY SYSTEM

- Removes waste materials
- Regulates fluid volume
- Maintains electrolytes, water, and acid balance
- Assists liver in detoxification

Organs (Figure 1-19)

Kidneys

Ureters

Urinary bladder

Urethra

Kidneys (Figure 1-20)

Electrolytes and fluid balance

Controls pH balance

Two organs located behind peritoneum (retroperitoneal space)

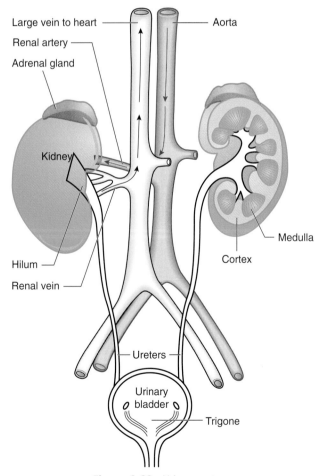

Figure 1-19 Urinary system.

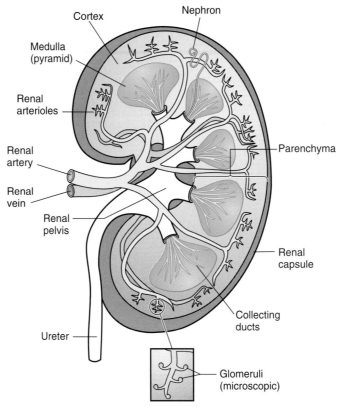

Figure 1-20 Kidney.

Cortex (outer layer)

Medulla (inner portion)

Pyramids (divisions of medulla)

Papilla (inner part of pyramids)

Pelvis (receptacle for urine within the kidney)

Calyces surround top of renal pelvis

Ureters

Narrow tubes connecting kidney and bladder

Urinary Bladder

Reservoir for urine

Shaped like an upside down pear with three surfaces

Posterior (base)

Anterior (neck)

Superior (peritoneum)

Trigone

Smooth area inside bladder

Formed by openings of the ureters and urethra

Urethra

Canal from bladder to exterior of body

Urinary meatus, outside opening of the urethra

COMBINING FORMS

1.	albumin/o	albumin
2.	azot/o	urea
3.	cyst/o	bladder
4.	glomerul/o	glomerulus
5.	glyc/o	sugar
6.	glycos/o	sugar
7.	hydr/o	water
8.	lith/o	stone
9.	meat/o	meatus
10.	nephr/o	kidney
11.	noct/i	night
12.	olig/o	scant
13.	pyel/o	renal pelvis
14.	ren/o	kidney
15.	son/o	sound
16.	ur/o	urine
17.	ureter/o	ureter
18.	urethr/o	urethra
19.	urin/o	urine
20.	vesic/o	bladder

PREFIXES

1.	dys-	painful
2.	peri-	surrounding
3.	poly-	many
4.	retro-	behind

SUFFIXES

1.	-eal	pertaining to
2.	-lithiasis	condition of stones
3.	-lysis	separation
4.	-plasty	repair
5.	-rrhaphy	suture
6.	-tripsy	crush

MEDICAL ABBREVIATIONS

1.	ARF	acute renal failure
2.	BUN	blood urea nitrogen
3.	ESRD	end-stage renal disease
4.	HD	hemodialysis
5.	IVP	intravenous pyelogram
6.	KUB	kidney, ureter, bladder
7.	pH	symbol for acid/base level
8.	sp gr	specific gravity
9.	UA	urinalysis
10.	UPJ	ureteropelvic junction
11.	UTI	urinary tract infection

MEDICAL TERMS

Bulbocavernosus	Muscle that constricts the vagina in a female and the urethra in a male
Bulbourethral	Gland with duct leading to the urethra
Calculus	Concretion of mineral salts, also called a stone
Calycoplasty	Surgical reconstruction of recess of renal pelvis
Calyx	Recess of renal pelvis
Cystolithectomy	Removal of a calculus (stone) from urinary bladder
Cystometrogram	Measurement of the pressures and capacity of the urinary bladder (CMG)
Cystoplasty	Surgical reconstruction of the bladder
Cystorrhaphy	Suture of the bladder
Cystoscopy	Use of a scope to view the bladder
Cystostomy	Surgical creation of an opening into the bladder
Cystotomy	Incision into the bladder
Cystourethroplasty	Surgical reconstruction of the bladder and urethra
Cystourethroscopy	Use of a scope to view the bladder and urethra
Dilation	Stretching
Dysuria	Painful urination
Endopyelotomy	Procedure involving the bladder and ureters, including the insertion of a stent into the renal pelvis
Extracorporeal	Occurring outside of the body
Fundoplasty	Repair of the bottom the bladder
Hydrocele	Sac of fluid
Kock pouch	Surgical creation of a urinary bladder from a segment of the ileum

Nephrocutaneous fistula	A channel from the kidney to the skin
Nephrolithotomy	Removal of a kidney stone through an incision made into the kidney
Nephrorrhaphy	Suturing of the kidney
Nephrostomy	Creation of a channel into the renal pelvis of the kidney
Transureteroureterostomy	Surgical connection of one ureter to the other ureter
Transvesical ureterolithotomy	Removal of a ureter stone (calculus) through the bladder
Ureterectomy	Surgical removal of a ureter, either totally or partially
Ureterocutaneous fistula	Channel from ureter to exterior skin
Ureteroenterostomy	Creation of a connection between the intestine and the ureter
Ureterolithotomy	Removal of a stone from the ureter
Ureterolysis	Freeing of adhesions of the ureter
Ureteroneocystostomy	Surgical connection of the ureter to a new site on the bladder
Ureteropyelography	Ureter and renal pelvis radiography
Ureterotomy	Incision into the ureter
Urethrocystography	Radiography of the bladder and urethra
Urethromeatoplasty	Surgical repair of the urethra and meatus
Urethropexy	Fixation of the urethra by means of surgery
Urethroplasty	Surgical repair of the urethra
Urethrorrhaphy	Suturing of the urethra
Urethroscopy	Use of a scope to view the urethra
Vesicostomy	Surgical creation of a connection of the viscera of the bladder to the skin

URINARY SYSTEM QUIZ

1. The outer covering of the kidney:
   a. medulla
   b. pyramids
   c. cortex
   d. papilla

2. Which is not a division of the kidneys:
   a. pelvis
   b. pyramids
   c. cortex
   d. trigone

3. The inner portion of the kidneys:
   a. medulla
   b. pyramids
   c. cortex
   d. papilla

4. The smooth area inside the bladder:
   a. pyramids
   b. calyces
   c. trigone
   d. cystocele

5. The narrow tube connecting the kidney and bladder:
   a. urethra
   b. ureter
   c. meatus
   d. trigone

6. Which of the following is NOT a surface of the urinary bladder:
   a. posterior
   b. anterior
   c. superior
   d. inferior

7. Combining form that means stone:
   a. azot/o
   b. cyst/o
   c. lith/o
   d. olig/o

8. Term meaning painful urination:
   a. pyuria
   b. dysuria
   c. diuresis
   d. hyperemia

9. Combining form meaning scant:
   a. glyc/o
   b. hydr/o
   c. meat/o
   d. olig/o

10. Term that describes renal failure that is acute:
    a. ARF
    b. ESRD
    c. HD
    d. BPH

DIGESTIVE SYSTEM

Function: digestion, absorption, and elimination

Includes gastrointestinal tract (alimentary canal) and accessory organs

Mouth (Figure 1-21)

Roof: hard palate, soft palate, uvula (projection at back of mouth)

Floor contains tongue (Figure 1-22), muscles, taste buds, and lingual frenulum, which anchors tongue to floor of mouth

Teeth

Thirty-two teeth (permanent)

Names of teeth: incisor, cuspid, bicuspid, and tricuspid

Tooth has crown (outer portion), neck (narrow part below gum line), root (end section), and pulp cavity (core)

Salivary Glands (Figure 1-23)

Surround the mouth and produce saliva

Parotid

Submandibular

Sublingual

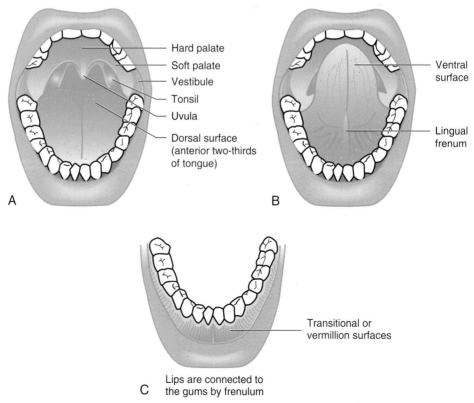

Figure 1-21   Anatomical structures of the mouth.

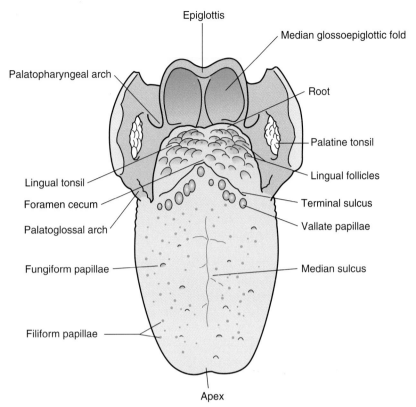

Figure 1-22   Dorsum of the tongue.

Pharynx or Throat (Figure 1-24)

Muscular tube through which air and food/water travel

Epiglottis covers larynx when swallowing

Esophagus

Muscular tube that carries food to stomach by means of peristalsis (rhythmic contractions)

Stomach

Sphincters (ring of muscles) at entry into stomach (gastroesophageal or cardiac)

Three parts of stomach: fundus (upper part), body (middle part), antrum/pylorus (lower part)

Lined with rugae (folds of mucosal membrane)

Pyloric sphincter opens to allow food to leave stomach and enter small intestine

Small Intestine

Duodenum

Jejunum

Ileum

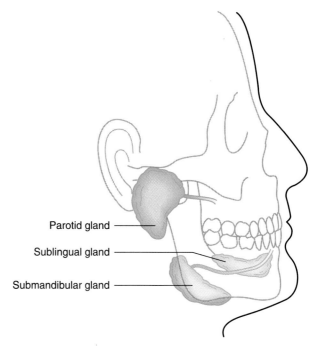

Figure 1-23 Major salivary glands.

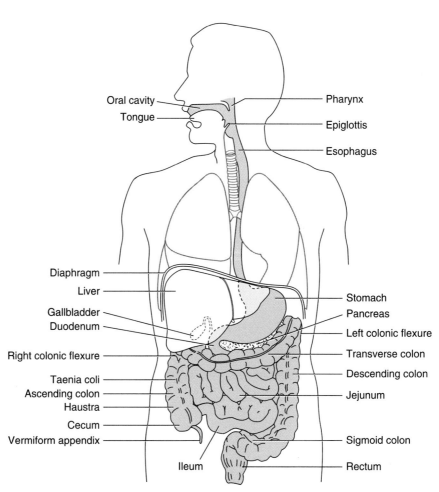

Figure 1-24 Digestive system.

Large Intestine

Extends from ileum to anus

Cecum, from which appendix extends, connects ileum and colon

Colon, divided into ascending, transverse, descending, and sigmoid

Sigmoid colon, connected to rectum that terminates at anus

Accessory Organs

Liver produces bile, sent to gallbladder via hepatic duct and cystic duct

Gallbladder stores bile, sent to duodenum via common bile duct

Pancreas produces enzymes sent through pancreatic duct to common bile duct then to duodenum

Islets of Langerhans produce insulin and glucagon

Peritoneum

Serous membrane lines abdominal cavity and maintains organs in correct anatomical place

COMBINING FORMS

1.	abdomin/o	abdomen
2.	an/o	anus
3.	appendic/o	appendix
4.	bil/i	bile
5.	bilirubin/o	bile pigment
6.	cec/o	cecum
7.	celi/o	abdomen
8.	chol/e	gall/bile
9.	cholangio/o	bile duct
10.	cholecyst/o	gallbladder
11.	choledoch/o	common bile duct
12.	col/o	colon
13.	dent/i	tooth
14.	diverticul/o	diverticulum
15.	duoden/o	duodenum
16.	enter/o	small intestine
17.	esophag/o	esophagus
18.	gastr/o	stomach
19.	gingiv/o	gum

20. gloss/o   tongue
21. hepat/o   liver
22. herni/o   hernia
23. ile/o   ileum
24. jejun/o   jejunum
25. lapar/o   abdomen
26. lingu/o   tongue
27. lip/o   fat
28. lith/o   stone
29. or/o   mouth
30. palat/o   palate
31. pancreat/o   pancreas
32. peritone/o   peritoneum
33. polyp/o   polyp
34. proct/o   rectum
35. pylor/o   pylorus
36. rect/o   rectum
37. sial/o   saliva
38. sigmoid/o   sigmoid colon
39. steat/o   fat
40. stomat/o   mouth
41. uvul/o   uvula

SUFFIXES

1. -phagia   eating
2. -cele   hernia
3. -chezia   defecation

MEDICAL ABBREVIATIONS

1. EGD   esophagogastroduodenoscopy
2. EGJ   esophagogastric junction
3. ERCP   endoscopic retrograde cholangiopancreatography
4. GERD   gastroesophageal reflux disease
5. GI   gastrointestinal

| 6. HJR | hepatojugular reflux |
| 7. PEG | percutaneous endoscopic gastrostomy |

MEDICAL TERMS

Anastomosis	Surgical connection of two tubular structures, such as two pieces of the intestine
Biliary	Refers to gallbladder, bile, or bile duct
Cholangiography	Radiographic recording of the bile ducts
Cholecystectomy	Surgical removal of the gallbladder
Cholecystoenterostomy	Creation of a connection between the gallbladder and intestine
Colonoscopy	Fiberscopic examination of the entire colon that may include part of the terminal ileum
Colostomy	Artificial opening between the colon and the abdominal wall
Diverticulum	Protrusion in the wall of an organ
Dysphagia	Difficulty swallowing
Enterolysis	Releasing of adhesions of intestine
Eventration	Protrusion of the bowel through an opening in the abdomen
Evisceration	Pulling the viscera outside of the body through an incision
Exstrophy	Condition in which an organ is turned inside out
Fulguration	Use of electric current to destroy tissue
Gastrointestinal	Pertaining to the stomach and intestine
Gastroplasty	Operation on the stomach for repair or reconfiguration
Gastrostomy	Artificial opening between the stomach and the abdominal wall
Hernia	Organ or tissue protruding through the wall or cavity that usually contains it
Ileostomy	Artificial opening between the ileum and the abdominal wall
Imbrication	Overlapping
Incarcerated	Regarding hernias, a constricted, irreducible hernia that may cause obstruction of an intestine
Intussusception	Slipping of one part of the intestine into another part
Jejunostomy	Artificial opening between the jejunum and the abdominal wall
Laparoscopy	Exploration of the abdomen and pelvic cavities using a scope placed through a small incision in the abdominal wall
Lithotomy	Incision into an organ or a duct for the purpose of removing a stone
Lithotripsy	Crushing of a gallbladder or urinary bladder stone followed by irrigation to wash the fragment out
Paraesophageal hiatus hernia	Hernia that is near the esophagus
Perinephric cyst	Cyst in the tissue around the kidney
Perirenal	Around the kidney

Proctosigmoidoscopy	Fiberscopic examination of the sigmoid colon and rectum
Sialolithotomy	Surgical removal of a stone of the salivary gland or duct
Varices	Varicose vein
Volvulus	Twisted section of the intestine

DIGESTIVE SYSTEM QUIZ

1. NOT a part of the small intestine:
   a. ileum
   b. cecum
   c. duodenum
   d. jejunum

2. Term meaning a ring of muscles:
   a. pyloric
   b. parotid
   c. epiglottis
   d. sphincter

3. The throat is also known as the:
   a. larynx
   b. epiglottis
   c. esophagus
   d. pharynx

4. The three parts of the stomach:
   a. pyloric, rugae, fundus
   b. fundus, body, antrum
   c. antrum, pyloric, rugae
   d. ilium, fundus, pyloric

5. The projection at the back of the mouth:
   a. palate
   b. sublingual
   c. uvula
   d. parotid

6. Mucosal membrane that lines the stomach:
   a. cecum
   b. rugae
   c. frenulum
   d. fundus

7. The parts of the colon are:
   a. ascending, transverse, descending, sigmoid
   b. ascending, descending, sigmoid
   c. transverse, descending, sigmoid
   d. descending, sigmoid

8. Combining form meaning abdomen:
   a. an/o
   b. cec/o
   c. celi/o
   d. col/o

9. Term that means tying together of two ends of a tube:
   a. anastomosis
   b. amylase
   c. aphthous stomatitis
   d. atresia

10. Abbreviation that means a scope placed through the esophagus, into the stomach, and to the duodenum:
    a. ERCP
    b. EGD
    c. GERD
    d. PEG

MEDIASTINUM AND DIAPHRAGM

Not an organ system

Mediastinum

That area between lungs that a median (partition) divides (Figure 1-25) into:
* superior
* anterior
* posterior
* middle

Diaphragm

A dome-shaped muscular partition that separates abdominal cavity from thoracic cavity

Assists in breathing

Expands to assist lungs in exhalation/relaxation of the diaphragm

Flattens out during inspiration/contraction of diaphragm

Diaphragmatic hernia: esophageal hernia

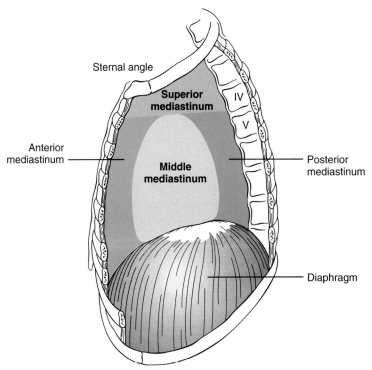

Figure 1-25   Mediastinum and diaphragm.

MEDIASTINUM AND DIAPHRAGM QUIZ

1. The mediastinum is not an organ system:
   a. true
   b. false

2. The mediastinum is divided into:
   a. superior, anterior, posterior
   b. superior, anterior, posterior, middle
   c. anterior, posterior, middle
   d. middle, anterior, superior

3. During inspiration, the diaphragm:
   a. expands
   b. moves upward
   c. collapses
   d. flattens out

4. The term means partition:
   a. middle
   b. medium
   c. median
   d. diaphragm

5. The diaphragm is said to be this shape:
   a. square
   b. flat
   c. dome
   d. round

6. This separates the abdominal cavity from the thoracic cavity:
   a. mediastinum
   b. diaphragm
   c. superior
   d. inferior

7. This is the area between the lungs:
   a. mediastinum
   b. diaphragm
   c. superior
   d. inferior

8. This is an esophageal hernia:
   a. mediastinal
   b. diaphragmatic
   c. paraesophageal
   d. hiatal

9. A diaphragmatic hernia is also known as:
   a. esophageal
   b. epiglottis
   c. partitional
   d. medial

10. The diaphragm assists in:
    a. percussion
    b. auscultation
    c. contraction
    d. breathing

HEMIC AND LYMPHATIC SYSTEM

Hemic refers to blood

Lymphatic system removes excess tissue fluid
- Located throughout body
- Composed of lymph, vessels, and organs

Lymph

Colorless fluid containing lymphocytes and monocytes

Originates in blood and after filtering, returns to blood

Transports fluids and proteins that have leaked from blood system back to veins

Absorbs and transports fats from villi of small intestine to blood system

Assists in immune function

Lymph Vessels

Similar to veins

Scattered throughout body

Lymph Organs

Lymph nodes, spleen, bone marrow, thymus, and tonsils

Lymph nodes, areas of concentrated tissue (Figure 1-26)

Spleen, located in upper left quadrant (ULQ) of abdomen

   Composed of lymph tissue

      Function is to filter blood; activates lymphocytes and B-cells to filter or attach antigens

      Stores blood

Bone marrow, contains tissue that produces RBCs and platelets

   Produces stem cells

Thymus secretes thymosin causing T-cells to mature

   Larger in infants and shrinks with age

Tonsils

   Palatine tonsils

   Pharyngeal tonsils/adenoids

COMBINING FORMS

1.	adeno or adnen/o	gland
2.	adenoid/o	adenoids
3.	axill/o	armpit
4.	cervic/o	neck/cervix
5.	immun/o	immune
6.	inguin/o	groin

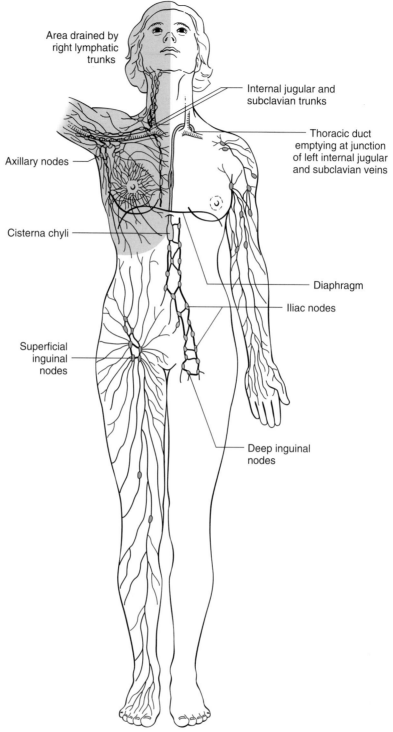

Area drained by
right lymphatic
trunks

Internal jugular and
subclavian trunks

Axillary nodes

Thoracic duct
emptying at junction
of left internal jugular
and subclavian veins

Cisterna chyli

Diaphragm

Iliac nodes

Superficial
inguinal
nodes

Deep inguinal
nodes

Figure 1-26 Lymphatic system.

7.	lymph/o	lymph
8.	lymphaden/o	lymph gland
9.	splen/o	spleen
10.	thym/o	thymus gland

11. tonsill/o   tonsil

12. tox/o   poison

PREFIXES

1. hyper-   excess

2. inter-   between

3. retro-   behind

SUFFIXES

1. -ectomy   removal

2. -edema   swelling

3. -itis   inflammation

4. -megaly   enlargement

5. -oid   resembling

6. -oma   tumor

7. -penia   deficient

8. -pexy   fixation

9. -phylaxis   protection

10. -poiesis   production

MEDICAL TERMS

Axillary nodes	Lymph nodes located in the armpit
Cloquet's node	Also called a gland; it is the highest of the deep groin lymph nodes
Inguinofemoral	Referring to the groin and thigh
Jugular nodes	Lymph nodes located next to the large vein in the neck
Lymph node	Station along the lymphatic system
Lymphadenectomy	Excision of a lymph node or nodes
Lymphadenitis	Inflammation of a lymph node
Lymphangiotomy	Incision into a lymphatic vessel
Parathyroid	Produces a hormone to mobilize calcium from the bones to the blood
Splenectomy	Excision of the spleen
Splenoportography	Radiographic procedure to allow visualization of the splenic and portal veins of the spleen
Stem cell	Immature blood cell
Thoracic duct	Collection and distribution point for lymph, and the largest lymph vessel located in the chest
Transplantation	Grafting of tissue from one source to another

HEMIC AND LYMPHATIC SYSTEM QUIZ

1. The spleen is located in this quadrant of the abdomen:
   a. URQ
   b. ULQ
   c. LLQ
   d. LRQ

2. Produces RBCs and platelets:
   a. thymus
   b. tonsils
   c. lymph node
   d. bone marrow

3. Which of the following is NOT a lymph organ:
   a. adrenal
   b. spleen
   c. thymus
   d. tonsil

4. Lymph transports fluids and _____ that have leaked from the blood system back to veins.
   a. stem cells
   b. lymphocytes
   c. B-cells
   d. proteins

5. This is largest in infants and shrinks with age:
   a. tonsils
   b. spleen
   c. thymus
   d. bone marrow

6. Combining form meaning gland:
   a. axill/o
   b. thym/o
   c. aden/o
   d. tox/o

7. Prefix meaning excess:
   a. hyper-
   b. hypo-
   c. inter-
   d. retro-

8. Suffix meaning enlargement:
   a. -edema
   b. -poiesis
   c. -penia
   d. -megaly

9. Lymph node located on neck:
   a. thoracic
   b. jugular
   c. Cloquet's
   d. axillary

10. These cells originate in the bone marrow:
    a. leucocytes
    b. erythrocytes
    c. monocytes
    d. stem cells

ENDOCRINE SYSTEM

- Regulates body through hormones
- Affects growth, development, and metabolism

Nine Glands (Figure 1-27)

Pituitary (hypophysis): master gland

Located at base of brain in a depression in skull (sella turcica)

Anterior pituitary (adenohypophysis)

Adrenocorticotropic hormone (ACTH)—stimulates adrenal cortex

Follicle-stimulating hormone (FSH)—males, stimulates sperm production; females, stimulates secretion of estrogen and stimulates follicle development

Growth hormone (GH or somatotropin)—stimulates growth and fat metabolism, and maintains blood glucose levels

Luteinizing hormone (LH)—male, stimulates testosterone; females, stimulates secretion of progesterone and estrogen

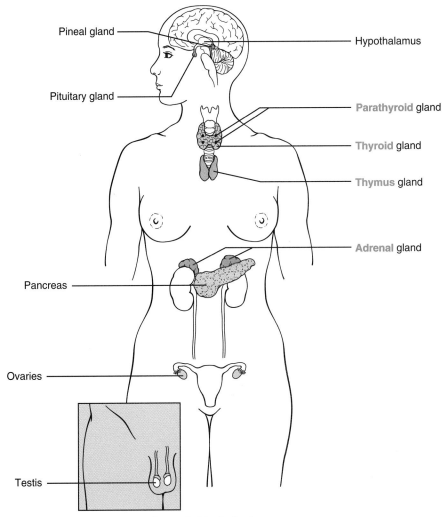

Figure 1-27   Endocrine system.

Melanocyte-stimulating hormone (MST)—increases pigmentation

Prolactin (PRL)—stimulates milk production and breast development

Thyroid-stimulating hormone (TSH or thyrotropin)—stimulates thyroid gland

Posterior pituitary (neurohypophysis)—stores hormones

Antidiuretic hormone (ADH)—stimulates reabsorption of water by kidney tubules

Oxytocin—stimulates contractions during childbirth and release of milk

Thyroid

Two lobes overlying trachea (Adam's apple)

Secretes two hormones that increase metabolism—thyroxine (T_4) and triiodothyronine (T_3)

Secretes one hormone that decreases blood calcium—thyrocalcitonin

Parathyroid (4)

Located on posterior side of thyroid

Secretes PTH (parathyroid hormone)

Mobilizes calcium from bones

Adrenal (pair)

Located on top of each kidney

Adrenal cortex—outer region that secretes corticosteroids

Cortisol—increases blood glucose

Aldosterone—increases reabsorption of sodium (salt)

Androgen, estrogen, progestin—sexual characteristics

Adrenal medulla—inner region that secretes catecholamines (epinephrine and norepinephrine)

Pancreas

Located behind stomach

Contains specialized cells (islet of Langerhans) that produce hormones

Produces: insulin (decreases blood glucose), glucagon (converts glycogen to glucose), and somatostatin (regulates other cells of pancreas)

Thymus

Located behind sternum

Atrophies during adolescence

Produces thymosin—stimulates T-lymphocytes

Hypothalamus (part of brain)

Located below thalamus

Stimulates pituitary to release hormones

Pineal

Located behind hypothalamus

Secretes melatonin—affects brain and releases of hormones

Ovaries (pair, females)

Estrogen—female sex characteristics

Progesterone—maintains pregnancy

Placenta

Produces HCG (human chorionic gonadotropin) during pregnancy

Testes (pair, males)

Testosterone—male sex characteristics

COMBINING FORMS

1.	aden/o	gland
2.	adren/o	adrenal gland
3.	adrenal/o	adrenal gland
4.	andr/o	male
5.	calc/o or calci/i	calcium
6.	cortic/o	cortex
7.	crin/o	secrete
8.	dips/o	thirst
9.	estr/o	female
10.	gluc/o	sugar
11.	glyc/o	sugar
12.	gonad/o	ovaries and testes
13.	home/o	same
14.	hormon/o	hormone
15.	kal/i	potassium
16.	lact/o	milk
17.	myx/o	mucus
18.	natr/o	sodium
19.	pancreat/o	pancreas
20.	phys/o	growing
21.	pituitar/o	pituitary gland
22.	somat/o	body
23.	ster/o or stere/o	solid, having three dimensions

24. thyroid/o   thyroid gland

25. toxic/o   poison

PREFIXES

1. eu-   good/normal

2. oxy-   sharp

3. pan-   all

4. tetra-   four

5. tri-   three

6. tropin-   act upon

SUFFIXES

1. -agon   assemble

2. -drome   run

3. -in   a substance

4. -ine   a substance

5. -tropin   act upon

6. -uria   urine

MEDICAL TERMS

Adrenal	Glands, located at the top of the kidneys, that produce steroid hormones
Contralateral	Opposite side
Hormone	Chemical substance produced by the body
Isthmus	Connection of two regions or structures
Isthmus, thyroid	Tissue connection between right and left thyroid lobes
Isthmusectomy	Surgical removal of the isthmus
Lobectomy	Removal of a lobe
Thymectomy	Surgical removal of the thymus
Thymus	Gland that produces hormones important to the immune response
Thyroglossal duct	Connection between the thyroid and the tongue
Thyroid	Part of the endocrine system that produces hormones that regulate metabolism
Thyroidectomy	Surgical removal of the thyroid

ENDOCRINE SYSTEM QUIZ

1. Which of the following is NOT affected by the endocrine system:
   a. growth
   b. development
   c. progesterone
   d. metabolism

2. Gland that overlies the Adam's apple:
   a. parathyroid
   b. adrenal
   c. pancreas
   d. thyroid

3. Gland that is located on the top of each kidney:
   a. parathyroid
   b. adrenal
   c. pancreas
   d. thyroid

4. The outer region of the adrenal gland that secretes corticosteroids:
   a. cortex
   b. medulla
   c. sternum
   d. medullary

5. Located on the thyroid:
   a. hypophysis
   b. thymus
   c. pineal
   d. parathyroid

6. Located at the base of the brain in a depression in the skull:
   a. pituitary
   b. thymus
   c. adrenal
   d. pineal

7. Stimulates contractions during childbirth:
   a. cortisol
   b. PTH
   c. ADH
   d. oxytocin

8. Produced only during pregnancy by the placenta:
   a. human chorionic gonadotropin
   b. melatonin
   c. thymosin
   d. adrenocorticotropic hormone

9. Combining form meaning secrete:
   a. dips/o
   b. crin/o
   c. gluc/o
   d. kal/i

10. Prefix meaning good:
    a. tri-
    b. tropin-
    c. pan-
    d. eu-

NERVOUS SYSTEM

- Controlling, regulating, and communicating system
- Organization
    - Central nervous system (CNS), brain and spinal cord
    - Peripheral nervous system (PNS), cranial and spinal nerves

Cells of the Nervous System (Figure 1-28)

Neurons

Classified according to function:

Dendrites (receives signals)

Cell body (nucleus, within cell body)

Axon (carries signals from cell body)

Myelin sheath (insulation around axon)

Glia

Astrocytes

Microglia

Oligodendrocytes

Divisions (Figure 1-29)

Brain

Brainstem

Medulla oblongata

Pons

Midbrain

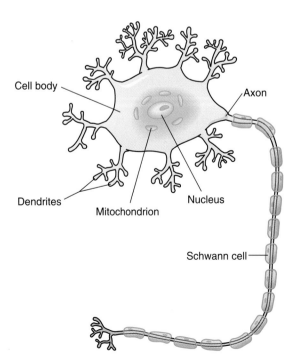

Figure 1-28   Myelinated axon.

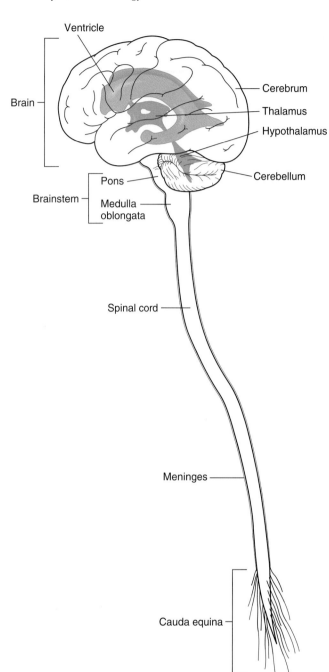

Figure 1-29   Brain and spinal cord.

Diencephalon

   Hypothalamus controls ANS

   Thalamus relays impulses to cerebral cortex

Cerebellum

   Controls muscle contractions

   Balance

Cerebrum

    Largest part of brain

    Mental processes

    Two hemispheres

    Right controls left side of body

    Left controls right side of body

    Divided into five lobes

        Frontal

        Parietal

        Temporal

        Occipital

        Insula

Spinal Cord

    Coverings

    Cranial bones and vertebrae

    Spinal and cerebral meninges

    Fluid spaces containing cerebrospinal fluid

    Subarachnoid spaces

    Ventricles

Peripheral Nervous System (PNS)

    Cranial nerves, 12 pair

    Spinal nerves, 31 pair

Autonomic Nervous System (ANS)

    Two divisions

        Sympathetic system

        Parasympathetic system

COMBINING FORMS

1.	cephal/o	head
2.	cerebell/o	cerebellum
3.	cerebr/o	cerebrum
4.	crani/o	cranium
5.	dur/o	dura mater
6.	encephal/o	brain

7.	gangli/o	ganglion
8.	ganglion/o	ganglion
9.	mening/o	meninges
10.	meningi/o	meninges
11.	ment/o	mind
12.	mon/o	one
13.	myel/o	spinal cord
14.	neur/o	nerve
15.	phas/o	speech
16.	phren/o	mind
17.	poli/o	gray matter
18.	pont/o	pons
19.	psych/o	mind
20.	quadr/i	four
21.	radic/o	nerve root
22.	radicul/o	nerve root
23.	rhiz/o	nerve root

PREFIXES

1.	hemi-	half
2.	per-	through
3.	quadri-	four
4.	tetra-	four

SUFFIXES

1.	-algesia	pain sensation
2.	-algia	pain
3.	-cele	hernia
4.	-esthesia	feeling
5.	-iatry	medical treatment
6.	-ictal	pertaining to
7.	-paresis	incomplete paralysis
8.	-plegia	paralysis

MEDICAL ABBREVIATIONS

1.	ANS	autonomic nervous system
2.	CNS	central nervous system

3. CSF   stroke/cerebrovascular accident

4. EEG   electroencephalogram

5. LP   lumbar puncture

6. PNS   peripheral nervous system

7. TENS   transcutaneous electrical nerve stimulation

8. TIA   transient ischemic attach

MEDICAL TERMS

Burr	Drill used to create an entry into the cranium
Central nervous system	Brain and spinal cord
Craniectomy	Permanent, partial removal of skull
Craniotomy	Opening of the skull
Cranium	That part of the skeleton that encloses the brain
Diskectomy	Removal of a vertebral disk
Electroencephalography	Recording of the electric currents of the brain by means of electrodes attached to the scalp
Laminectomy	Surgical excision of the lamina
Peripheral nerves	12 pairs of cranial nerves, 31 pairs of spinal nerves, and autonomic nervous system; connects peripheral receptors to the brain and spinal cord
Shunt	Divert or make an artificial passage
Skull	Entire skeletal framework of the head
Somatic nerve	Sensory or motor nerve
Stereotaxis	Method of identifying a specific area or point in the brain
Sympathetic nerve	Part of the peripheral nervous system that controls automatic body function and sympathetic nerves activated under stress
Trephination	Surgical removal of a disk of bone
Vertebrectomy	Removal of vertebrae

NERVOUS SYSTEM QUIZ

1. Portion of the nervous system contains the cranial and spinal nerves:
   a. central
   b. peripheral
   c. autonomic
   d. parasympathetic

2. The part of the neuron that receives signals:
   a. dendrites
   b. cell body
   c. axon
   d. myelin sheath

3. NOT associated with glia:
   a. monocytes
   b. astrocytes
   c. microglia
   d. oligodendrocytes

4. Largest part of the brain:
   a. cerebellum
   b. cerebrum
   c. cortex
   d. pons

5. Divided into two hemispheres:
   a. cerebellum
   b. cerebrum
   c. cortex
   d. pons

6. The number of pairs of cranial nerves:
   a. 10
   b. 11
   c. 12
   d. 13

7. Controls the right side of the body:
   a. left cerebrum
   b. right cerebrum
   c. right cortex
   d. left cortex

8. Combining form that means brain:
   a. mening/o
   b. mon/o
   c. esthesi/o
   d. encephal/o

9. Prefix that means four:
   a. per-
   b. tetra-
   c. para-
   d. bi-

10. Combining form that means speech:
    a. phas/o
    b. rhiz/o
    c. poli/o
    d. myel/o

SENSES

- Sight   Eyes
- Hearing   Ears
- Smell   Nose
- Taste   Tongue
- Touch   Skin

Sight: Three Layers (Figure 1-30)

Sclera (outer layer)

White of eye

Cornea, front transparent portion of sclera

Lies over iris

Choroid (middle layer)

Pigment layer

Ciliary muscle and iris on front portion of layer

Contracts

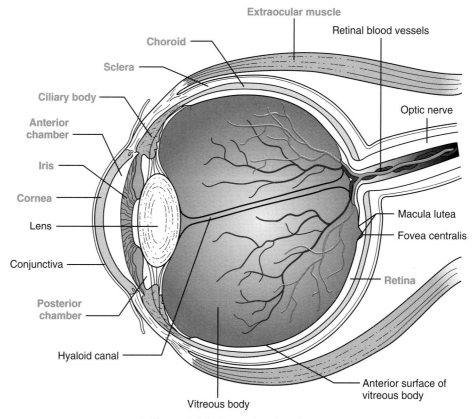

Figure 1-30   Eye and ocular adnexa.

Retina (inner layer)

Contains rods and cones

Rods provide night vision

Cones provide day and color vision

Conjunctivae

Covers front of sclera and lines eyelids

Lens

Behind pupils

Focuses light

Fluids

Aqueous humor (front of lens)

Vitreous humor (behind lens)

Hearing, Three Divisions

External Ear

Auricle (pinna)

External auditory canal

Middle Ear

Ossicles

Malleus

Incus

Stapes

Eustachian tube—leads to pharynx

Inner Ear

Vestibule

Semicircular canals/vestibular apparatus

Cochlea

Smell

Olfactory Sense Receptors

Located in nasal cavity

Closely related to sense of taste

Cranial nerve I

Taste

Gustatory sense

Taste buds located on tongue

Cranial nerves VII and IX

Touch

Mechanoreceptors

Widely distributed throughout body

Reacts to touch and pressure

Meissner corpuscles (touch)

Pacinian corpuscles (pressure)

Proprioceptors

Position and orientation

Thermoreceptors

Under skin

Senses temperature changes

Nociceptors

Pain sensors

In skin and internal organs

COMBINING FORMS

1.	ambly/o	dim
2.	aque/o	water
3.	audi/o	hearing
4.	blephar/o	eyelid
5.	conjunctiv/o	conjunctiva
6.	cor/o or coreo	pupil
7.	corne/o	cornea
8.	cycl/o	ciliary body
9.	dacry/o	tear
10.	essi/o	sensation
11.	ir/o	iris
12.	irid/o	iris
13.	kerat/o	cornea
14.	lacrim/o	tear

15.	ocul/o	eye
16.	ophthalm/o	eye
17.	opt/o	eye
18.	optic/o	eye
19.	ot/o	ear
20.	palpebr/o	eyelid
21.	papill/o	optic nerve
22.	phac/o	eye lens
23.	phak/o	eye lens
24.	pupill/o	pupil
25.	retin/o	retina
26.	scler/o	sclera
27.	staped/o	stapes
28.	tympan/o	ear drum
29.	uve/o	uvea
30.	vitre/o	glassy

PREFIXES

1.	audi-	hearing
2.	eso-	inward
3.	exo-	outward

SUFFIXES

1.	-opia	vision
2.	-tropia	to turn

MEDICAL ABBREVIATIONS

1.	AD	right ear
2.	AS	left ear
3.	AU	both ears
4.	H or E	hemorrhage or exudate
5.	IO	intraocular
6.	OD	right eye
7.	OS	left eye
8.	OU	each eye
9.	PERL	pupils equal and reactive to light
10.	PERRL	pupils equal, round, and reactive to light
11.	PERRLA	pupils equal, round, and reactive to light and accommodation

12. TM   tympanic membrane

13. REM   rapid eye movement

MEDICAL TERMS

Anterior segment	Those parts of the eye in the front of and including the lens, orbit, extraocular muscles, and eyelid
Apicectomy	Excision of a portion of the temporal bone
Astigmatism	Condition in which the refractive surfaces of the eye are unequal
Aural atresia	Congenital absence of the external auditory canal
Cataract	Opaque covering on or in the lens
Cholesteatoma	Tumor that forms in middle ear
Conjunctiva	The lining of the eyelids and the covering of the sclera
Dacryostenosis	Narrowing of the lacrimal duct
Enucleation	Removal of an organ or organs from a body cavity
Episclera	Connective covering of sclera
Exenteration	Removal of an organ all in one piece
Exophthalmos	Protrusion of the eyeball
Exostosis	Bony growth
Fenestration	Creation of a new opening in the inner wall of the middle ear
Glaucoma	Eye diseases that are characterized by an increase of intraocular pressure
Hyperopia	Farsightedness, eyeball is too short from front to back
Keratomalacia	Softening of the cornea associated with a deficiency of vitamin A
Keratoplasty	Surgical repair of the cornea
Labyrinth	Inner connecting cavities, such as the internal ear
Labyrinthitis	Middle ear inflammation
Lacrimal	Related to tears
Ménière's disease	Condition that causes dizziness, ringing in the ears, and deafness
Myopia	Nearsightedness, eyeball too long from front to back
Myringotomy	Incision into tympanic membrane
Ocular adnexa	Orbit, extraocular muscles, and eyelid
Ophthalmoscopy	Examination of the interior of the eye by means of a scope, also known as funduscopy
Otitis media	Noninfectious inflammation of the ear, serous otitis media produces liquid drainage (not purulent) and suppurative otitis media is purulent (pus) matter
Otoscope	Instrument used to examine the ear
Papilledema	Swelling of the optic disk (papilla)
Posterior segment	Those parts of the eye behind the lens

Sclera	Outer covering of the eye
Simple mastoidectomy	Removal of the mastoid bone
Strabismus	Extraocular muscle deviation resulting in unequal visual axes
Tarsorrhaphy	Suturing together of eyelids
Tinnitus	Ringing in the ears
Transmastoid	Creates an opening in mastoid for drainage antrostomy
Tympanolysis	Freeing of adhesions of the tympanic membrane
Tympanostomy	Insertion of ventilation tube into tympanum
Uveal	Vascular tissue of the choroid, ciliary body, and iris
Vertigo	Dizziness

SENSES QUIZ

1. The middle layer of the eye:
   a. sclera
   b. retina
   c. episclera
   d. choroid

2. The covering of the front of sclera and lining of eyelid:
   a. aqueous humor
   b. ossicles
   c. vitreous
   d. conjunctivae

3. Which of the following is NOT a bone of the middle ear:
   a. cochlear
   b. stapes
   c. malleus
   d. incus

4. This cranial nerve controls the sense of smell:
   a. I
   b. II
   c. III
   d. IV

5. Which of the following is NOT part of the inner ear:
   a. pinna
   b. vestibule
   c. semicircular canals
   d. cochlea

6. These receptors react to touch:
   a. nociceptors
   b. mechanoreceptors
   c. proprioceptors
   d. thermoreceptors

7. These react to position and orientation:
   a. nociceptors
   b. mechanoreceptors
   c. proprioceptors
   d. thermoreceptors

8. Combining form meaning eyelid:
   a. aque/o
   b. blephar/o
   c. optic/o
   d. uve/o

9. Combining form meaning eye lens:
   a. cor/o
   b. irid/o
   c. ocul/o
   d. phak/o

10. Abbreviation meaning the pupils are round, reactive to light, equal, and reactive to accommodation:
    a. PERRLA
    b. PERRL
    c. PERL
    d. PURL

ANATOMY AND TERMINOLOGY QUIZ ANSWERS

INTEGUMENTARY SYSTEM QUIZ

1. c
2. d
3. a
4. b
5. d

6. c
7. d
8. b
9. c
10. c

MUSCULOSKELETAL SYSTEM QUIZ

1. b
2. c
3. a
4. c
5. a

6. d
7. b
8. d
9. a
10. c

RESPIRATORY SYSTEM QUIZ

1. b
2. d
3. c
4. a
5. a

6. c
7. c
8. b
9. d
10. d

CARDIOVASCULAR SYSTEM QUIZ

1. d
2. a
3. c
4. a
5. d

6. b
7. d
8. a
9. d
10. d

FEMALE GENITAL AND PREGNANCY QUIZ

1. d
2. a
3. a
4. b
5. c

6. a
7. b
8. b
9. c
10. d

MALE GENITAL QUIZ

1. c
2. a
3. d
4. b
5. a

6. a
7. a
8. d
9. d
10. b

URINARY SYSTEM QUIZ

1. c
2. d
3. a
4. c
5. b

6. d
7. c
8. b
9. d
10. a

DIGESTIVE SYSTEM QUIZ

1. b
2. d
3. d
4. b
5. c

6. b
7. a
8. c
9. a
10. b

MEDIASTINUM AND DIAPHRAGM QUIZ

1. a
2. b
3. d
4. c
5. c

6. b
7. a
8. b
9. a
10. d

HEMIC AND LYMPHATIC SYSTEM QUIZ

1. b
2. d
3. a
4. d
5. c

6. c
7. a
8. d
9. b
10. d

ENDOCRINE SYSTEM QUIZ

1. c
2. d
3. b
4. a
5. d

6. a
7. d
8. a
9. b
10. d

NERVOUS SYSTEM QUIZ

1. b
2. a
3. a
4. b
5. b

6. c
7. a
8. d
9. b
10. a

SENSES QUIZ

1. d	6. b
2. d	7. c
3. a	8. b
4. a	9. d
5. a	10. a

UNIT II

Reimbursement Issues

REIMBURSEMENT ISSUES

Your Responsibility

Ensure accurate coding data

Obtain correct reimbursement for services rendered

Upcoding (maximizing) never appropriate

Population Changing

Elderly fastest growing patient segment

By 2030, one elderly person for each person younger than 19 years

Medicare primarily for elderly

Medicare

Getting Bigger All the Time!

- By 2008, Medicare spending will exceed $364 billion
- Health care will continue to expand to meet enormous future demands
  - Job security for coders!

Basic Structure

Medicare program established in 1965

Part A: Hospital insurance

Part B: Supplemental—nonhospital

   Example: Physician services and medical equipment

Part C: Medicare + Choice—health care options (Added later)

Those Covered

Originally established for those 65 and older

Later disabled and ESRD added

Persons covered "beneficiaries"

Officiating Office

Department of Health and Human Services (DHHS)

Delegated to Centers for Medicare and Medicaid Services (CMS)

- CMS runs Medicare and Medicaid
- CMS delegates daily operation to fiscal intermediaries (FI)
- FI usually insurance companies

Funding for Medicare

- Social security taxes
- Equal match from government
- CMS sends money to FI
- FI handle paperwork and pay claims

Medicare Covers

Beneficiary pays

- 20% of cost of service
- Plus annual deductible

Medicare pays

- 80% covered services

Participating Providers

Signed agreement with FI

Provider agrees to accept what FI pays as payment in full

- Accepting assignment

Block 27 on CMS-1500 **(Figure 2-1)**

Good Reasons to Participate

FI usually do not pay charges provider submits
- Significant decrease

Participating providers (PARs) receive 5% more than non-PARs

Check sent directly from FI to PAR

Faster claims processing

Provider names listed in PARs directory
- Sent to all beneficiaries

Part A, Hospital

Hospitals submit charges on UB92 form

ICD-9-CM codes basis for payment

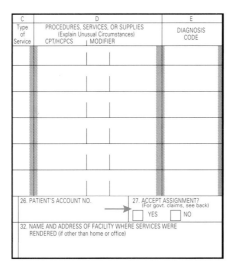

Figure 2-1 Block 27, Accept Assignment on the CMS-1500 Health Insurance Claim Form. *(Courtesy U.S. Department of Health and Human Services, Centers for Medicare and Medicaid Services.)*

Covered In-Hospital Expenses

Semiprivate room

Meals and special diets in hospital

All medically necessary services

Noncovered In-Hospital Expenses

Personal convenience items

Example: Slippers, TV

Not medically necessary

Types of Covered Expenses

Rehabilitation

Skilled-nursing

Some personal convenience items for long-term illness or disabilities

Home health visits

Hospice care

Not automatically covered
- Must meet certain criteria

Part B, Supplemental

Part B pays services and supplies not covered under Part A

Not automatic

Beneficiaries purchase
- Pay monthly premiums

Type of Items Covered Part B

Physician services

Outpatient hospital services

Home health care

Medically necessary supplies and equipment

Coding for Medicare Part B Services

Three coding systems used to report Part B:
- CPT
- HCPCS
- ICD-9-CM

FEDERAL REGISTER

Government publishes changes in laws **(Figure 2-2)**

November and December issues contain outpatient facility changes

PEER REVIEW ORGANIZATION (PRO)

Social Security Act was amended to establish PRO

Also known as Quality Improvement Organizations

Purpose: Ensure hospitals adhered to payment system

PRO Reviews

Admission

Discharge

Quality

DRG validation

Coverage

Procedure

The Review

Begins with nurse who screens records based on PRO guidelines

Out-of-compliance cases forwarded to physician reviewer

Violations can result in severe sanctions

RESOURCE-BASED RELATIVE VALUE SCALE (RBRVS)

Physician payment reform implemented in 1992

Paid physicians lowest of
- Physician's charge for service
- Physician's customary charge
- Prevailing charge in locality

National Fee Schedule

Replaced RBRVS

Termed Medicare Fee Schedule (MFS)

Payment 80% of MFS, after patient deductible

Used for physicians and suppliers

Relative Value Unit

Assigns national unit values to each CPT code

Local adjustments made:
- Work and skill required

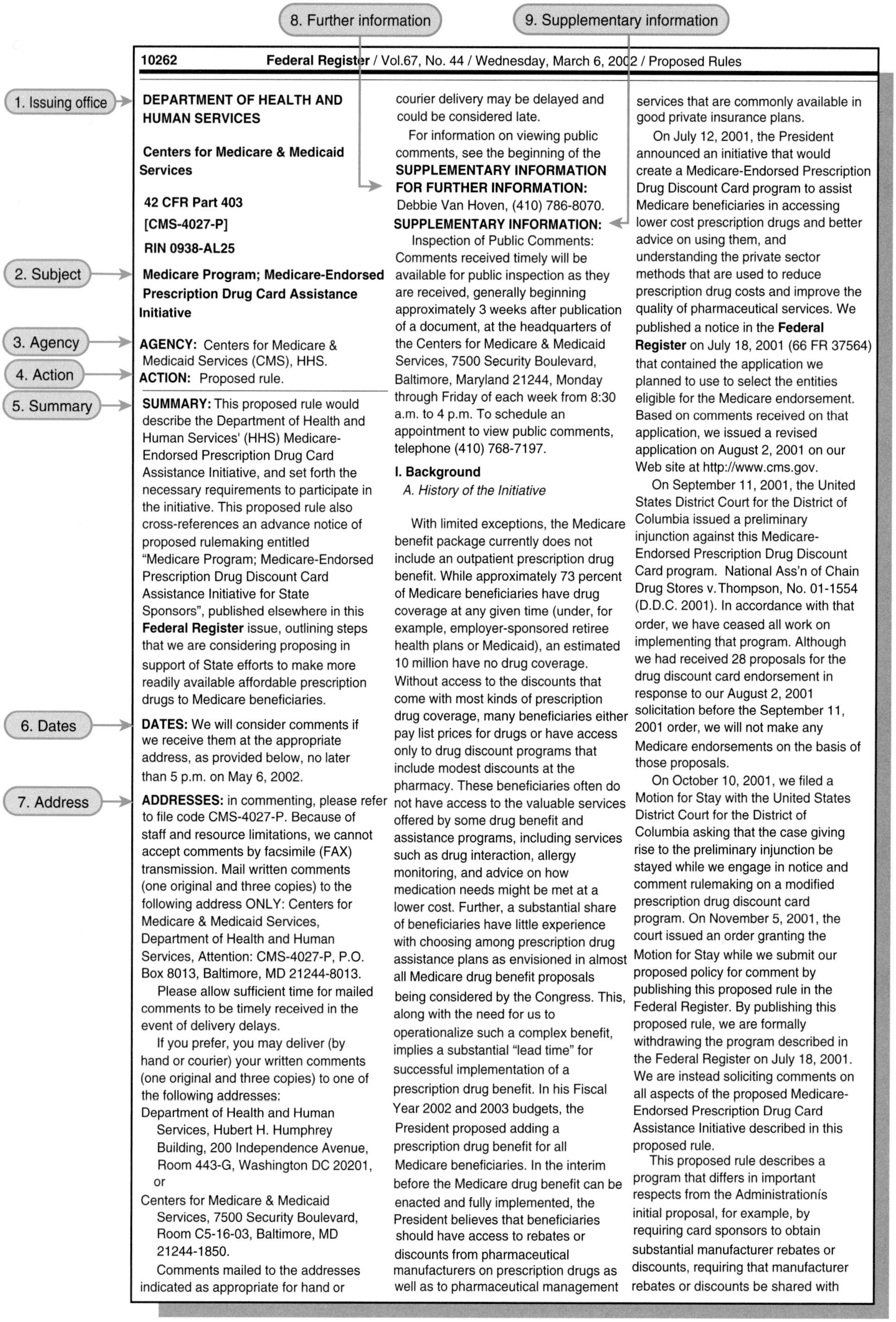

1. Issuing office →

DEPARTMENT OF HEALTH AND HUMAN SERVICES

Centers for Medicare & Medicaid Services

42 CFR Part 403

[CMS-4027-P]

RIN 0938-AL25

2. Subject →

Medicare Program; Medicare-Endorsed Prescription Drug Card Assistance Initiative

3. Agency →

AGENCY: Centers for Medicare & Medicaid Services (CMS), HHS.

4. Action →

ACTION: Proposed rule.

5. Summary →

SUMMARY: This proposed rule would describe the Department of Health and Human Services' (HHS) Medicare-Endorsed Prescription Drug Card Assistance Initiative, and set forth the necessary requirements to participate in the initiative. This proposed rule also cross-references an advance notice of proposed rulemaking entitled "Medicare Program; Medicare-Endorsed Prescription Drug Discount Card Assistance Initiative for State Sponsors", published elsewhere in this **Federal Register** issue, outlining steps that we are considering proposing in support of State efforts to make more readily available affordable prescription drugs to Medicare beneficiaries.

6. Dates →

DATES: We will consider comments if we receive them at the appropriate address, as provided below, no later than 5 p.m. on May 6, 2002.

7. Address →

ADDRESSES: in commenting, please refer to file code CMS-4027-P. Because of staff and resource limitations, we cannot accept comments by facsimile (FAX) transmission. Mail written comments (one original and three copies) to the following address ONLY: Centers for Medicare & Medicaid Services, Department of Health and Human Services, Attention: CMS-4027-P, P.O. Box 8013, Baltimore, MD 21244-8013.

Please allow sufficient time for mailed comments to be timely received in the event of delivery delays.

If you prefer, you may deliver (by hand or courier) your written comments (one original and three copies) to one of the following addresses:
Department of Health and Human
   Services, Hubert H. Humphrey
   Building, 200 Independence Avenue,
   Room 443-G, Washington DC 20201,
   or
Centers for Medicare & Medicaid
   Services, 7500 Security Boulevard,
   Room C5-16-03, Baltimore, MD
   21244-1850.

Comments mailed to the addresses indicated as appropriate for hand or courier delivery may be delayed and could be considered late.

For information on viewing public comments, see the beginning of the **SUPPLEMENTARY INFORMATION FOR FURTHER INFORMATION:** Debbie Van Hoven, (410) 786-8070.

SUPPLEMENTARY INFORMATION: Inspection of Public Comments: Comments received timely will be available for public inspection as they are received, generally beginning approximately 3 weeks after publication of a document, at the headquarters of the Centers for Medicare & Medicaid Services, 7500 Security Boulevard, Baltimore, Maryland 21244, Monday through Friday of each week from 8:30 a.m. to 4 p.m. To schedule an appointment to view public comments, telephone (410) 768-7197.

I. Background

A. History of the Initiative

With limited exceptions, the Medicare benefit package currently does not include an outpatient prescription drug benefit. While approximately 73 percent of Medicare beneficiaries have drug coverage at any given time (under, for example, employer-sponsored retiree health plans or Medicaid), an estimated 10 million have no drug coverage. Without access to the discounts that come with most kinds of prescription drug coverage, many beneficiaries either pay list prices for drugs or have access only to drug discount programs that include modest discounts at the pharmacy. These beneficiaries often do not have access to the valuable services offered by some drug benefit and assistance programs, including services such as drug interaction, allergy monitoring, and advice on how medication needs might be met at a lower cost. Further, a substantial share of beneficiaries have little experience with choosing among prescription drug assistance plans as envisioned in almost all Medicare drug benefit proposals being considered by the Congress. This, along with the need for us to operationalize such a complex benefit, implies a substantial "lead time" for successful implementation of a prescription drug benefit. In his Fiscal Year 2002 and 2003 budgets, the President proposed adding a prescription drug benefit for all Medicare beneficiaries. In the interim before the Medicare drug benefit can be enacted and fully implemented, the President believes that beneficiaries should have access to rebates or discounts from pharmaceutical manufacturers on prescription drugs as well as to pharmaceutical management services that are commonly available in good private insurance plans.

On July 12, 2001, the President announced an initiative that would create a Medicare-Endorsed Prescription Drug Discount Card program to assist Medicare beneficiaries in accessing lower cost prescription drugs and better advice on using them, and understanding the private sector methods that are used to reduce prescription drug costs and improve the quality of pharmaceutical services. We published a notice in the **Federal Register** on July 18, 2001 (66 FR 37564) that contained the application we planned to use to select the entities eligible for the Medicare endorsement. Based on comments received on that application, we issued a revised application on August 2, 2001 on our Web site at http://www.cms.gov.

On September 11, 2001, the United States District Court for the District of Columbia issued a preliminary injunction against this Medicare-Endorsed Prescription Drug Discount Card program. National Ass'n of Chain Drug Stores v. Thompson, No. 01-1554 (D.D.C. 2001). In accordance with that order, we have ceased all work on implementing that program. Although we had received 28 proposals for the drug discount card endorsement in response to our August 2, 2001 solicitation before the September 11, 2001 order, we will not make any Medicare endorsements on the basis of those proposals.

On October 10, 2001, we filed a Motion for Stay with the United States District Court for the District of Columbia asking that the case giving rise to the preliminary injunction be stayed while we engage in notice and comment rulemaking on a modified prescription drug discount card program. On November 5, 2001, the court issued an order granting the Motion for Stay while we submit our proposed policy for comment by publishing this proposed rule in the Federal Register. By publishing this proposed rule, we are formally withdrawing the program described in the Federal Register on July 18, 2001. We are instead soliciting comments on all aspects of the proposed Medicare-Endorsed Prescription Drug Card Assistance Initiative described in this proposed rule.

This proposed rule describes a program that differs in important respects from the Administration's initial proposal, for example, by requiring card sponsors to obtain substantial manufacturer rebates or discounts, requiring that manufacturer rebates or discounts be shared with

Figure 2-2 Example of page from the *Federal Register. (From* Federal Register, *October 11, 2000, vol. 65 [197]: 60366.)*

- Overhead costs
- Malpractice costs

Often referred to as fee schedule

Annually, CMS updates RVU based on national and local factors

MEDICARE FRAUD AND ABUSE

Program established by Medicare
- To decrease fraud and abuse

Beneficiary signatures on file
- Service, charges submitted without need for patient signature

Presents opportunity for fraud

Fraud

Intentional deception to benefit

Example: Submitting for services not provided

Anyone who submits for Medicare services can be violator
- Physicians
- Hospitals

Laboratories

Billing services

YOU

Fraud Can Be

Billing for services not provided

Misrepresenting diagnosis

Kickbacks

Unbundling services

Falsifying medical necessity

Consistent waiver of copayment

Office of the Inspector General (OIG)

Each year develops work plan

Outlines Medicare monitoring program

FI monitors those areas identified in plan

Complaints of Fraud or Abuse

Submitted orally or in writing to FI

Allegations made by anyone against anyone

Allegations followed up by FI

Abuse

Generally involves
- Impropriety
- Lack of medical necessity for services reported

Review takes place after claim submitted
- FI go back and do historical review of claims

Kickbacks

Bribe or rebate for referring patient for any service covered by Medicare

Any personal gain kickback

A felony
- 25,000 fine or
- 5 years in jail or
- Both

Protect Yourself

Use your common sense

Submit only truthful and accurate claims

If you are unsure about charges
- Check with physician or supervisor

MANAGED HEALTH CARE

Network health care providers that offer health care services under one organization

Group hospitals, physicians, or other providers

90% of people with health care coverage have organization (e.g., HMO)

Managed Care Organizations

Responsible for health care services to an enrolled group or person

Coordinate various health care services

Negotiate with providers

Preferred Provider Organization

Providers form network to offer health care services as group

Enrollees who seek health care outside PPO pay more

Health Maintenance Organization

Total package health care

Out-of-pocket expenses minimal

Assigned physician acts as gatekeeper to refer patient outside organization

REIMBURSEMENT TERMINOLOGY

Advance Beneficiary Notice	ABN, notification in advance of services as to the amount of reimbursement from Centers for Medicare and Medicaid Services
Ancillary Service	A service that is supportive of care of a patient, such as laboratory services
Assignment	A legal agreement that allows the provider to receive direct payment from a payer and the provider to accept payment as payment in full for covered services
Attending Physician	The physician legally responsible for oversight of an inpatient's care
Beneficiary	The person who benefits from insurance coverage; also known as subscriber, dependent, enrollee, member, or participant
Birthday Rule	When both parents have insurance coverage, the parent with the birthday earliest in the year is the primary coverage for a dependent
Certified Registered Nurse Anesthetist	CRNA, an individual with specialized training and certification in nursing and anesthesia
Coinsurance	Cost-sharing of covered services
Compliance Plan	Written strategy developed by medical facilities to ensure appropriate, consistent documentation within the medical record and ensure compliance with third-party payer guidelines
Concurrent Care	More than one physician providing care to a patient at the same time
Coordination of Benefits	COB, management of multiple third-party payments to ensure overpayment does not occur
Co-payment	Cost-sharing between beneficiary and payer
Deductible	That portion of covered services paid by the beneficiary before third-party payment begins
Documentation	Detailed chronology of facts and observations regarding a patient's health
Durable Medical Equipment	DME, medically related equipment that is not disposable, such as wheelchairs, crutches, and vaporizers
Electronic Data Interchange	EDI, computerized submission of health care insurance information exchange
Employer Identification Number	EIN, an Internal Revenue Services (IRS)–issued identification number used on tax documents
Encounter Form	Medical document that contains information regarding a patient visit for health care services
Explanation of Benefits	EOB, written, detailed listing of medical service payments by third-party payer to inform beneficiary and provider of payment
Fee Schedule	Established list of established payment for medical services

Follow-up Days	FUD, established by third-party payers and listing the number of days after a procedure for which a provider must provide services to a patient for no fee
Group Provider Number	GPN, numeric designation for a group of providers that is used instead of the individual provider number
Invalid Claim	Claim that is missing necessary information and cannot be processed or paid
Medical Record	Documentation about the health care of a patient
Noncovered Services	Any service not included by a third-party payer in the list of services for which payment is made
National Provider Identifier	NPI, 10-digit number assigned to provider and used for identification purposes when submitting services to third-party payers
Prior Authorization	Also known as preauthorization, which is a requirement by payer to receive written permission prior to patient services if the service is to be considered for payment by the payer
Provider Identification Number	PIN, or UPIN, number assigned by the third-party payer to providers to be used for identification purposes when submitting services to third-party payers
Reimbursement	Payment from a third-party payer for services rendered to a patient covered by the payer's health care plan
Resource-based Relative Value Scale	RBRVS, a list of physician services with units of monetary value
State License Number	Identification number issued by a state to a physician who has been granted the right to practice in that state
Usual, Customary, and Reasonable	UCR, used by third-party payers to establish a payment rate for a service in an area with the usual (standard fee in area), customary (standard fee by the physician), and reasonable (as determined by payer)

REIMBURSEMENT QUIZ

1. Any person who is identified as receiving life or medical benefits:
   a. primary
   b. beneficiary
   c. participant
   d. recipient

2. According to the Birthday Rule, if both parents are covered by an employer-provided health policy, the insurance policy that would be primary for reporting their child's health services is:
   a. parent with the birthday earliest in the year
   b. parent with the birthday latest in the year
   c. either parent
   d. whichever parent the child's birthday is closest to

3. Abbreviation for medical equipment that is able to be reused:
   a. DRG
   b. CRN
   c. DME
   d. DIM

4. Management of multiple third-party payments to ensure that overpayment does not occur:
   a. PRO
   b. COB
   c. DME
   d. FUD

5. CMS delegates the daily operation of the Medicare program to:
   a. DHHS
   b. PRO
   c. RVU
   d. FI

6. A PAR physician is one who:
   a. signs an agreement with the FI
   b. submits charges directly to CMS
   c. receives 5% less than some other physicians
   d. can bill the patient after payment from Medicare

7. This part of Medicare covers the hospital portion:
   a. Part A
   b. Part B
   c. Part C
   d. Part D

8. This issue of the *Federal Register* contains outpatient facility changes for CMS programs for the coming year:
   a. October/November
   b. November/December
   c. December/October
   d. November/August

9. This replaced the RBRVS:
   a. RAI
   b. OPPS
   c. APC
   d. NFS

10. Entity responsible for development of the plan that outlines monitoring of the Medicare program:
    a. FI
    b. OIG
    c. DHSS
    d. HEW

REIMBURSEMENT QUIZ ANSWERS

1. b		6. a	
2. c		7. a	
3. c		8. b	
4. b		9. d	
5. d		10. b	

UNIT III

Overview of CPT, ICD-9-CM, and HCPCS Coding

INTRODUCTION TO MEDICAL CODING

- Transforms services/procedures/supplies/drugs into CPT/HCPCS codes
- Transforms diagnosis into ICD-9-CM codes

Three Levels of Service Codes

1. Level I CPT
2. Level II HCPCS, National Codes
3. Level III Local Codes—phased out

Diagnosis Codes, ICD-9-CM

ICD-9-CM, Volumes 1 and 2, *International Classification of Disease*, 9th ed., Clinical Modification

1. Classification system
2. Changes diagnoses into codes
3. Diabetes becomes 250.XX

CPT

Developed by the AMA in 1966

Five-digit codes to report services provided to patients

Updated in November for use January 1

Types of CPT Codes

1. Medical
2. Surgical
3. Diagnostic services
4. Anesthesia

CPT Codes

Allow communication that is both effective and efficient

Informs third-party payers of services/procedures provided

Are used as a basis of payment

Incorrect Coding

Results in providers being paid inappropriately (either too much or too little)

Outpatient Services

Reported on insurance form

CMS-1500 = universal form **(Figure 3-1)**

PLEASE
DO NOT
STAPLE
IN THIS
AREA

HEALTH INSURANCE CLAIM FORM

PICA ☐☐

PICA ☐☐	

1. MEDICARE   MEDICAID   CHAMPUS   CHAMPVA   GROUP HEALTH PLAN   FECA BLK LUNG   OTHER
  ☐ (Medicare #) ☐ (Medicaid #) ☐ (Sponsor's SSN) ☐ (VA File #) ☐ (SSN or ID) ☐ (SSN) ☐ (ID)

1a. INSURED'S I.D. NUMBER   (FOR PROGRAM IN ITEM 1)

2. PATIENT'S NAME (Last Name, First Name, Middle Initial)

3. PATIENT'S BIRTH DATE   MM   DD   YY   SEX   M ☐   F ☐

4. INSURED'S NAME (Last Name, First Name, Middle Initial)

5. PATIENT'S ADDRESS (No., Street)

6. PATIENT RELATIONSHIP TO INSURED   Self ☐ Spouse ☐ Child ☐ Other ☐

7. INSURED'S ADDRESS (No., Street)

CITY   STATE

8. PATIENT STATUS   Single ☐ Married ☐ Other ☐

CITY   STATE

ZIP CODE   TELEPHONE (Include Area Code)   (   )

Employed ☐   Full-Time Student ☐   Part-Time Student ☐

ZIP CODE   TELEPHONE (INCLUDE AREA CODE)   (   )

9. OTHER INSURED'S NAME (Last Name, First Name, Middle Initial)

10. IS PATIENT'S CONDITION RELATED TO:

11. INSURED'S POLICY GROUP OR FECA NUMBER

a. OTHER INSURED'S POLICY OR GROUP NUMBER

a. EMPLOYMENT? (CURRENT OR PREVIOUS)   ☐ YES   ☐ NO

a. INSURED'S DATE OF BIRTH   MM   DD   YY   SEX   M ☐   F ☐

b. OTHER INSURED'S DATE OF BIRTH   MM   DD   YY   SEX   M ☐   F ☐

b. AUTO ACCIDENT?   PLACE (State)   ☐ YES   ☐ NO

b. EMPLOYER'S NAME OR SCHOOL NAME

c. EMPLOYER'S NAME OR SCHOOL NAME

c. OTHER ACCIDENT?   ☐ YES   ☐ NO

c. INSURANCE PLAN NAME OR PROGRAM NAME

d. INSURANCE PLAN NAME OR PROGRAM NAME

10d. RESERVED FOR LOCAL USE

d. IS THERE ANOTHER HEALTH BENEFIT PLAN?   ☐ YES   ☐ NO   **If yes**, return to and complete item 9 a-d.

READ BACK OF FORM BEFORE COMPLETING & SIGNING THIS FORM.
12. PATIENT'S OR AUTHORIZED PERSON'S SIGNATURE I authorize the release of any medical or other information necessary to process this claim. I also request payment of government benefits either to myself or to the party who accepts assignment below.

SIGNED _____   DATE _____

13. INSURED'S OR AUTHORIZED PERSON'S SIGNATURE I authorize payment of medical benefits to the undersigned physician or supplier for services described below.

SIGNED _____

14. DATE OF CURRENT: MM   DD   YY   ◀ ILLNESS (First symptom) OR INJURY (Accident) OR PREGNANCY(LMP)

15. IF PATIENT HAS HAD SAME OR SIMILAR ILLNESS. GIVE FIRST DATE   MM   DD   YY

16. DATES PATIENT UNABLE TO WORK IN CURRENT OCCUPATION   MM   DD   YY   FROM   TO   MM   DD   YY

17. NAME OF REFERRING PHYSICIAN OR OTHER SOURCE

17a. I.D. NUMBER OF REFERRING PHYSICIAN

18. HOSPITALIZATION DATES RELATED TO CURRENT SERVICES   MM   DD   YY   FROM   TO   MM   DD   YY

19. RESERVED FOR LOCAL USE

20. OUTSIDE LAB?   ☐ YES   ☐ NO $ CHARGES

21. DIAGNOSIS OR NATURE OF ILLNESS OR INJURY. (RELATE ITEMS 1,2,3 OR 4 TO ITEM 24E BY LINE)
1. |___.__   3. |___.__
2. |___.__   4. |___.__

22. MEDICAID RESUBMISSION CODE   ORIGINAL REF. NO.

23. PRIOR AUTHORIZATION NUMBER

24. A DATE(S) OF SERVICE						B Place of Service	C Type of Service	D PROCEDURES, SERVICES, OR SUPPLIES (Explain Unusual Circumstances) CPT/HCPCS MODIFIER	E DIAGNOSIS CODE	F $ CHARGES	G DAYS OR UNITS	H EPSDT Family Plan	I EMG	J COB	K RESERVED FOR LOCAL USE
From MM	DD	YY	To MM	DD	YY										
1															
2															
3															
4															
5															
6															

25. FEDERAL TAX I.D. NUMBER   SSN ☐ EIN ☐

26. PATIENT'S ACCOUNT NO.

27. ACCEPT ASSIGNMENT? (For govt. claims, see back)   ☐ YES   ☐ NO

28. TOTAL CHARGE $

29. AMOUNT PAID $

30. BALANCE DUE $

31. SIGNATURE OF PHYSICIAN OR SUPPLIER INCLUDING DEGREES OR CREDENTIALS (I certify that the statements on the reverse apply to this bill and are made a part thereof.)

SIGNED _____   DATE _____

32. NAME AND ADDRESS OF FACILITY WHERE SERVICES WERE RENDERED (If other than home or office)

33. PHYSICIAN'S, SUPPLIER'S BILLING NAME, ADDRESS, ZIP CODE & PHONE #

PIN#   GRP#

(APPROVED BY AMA COUNCIL ON MEDICAL SERVICE 8/88)   **PLEASE PRINT OR TYPE**   APPROVED OMB-0938-0008 FORM CMS-1500 (12-90),   FORM RRB-1500,
APPROVED OMB-1215-0055 FORM OWCP-1500,   APPROVED OMB-0720-0001 (CHAMPUS)

(vertical right margin labels: CARRIER — PATIENT AND INSURED INFORMATION — PHYSICIAN OR SUPPLIER INFORMATION)

Figure 3-1   Block 27, Accept Assignment on the CMS-1500 Health Insurance Claim Form. *(Courtesy U.S. Department of Health and Human Services, Centers for Medicare and Medicaid Services.)*

CPT Format

Five symbols. Used to convey information

1. • Bullet = New code symbol

2. ▲ Triangle = Description change

3. ►◄ Right and left triangles = Beginning and ending of text change

4. + Plus = Add-on code
   - Can only be used with another specific code
   - Never used alone
   - Full list in Appendix D of CPT

5. ⊘ Circle with line = -51 cannot be used with these codes
   - Full list in Appendix E of CPT

Six CPT Sections

1. Evaluation & Management (E/M)

2. Anesthesia

3. Surgery

4. Radiology

5. Pathology and Laboratory

6. Medicine

Categorized By

Sections

Subsections

Subheadings

Categories

Anatomy

Knee or Shoulder

Procedure

Incision or Excision

Condition

Fracture or Dislocation

Description

Cast or Strap

Surgical approach

Anterior Cranial Fossa or Middle Cranial Fossa

Guidelines

- Section-specific information begins each section
- Must reading

Notes

- Located throughout CPT

Two Types of Codes

1. Stand-alone: Full description

2. Indented: Dependent on preceding stand-alone for meaning

Semicolon

1. Indicates full description in preceding code

2. You must return to stand-alone for full description

Modifiers Add Information

CPT Modifier

Example of Modifier

43820 gastrojejunostomy
- -62 two surgeons
- 43820-62 two surgeons performed a gastrojejunostomy

Level II HCPCS Modifiers

- "-AS" physician's assistant
- "-F1" Left hand, second digit

All modifiers used on CPT or HCPCS codes

Modifiers are placed in 24D modifier on CMS-1500 (see Figure 3-1)

Unlisted Services

Codes end in "99" = "no specific code"

Equals = Miscellaneous

Used if no more specific code

Written report must accompany indicating

1. Nature

2. Extent

3. Need

4. Time

5. Effort

6. Equipment used

Category III Codes—New Technology

- Temporary codes—up to 3 years
- Identify emerging technology, services, and procedures
- Located after Medicine Section
- Alphanumeric (0012T)

1. May or may not receive future Category I code status
   - Category I codes (00100-99600)

1. Approved by AMA and the Food and Drug Administration

2. Proven clinical effectiveness
   - Category III have not been approved and have no proven clinical effectiveness.
   - Use Category III code instead of unlisted code.
   - Use unlisted code if no Category III code.

The Index

Used to locate service/procedure terms and codes

Speeds up code location

Like a dictionary

- First entries and last entries on top of page
- Code display in index:
  *Single code: 38115
  *Multiple codes: 26645, 26650
  *Range of codes: 22305-22325

Location Methods

Service/procedure: Repair, excision

Anatomic site: Medial nerve, elbow

Condition or disease: Cleft lip, clot

Synonym: Toe and interphalangeal joint

Eponym: Jones Procedure, Heller Operation

Abbreviation: ECG, PEEP (Pressure Breathing, Positive)

"See" in Index

Cross-reference terms: "Look here for code"

Index: Stem, Brain: *See* Brainstem

Appendices of CPT

1. Appendix A: Modifiers

2. Appendix B: Additions, deletions, revision

3. Appendix C: Clinical examples, E/M codes

4. Appendix D: Add-on codes

5. Appendix E: -51 Exempt codes

EVALUATION AND MANAGEMENT (E/M) SECTION (99201-99499)

> **Your job is to code what is documented in medical record**
> **Optimize—never maximize**
> **Accurately report documented services**
> **Coding for services not provided is a CRIME**

- Subsections by type of service
- Types of service:
  1. Consultation
  2. Office Services
  3. Hospital Services, etc.

Three Factors of E/M Codes

Place of Service

Explains setting of service:

*Office

*Emergency Department

*Nursing Home

Type of Service

Physicians provide many types of services:
- Consultations
- Admissions
- Office visits, etc.

Patient Status

The four status types are:

1. New patient

2. Established patient

3. Outpatient

4. Inpatient

New Patient

- Has not received service in last 3 years from the same physician or another physician in same specialty in same group
- New patients are more labor intensive for physician and staff

Established Patient

- Has received services in last 3 years from the same physician or another physician of the same specialty in the same group
- Medical record available with current, relevant information

Outpatient

One who has not been admitted to a health care facility

> **Example:** Patient receives services at clinic or same-day surgery center

Inpatient

*One who has been formally admitted to a health care facility

*Physician dictates:

Admission orders

H&P

Requests consultations

On certification examinations, the level of E/M service is indicated.
- DO NOT challenge the indicated levels.

Levels of E/M Service Based on

- Skill required to provide service
- Time spent
- Level of knowledge necessary
- Effort required
- Responsibility required

E/M Levels Are Divided Based on

Key Components (KC)

1. History

2. Examination

3. Medical decision making

Contributing Factors (CF)

1. Counseling

2. Coordination of care

3. Nature of presenting problem

4. Time

Every Encounter Contains Varying Amount of KC and CF

1. More of each component/factor
   - Higher level of service

2. Less of each component/factor
   - Lower level of service

KEY COMPONENTS

Four Elements of a History

1. Chief Complaint (CC)

2. History of Present Illness (HPI)

3. Review of Systems (ROS)

4. Past, Family, or Social History (PFSH)

Chief Complaint (CC)—Subjective

- Reason for encounter: patient's current complaint
- Documented in medical record for each encounter

History of Present Illness (HPI)—Subjective

- Description of development of current illness, e.g., date of onset
- Patient describes HPI

PHYSICIAN AND PATIENT DIALOGUE

Development of a CC of Abdominal Pain:

"Started Thursday night and was mild. During the night, it got worse. Friday morning I went to work but had to leave because the pain got so bad."
Location. Specific source of pain
"Pain was in lower left-hand side, a little toward back."
Quality. Is pain sharp, intermittent, burning?
"Pain is really sharp and constant."
Severity. Is pain intense, moderate, mild?
"Pain is terrible, worst pain I have ever had." (intense)
Duration. How long has pain been present?
"Pain has been going on now for three days."
Timing. Is pain present all of time or does it come and go?
"Pain just continues. It just doesn't go away."
Context. When does it hurt most?
"Pain is just there, it doesn't matter what I am doing."
Modifying factors. Does anything make it better or worse?
"Nothing I do makes it any better or any worse."
Associated signs and symptoms. Does anything else feel different when pain is present?
"Yes, I have nausea when pain is worst."

Review of Systems (ROS): Subjective

Body Areas. e.g., the back, arm, leg
Organ Systems. e.g., respiratory system, cardiovascular system

Extent of ROS depends on CC

ROS Elements

1. Constitutional—General, Fever, Weight

2. Eyes—Organ System (OS)

3. Ears, Nose, Mouth, Throat (OS)

4. Cardiovascular (OS)

5. Respiratory (OS)

6. Gastrointestinal (OS)

7. Genitourinary (OS)

8. Musculoskeletal (OS)

9. Integumentary (OS)

10. Neurologic (OS)

11. Psychiatric (OS)

12. Endocrine (OS)

13. Hematologic (OS)

14. Allergic/Immunologic (OS)

Past, Family, and Social History (PFSH)

Past and Social History. Contains relevant information about past:

1. Major illnesses/injuries

2. Operations

3. Hospitalizations

4. Allergies

5. Immunizations

6. Dietary status

7. Sexual history

8. Other relevant social factors

Family History

1. Health status of family members:
   - Parents
   - Siblings
   - Children

2. Family history items related to CC

Four History Levels

1. Problem Focused

2. Expanded Problem Focused

3. Detailed

4. Comprehensive

Problem Focused History

1. Brief history focused on CC

2. HPI

3. No PFSH

4. No ROS

Expanded Problem Focused History

1. Brief history focused on CC

2. HPI

3. No PFSH

4. ROS as it pertains to Presenting Problem

Detailed History

1. Extended history

2. HPI

3. Pertinent PFSH

4. Extended ROS

Comprehensive History

1. Extended history

2. HPI

3. Complete PFSH

4. Comprehensive ROS

Summary of elements required for each level of history **(Figure 3-2)**

Four Examination Levels

Problem Focused Examination

1. Affected body area or organ system

Expanded Problem Focused Examination

1. Affected body area or organ system

2. Other related body area(s) or organ system(s)

Detailed Examination

1. Extended examination of affected body area(s) or related organ system(s)

Comprehensive Examination

1. Complete single specialty or complete multisystem examination

Summary of elements required for each level of examination **(Figure 3-3)**

History Elements

Chief Complaint (CC)
Reason for the encounter in the patient's words

History of Present Illness (HPI)
Location
Quality
Severity
Duration
Timing
Context
Modifying factors
Associated signs and symptoms

Review of Systems (ROS)
Constitutional symptoms
Ophthalmologic (eyes)
Otolaryngologic (ears, nose, mouth, throat)
Cardiovascular
Respiratory
Gastrointestinal
Genitourinary
Musculoskeletal
Integumentary
Neurologic
Psychiatric
Endocrine
Hematologic/Lymphatic
Allergic/Immunologic

Past, Family, and/or Social History (PFSH)
Past illnesses, operations, injuries, and treatments
Family medical history for heredity and risk
Social activities, both past and current

Elements Required for Each Level of History

History	Problem Focused	Expanded Problem Focused	Detailed	Comprehensive
	CC	CC	CC	CC
	Brief HPI	Brief HPI	Extended HPI	Extended HPI
		Problem-pertinent ROS	Extended ROS	Complete ROS
			Pertinent PFSH	Complete PFSH

Figure 3-2 History elements required for each level of history.

Medical Decision Making Complexity (MDM)

Management Options

1. Based on number of possible diagnoses or various ways condition can be treated

2. Levels: Minimal, limited, multiple, or extensive

Data Reviewed

1. Laboratory, radiology; any test/procedure results are documented in medical record

2. A review of results should be documented in the medical record:

   "Hemoglobin within normal limits."

   "Chest x-ray, negative."

3. Old medical records (data) from others may be requested and reviewed

4. Levels: minimal, limited, multiple, or extensive

Examination Elements

General
Constitutional

Body Areas (BA)
Head (including the face)
Neck
Chest (including breasts and axillae)
Abdomen
Genitalia, groin, buttocks
Back
Each extremity

Organ System (OS)
Ophthalmologic (eyes)
Otolaryngologic (ears, nose, mouth, throat)
Cardiovascular
Respiratory
Gastrointestinal
Genitourinary
Musculoskeletal
Integumentary
Neurologic
Psychiatric
Hematologic/Lymphatic/Immunologic

Elements Required for Each Level of Examination

	Problem Focused	Expanded Problem Focused	Detailed	Comprehensive
Examination	Limited to affected BA or OS	Limited to affected BA or OS and other related OS(s)	Extended of affected BA(s) and other related OS(s)	General multi-system or complete single OS

Figure 3-3 Examination elements required for each level of examination.

Risks

1. Risks of morbidity (poor outcome), complications, or mortality (death) with problem and/or treatment

2. Other diseases or factors:
   Diabetes
   Extreme age

3. Urgency relates to risks:

   Myocardial infarction

   Ruptured appendix

4. Levels: minimal, low, moderate, or high

Four Risk Levels

Minimal

Self-limited
• Wasp bite

Low

Several minimal levels or one level that is more than minimal
• Multiple wasp bites

Moderate

- One chronic condition
  - Diabetes
- Two or more stable but chronic conditions
  - Controlled high blood pressure and diabetes
- Undiagnosed condition with unknown prognosis
  - Breast lump
- Acute illness
  - Pneumonia

High

- One or more chronic illnesses with current exacerbation
  - Malignant hypertension and uncontrolled diabetes
- Illness or injury that is life threatening
  - Myocardial infarction
  - Cardiac arrest

Four Levels of MDM Complexity

Straightforward MDM

1. Number of diagnosis or management options: minimal

2. Amount or complexity of data: minimal/none

3. Risk of complications or death: minimal

Low-Complexity MDM

1. Number of diagnosis or management options: limited

2. Amount and complexity of data: limited

3. Risk of complications or death: low

Moderate-Complexity MDM

1. Number of diagnosis or management options: multiple

2. Amount and complexity of data: moderate

3. Risk of complications or death: moderate

High-Complexity MDM

1. Number of diagnosis or management options: extensive

2. Amount and complexity of data: extensive

3. Risk of complications or death: high

Summary of elements required for each level of MDM **(Figure 3-4)**

Contributing Factors

Counseling

Provided to patient or family members

Discussion of diagnosis, test results, impressions, recommendations

Medical Decision-Making Elements

Number of Diagnoses or Management Options
Minimal
Limited
Multiple
Extensive

Amount or Complexity of Data to Review
Minimal/None
Limited
Moderate
Extensive

Risk of Complications or Death if Condition Goes Untreated
Minimal
Low
Moderate
High

Elements Required for Each Level of Medical Decision Making

	Straightforward	Low	Moderate	High
Number of diagnoses or management options	Minimal	Limited	Multiple	Extensive
Amount or complexity of data to review	Minimal/None	Limited	Moderate	Extensive
Risk	Minimal	Low	Moderate	High

Figure 3-4 Decision making elements required for each level of medical decision making.

Coordination of Care

Work done on behalf of patient by physician to provide care

Nature of Presenting Problem

Type of problem patient presents to physician with

Levels of Presenting Problem

Minimal Presenting Problem

May not require a physician

Example: A dressing change or removal of an uncomplicated suture

Self-Limiting Presenting Problem

Self-limiting problem are minor and with a good outcome predicted

Example: Sore throat or a slightly irritated skin tag

Low-Risk Presenting Problem

Without treatment, low risk

Example: A middle aged, healthy male with an upper respiratory infection

Moderate-Risk Presenting Problem

Without treatment, moderate risk

Example: An elderly male with pneumonia

High-Risk Presenting Problem

Without treatment, high risk

Example: An elderly male in very poor health with severe pneumonia

Time

- Direct face-to-face: Physician and patient together
  Example: Clinic visit or at bedside in hospital
- To use to assign code, beginning and ending times documented in medical record
- Unit/Floor: Time spent on patient's floor or unit, also at patient's bedside
  Example: Reviewing patient records or at chart desk and then with patient

Use of E/M Code

Codes are grouped by type of service

1. Consultation

2. Office visit

3. Hospital service

Different codes for various levels of service
    New patient (99201-99205) services to new patient in office or other outpatient setting

Established Patient (99211-99215)

99211, may not require a physician

No such code in New Patient category; all new patients are seen by physician

Hospital Observation Status (99217-99220, 99234-99239)

- Not officially admitted to a hospital
- Patient not ill enough to admit but is too ill not to be monitored
- Read notes at beginning of subsection
- Observation services are not codes for "inpatient" services
- Observation admission can only be reported for first day of service
- When patient admitted on observation status and discharged on same day:
  Use code from 99234-99236 (Observation or Inpatient Care Services category)
- Patient in hospital overnight for observation but less than 48 hours:
  1st day: 99218-99220 (Initial Observation Care)
  2nd day: 99217 (Observation Care Discharge Services)
- If observation stay longer than 48 hours:
  1st day: 99218-99220 (Initial Observation Care)
  2nd day: 99212-99215 (Established Pt, Office)
  3rd day: 99217 (Observation Care Discharge Services)

- Initial Observation Care
    - Beginning of observation care service
    - Does not require a specific hospital unit; can be a regular bed
        - Status specified as "observation"
- Services immediately prior to admission bundled into observation service
    - **Example:** Office visit prior to observation, bundled into observation service

Hospital Inpatient Services (99221-99239)

Officially admitted to a hospital setting

Total (all day and night)

Partial (all day and no night, or all night and no day, or a variation)

Types of Physician Status

Attending: Primary or admitting physician

Consultant: Physician whose opinion and advice requested by attending physician

Referring: Physician requesting a consultation from another physician regarding a patient's health status

Types of Care

Concurrent care given to patient by more than one physician

Example: Pulmonologist and cardiologist both treating patient for different conditions at same time

Three Types of Hospital Inpatient Services

Initial Hospital Care (99221-99223)

First service includes admission

Initial paperwork

Initial plans and orders

Used only once for each admission

Subsequent Hospital Care (99231-99233)

After initial service

Physician reviews patient's progress using documentation, information received from nursing staff, examination of patient

Hospital Discharge Services (99238, 99239)

Final day of hospital stay when patient in hospital more than one day

Documentation indicates final patient status

Final Status of Patient

1. Condition
2. Medications

3. Plan for return to physician

4. How hospital stay progressed

5. Discharged to home, nursing facility, etc.

6. Only attending physician can use discharge code

7. Code based on time spent in service

8. Beginning and ending time must be documented or use lowest level code

Consultation Services (99241-99275)

One physician requests another physician's opinion

Either inpatient or outpatient

Confirmatory consultations, requested to confirm or deny a diagnosis

May not know patient is seeking a confirmatory

Third-Party Payer Confirmatory Consultations

Request confirmation for:
* Past medical treatment
* Current condition
* Payers may request prior to approving procedure
* Report services with -32, mandatory services
Outpatient consultations include those provided in ER.

Emergency Department (ED) Services (99281-99288)

Codes for both new or established patients

Qualify as ED (ER) must be open 24 hours a day

Critical Care and ED Codes (99291, 99292)

ED services often require additional codes from Critical Care Services

Example: Multiple organ failure

Critical Care Services are provided to patients in life-threatening situations

Critical Care Services

99291 and 99292 to report length of time a physician spends caring for critically ill patient

99291: 30-74 minutes

99292: each additional 30 minutes

Pediatric Critical Care Patient Transport (99289-99290)

Physician, services to critically ill patients
* Face-to-face or work directly related to patient care

Codes divided on first 30-74 minutes
* Then each additional 30 minutes
* Additional time under 30 minutes not reported

Inpatient Neonatal & Pediatric Critical Care Services (99293-99299)

Reports services of physician directing care

Inpatient Pediatric Critical Care (99293, 99294)

31 days through 24 months

Reported per day

Inpatient Neonatal Critical Care (99295-99296)

1-30 days for critically ill

99295, reserved for date of admission

99296, subsequent care

Intensive (Non-Critical) Low Birth Weight Services (99298-99299)

Intensive care of VLBW (very low birth weight) or LBW (low birth weight) (<2500 g)
* 1000 g = 2.2 lb

Subsequent to admission based on VLBW (<1500 g) or LBW (1500-2500 g)

Reported per day

Nursing Facility Services (99301-99316)

Nonhospital settings with professional staff
* Provide continuous health care services to patients who are not acutely ill

Also known as: Skilled Nursing Facility (SNF)

Various Levels of Nursing Facility Services
* Intermediate care facility (ICD): lower level of care than hospital
* Long-term care facility (LTCF): lower level of care than ICD

Comprehensive Nursing Facility Assessment (99301-99303)

Provided at time of admission

Provided periodically during stay as established by facility regulations

Subsequent Nursing Facility Care codes 99311-99313 used if patient stable or condition unchanged

Domiciliary, Rest Home, or Custodial Care Services (99321-99333)

Health care services are not available on site

Types of services provided are lodging, meals, supervision, personal care, leisure activities

Residents cannot live independently

Codes for either new or established patients

Home Services (99341-99350)

Care provided in patient's home

Services based on key components and contributing facts

Prolonged Services (99354-99359)

Time codes for inpatient and outpatient

Codes for first 30-74 minutes

If less than 30 minutes, do not report service as prolonged

Physician Standby Service (99360)

Physician not caring for other patient to use these codes

Physician standing by only for that patient

Report in 30-minute increments

Less than 30 minutes—do not report

Can only report for subsequent 30 minutes if a full 30 minutes

Case Management Services (99361-99373)

Used to report coordination of care with other health professionals

Reported in increments of approximately 30 or 60 minutes

Team conferences or telephone calls

Most third-party payers will not pay for telephone calls

Care Plan Oversight Services (99374-99380)

Used to report physician supervision of patient care under home, domiciliary, or equivalent environment

Reported once for each 30-day period

Preventive Medicine Services (99381-99429)

Used to report services when patient is not currently ill

> **Example:** Annual checkup

Codes divided on new or established patient status, and age

If significant problem is encountered during preventive examination:

> *E/M code also reported

Counseling and/or Risk Factor Reduction Intervention (99401-99429)

Patient is seen specifically to promote health

> **Example:** Diet, exercise program

Patient does not have symptoms or an established diagnosis to use these codes

Codes based on:
- Time
- Individual or group
- Physician review of assessment data

Newborn Care Services (99431-99440)

Services are for normal newborns:
- Newborn H&P
- Physical exam of newborn
- Attendance at delivery to stabilize newborn requested by delivering physician

Special E/M Services (99450-99456)

Used for services provided insurance or disability assessments

Involves no treatment. Any treatment provided would be coded separately.

Codes divided on whether for work or nonwork

99455: Assessment by treating physician

99456: Assessment for non-treating physician

For new/established patients in any setting

Unlisted E/M Service (99499)

Seldom used

Require a written report with submission

ANESTHESIA SECTION (00100-01999)

Anesthesiologist

Doctor of medicine specialized in anesthesia

Usually outside practices, e.g., Anesthesia Associates, Inc. or Pain Clinic, Ltd.

Services reported separately

Uses of Anesthesia

Relieve pain

Manage unconscious patients, life functions, and resuscitation

Some Methods of Sedation

Endotracheal: Through mouth

Local: Application to area (injection or topical)

Epidural: Between vertebral spaces

Regional: Field or nerve

Patient-Controlled Analgesia (PCA)

Patient administers drug

Used to relieve chronic pain

Conscious Sedation

Decreased level of consciousness

Report with 99141 or 99142 (Medicine)

Administered by other than physician performing procedure

Anesthesia Formula

B + T + M

B Is for Basic Units

Published in RVG *(Relative Value Guide)* by American Society of Anesthesiologists

National unit values for anesthesia services based on complexity of service

T Is for Time

Patient record indicates time, e.g., 60 minutes

Usually, 15 minutes = 1 unit

   Example: 60 minutes = 4 units

Begins: Anesthesiologist begins to manage patient—preoperative

Continues throughout procedure—intraoperative

Ends: Patient no longer under care of anesthesiologist—postoperative

M Is for Modifying Unit

Physical condition indicated by modifiers

Physical Status Modifiers, P1-P6

Located in Anesthesia Guidelines

1. P1 Normal healthy
2. P2 Mild systemic disease
3. P3 Severe systemic disease
4. P4 Severe systemic disease and constant threat to life
5. P5 Not expected to survive
6. P6 Brain dead

Qualifying Circumstances Codes and Relative Value (99100-99140)

Anesthesia services provided under difficult circumstances

Located in both Anesthesia Guidelines and Medicine section

Listed in addition to primary anesthesia code

Summing Up Formula

Basic units (from RVG) based on CPT codes

Time units (15 min is usually a unit)

Modifiers [Qualifying Circumstances (99100-99140) and/or Physical Status (P1-P6)]

B + T + M = Total Units × $ = Anesthesia Payment

Conversion Factors

CMS anesthesia conversion factors

Sum of money allocated by payer, per unit for payment of anesthesia services

Anesthesia for Multiple Surgical Procedures

Once anesthetized, length of time not number of procedures performed during session

Report highest service units only

> **Example**: Two procedures during same session
> * One, 10 units; the other, 5 units
> * Report only 10 units

CPT MODIFIERS (-21 to -99)

Alters CPT or HCPCS code

Full list, CPT, Appendix A

Modifier Functions

Altered (i.e., more or less)

Bilateral

Multiple

Only portions of service

More than one surgeon

-21 PROLONGED E/M SERVICE

* Only used with highest level E/M codes (99205-99397)
* Indicates extended service above highest level in category

-22 UNUSUAL PROCEDURAL SERVICE

* Indicates services significantly greater than usual
* Accompanied by written report and supportive documentation

-23 UNUSUAL ANESTHESIA

* Use of general anesthesia where local or regional is norm
  Example: Highly agitated senile patient
* Only used with anesthesia codes
* Written report with submission of modifier

-24 UNRELATED E/M SERVICES BY SAME PHYSICIAN DURING A POSTOPERATIVE PERIOD

* Service not related to surgery

If E/M provided during post-operative global period, no payment without -24

-25 SIGNIFICANT, SEPARATELY IDENTIFIABLE E/M SERVICE, SAME PHYSICIAN/ AND DAY OF PROCEDURE/SERVICE

- Documentation must support service
  Example: Patient seen for sinus congestion, physician performs H&P, prescribes decongestant, notes lesion on back, and removes
- Code: Procedure + E/M-25

-26 PROFESSIONAL COMPONENT

- Professional component (physician, -26)
- Technical component (technician + equipment, -TC)

-32 MANDATED SERVICE

- Mandated by payer, workers' comp, or official body
- Not requests of patient, patient's family, or another physician
  Example: Worker's Compensation requests examination of person currently receiving disability benefits

-47 ANESTHESIA BY SURGEON

- Physician administers regional or general anesthesia
- Surgeon acts as both surgeon and anesthesiologist
- Only used with Surgery codes

-50 BILATERAL PROCEDURE

- Body is bilateral
  Example: Procedure on hands
- Caution: Some codes describe bilateral procedures

-51 MULTIPLE PROCEDURE—THREE TYPES

- Same Procedure, Different Sites
- Multiple Operation(s), Same Operative Session
- Same Procedure Performed Multiple Times
- List most resource intense first
- Next other procedure(s) + -51 (unless code is -51 exempt)
- Usual procedure payment: 1st 100%, 2nd 50%, 3rd 25%

-52 REDUCED SERVICES

- Service reduced from those in code description
- Physician directed reduction
- Documentation substantiates reduction
- Not for patient unable to pay

-53 DISCONTINUED PROCEDURE

- Surgical/diagnostic procedures
- Started then stopped due to patient's condition
- Does not apply to presurgical discontinuance
- DO NOT USE -53:
  When patient cancels scheduled procedure

With E/M codes
With time-based code

-54 SURGICAL CARE ONLY

- Physician provides only procedure (intraoperative)
- Documented patient transfer must be in record
  Some payers require copy of transfer

-55 POSTOPERATIVE MANAGEMENT ONLY

- Physician provides only the care after hospital discharge
- If transferred while patient hospitalized, report postop management with subsequent hospital codes 99231-99233
- Documentation of transfer in medical record

-56 PREOPERATIVE MANAGEMENT ONLY

- Physician provided only preoperative care
- Not acceptable for Medicare
  Requires E/M code
- Usual Reimbursement for portions, surgical package
  10% preoperative
  70% intraoperative
  20% postoperative
- Each payer determines portions

-57 DECISION FOR SURGERY USED WITH

- E/M, 99201-99499
- Medicine, 92012 and 92014 ophthalmologic services
- Medicare: Only for preop period of major surgery (day before or day of)

-58 STAGED/RELATED BY SAME PHYSICIAN DURING POSTOPERATIVE PERIOD

- Subsequent procedure planned at time of first surgery
  - During postop of previous surgery in series
    Example: Multiple skin grafts completed in several sessions
  - Do not use when code describes a session
    Example: 67208: lesion destruction of retina, one or more sessions

-59 DISTINCT PROCEDURAL SERVICE

- Different session or encounter
- Different procedure
- Different site
- Separate incision, excision, lesion, injury
  Example: Physician removes several lesions from patient's leg, also notes and removes mole on torso
  - Excision code for lesion removal + biopsy code for mole with -59
  - Indicates biopsy distinct procedure, not part of lesion removal

-62 TWO SURGEONS

- Both function as cosurgeons (equals)
- Usually different specialties
- Each reports same code + -62

-63 PROCEDURE PERFORMED ON INFANTS LESS THAN 4 KG

- Kilogram: 2.2 lb (4 kg = 8.8 lb)
- Small size increases complexity
- Use with all Surgery section codes except Integumentary

-66 SURGICAL TEAM

- Team: Several physicians with various specialties plus a technicians and other support personnel
- Very complex procedures
- Payers may increase payment 50%

-76 REPEAT PROCEDURE/SERVICE BY SAME PHYSICIAN

- Note: "Same Physician"
- Used to indicate necessary service
    Example: X-rays before and after fracture repair

-77 REPEAT PROCEDURE/SERVICE BY ANOTHER PHYSICIAN

- Note: "Another Physician"
- Performed by one physician, repeated by another physician
- Submitted with written report to establish medical necessity

-78 RETURN TO OPERATING ROOM FOR A RELATED PROCEDURE DURING POSTOPERATIVE PERIOD

- For complication of first procedure
    Example: Patient has outpatient procedure in morning, was returned to operating room in afternoon with severe hemorrhage
- Indicates not typographical error

-79 UNRELATED PROCEDURE OR SERVICE BY SAME PHYSICIAN DURING POSTOPERATIVE PERIOD

    Example: Several days after discharge for procedure, patient returns for unrelated office service
- Diagnosis code would also be different

-80 ASSISTANT SURGEON

- Reimbursed at 15% to 30%
- Payers identify procedures for which they reimburse assistant

-81 MINIMUM ASSISTANT SURGEON

- Services at a level less than that described in -80
- Reimbursed at 10%

-82 ASSISTANT SURGEON

- Teaching hospitals:
  Have residents who assist as part of education
  Must demonstrate no qualified resident available to use -82
  - Unavailability documented in written report

-90 REFERENCE (OUTSIDE) LABORATORY

- Physician has business relationship with outside lab
- Physician pays lab
- Physician bills payer for lab services

-91 REPEAT CLINICAL DIAGNOSTIC LABORATORY TEST

- Repeat same laboratory tests on same day for multiple test results
- Not tests rerun to confirm original test results
- Not malfunction of equipment or technician error

-99 MULTIPLE MODIFIERS

- Used when service needs more than one modifier but payer only allows for one modifier with each code
- Placement of modifier -99 on CMS-1500 **(Figure 3.5)**

SURGERY SECTION (10021-69990)

Largest CPT Section

Section Format

Divided by subspecialty, i.e., integumentary, cardiovascular

Notes and Guidelines

Throughout section

Information varied and extensive

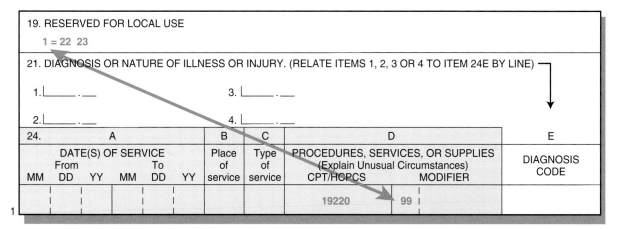

Figure 3-5 Placement of modifier -99 on the CMS-1500 Health Insurance Claim Form. *(Courtesy U.S. Department of Health and Human Services, Centers for Medicare and Medicaid Services.)*

"Must reading"

Subsection notes apply to entire subsection

Subheading notes apply to entire subheading

Category notes apply to entire category

Parenthetical information **(Figure 3-6)**

Unlisted Procedure Codes

Used only when more specific code found

Written report accompanies submission

Each unlisted code service paid on case-by-case basis

Separate Procedures

"(Separate procedure)" follows code description

Usually minor surgical procedure

Incidental to more major procedure
- Breast biopsy
- Before radical mastectomy would not be coded

Separate procedures reported when:
- Only procedure performed
- With another procedure
  - On different site
  - Unrelated to major procedure

First Major Guideline of Surgical Packages

Usually include

1. Preoperative (before, preop)

2. Intraoperative (during, intraop)

3. Postoperative (after—also known as global period, postop)

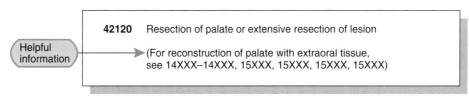

42120   Resection of palate or extensive resection of lesion

(For reconstruction of palate with extraoral tissue, see 14XXX–14XXX, 15XXX, 15XXX, 15XXX, 15XXX)

Helpful information

Figure 3-6 Parenthetical information in the CPT manual.

One bundle—one price

Each payer decides what is in bundle

Example
- Most payers specify 90 days after major surgery
- All services related to surgery in package
- Including preop, intraop, and postop

Reporting bundled items separately is unbundling

Second Major Guideline of Surgical Package

Minor Procedure: Preop and postop services are usually reported separately

Can be reported separately if specified by payer

Example
- Needle biopsy in office reported with starred procedure code
- Report:
  - Procedure (biopsy)
  - Supplies (surgical tray)

Surgical Tray

Starred procedures usually do not have supplies bundle, e.g., surgical tray: needles, suture materials, wipes, drugs

Report surgical tray with:

99070 CPT, Medicine section

A4550 HCPCS

GENERAL SUBSECTION (10021-10022)

Fine needle aspirations with or without (w/wo) imaging guidance
- Excludes bone marrow aspirations (38220)

Pathology 88172 and 88173 for aspirate evaluation

INTEGUMENTARY SYSTEM SUBSECTION (10040-19499)

Often used in all specialties of medicine

Not just surgeons or dermatologists, wide range of physicians

Subheadings of Integumentary Subsection

1. Skin, Subcutaneous, and Accessory Structures
2. Nails
3. Repair (Closure)
4. Destruction
5. Breast

Skin, Subcutaneous, and Accessory Structures (10040-11646)

Incision & Drainage (10040-10180)

- I&D of abscess, carbuncle, boil, cyst, infection, hematoma
  - Lancing (cutting of skin)
  - Aspiration (removal with needle)
- Gauze or tube may be inserted for continued drainage

Excision—Debridement (11000-11044)

Dead tissue cut away or washed away with saline

11000-11001 eczematous or infected skin

11010-11012 foreign material with fracture or dislocation

11040-11044 skin

Paring or Cutting (11055-11057)

- Removal by scraping or peeling, e.g., removal of corn or callus
- Codes indicate number: 1, 2-4, 4+

Biopsy (11100-11101)

- Skin, subcutaneous tissue, or mucous membrane biopsy
- Not all of lesion removed
  All lesion removed = excision
- Do not use modifier -51
  Codes indicate number: 1 or each additional

Skin Tag Removal (11200-11201)

- Benign lesions
- Removed with scissors, blade, chemicals, electrosurgery, etc.
- Do not use -51
  Codes indicate number: up to 15 or each additional

Shaving of Lesions (11300-11313)

- Based on:
  Size (e.g., 1.1-2 cm)
  Location (e.g., arm, hand, nose)
- Does not require suture closure
- Report most extensive lesion first with no modifier, then least extensive lesions with modifier -51

Benign/Malignant Lesions (11400-11646)

- Codes divided: Benign or malignant
- Physician assesses lesion as benign or malignant
- Codes include local anesthesia and simple closure
- Lesion size
  - Taken from physician's notes
    - Includes greatest diameter plus margins
    - Not pathology report—storage solution shrinks tissue
    - Margins (healthy tissue) are also taken for comparison with unhealthy tissue
- All excised tissue pathologically examined
- Destroyed lesions have no pathology samples
  Example: Laser or chemical
- Lesion closure
  - Simple or subcutaneous closure included in removal
  - Reported separately
    - Layered or intermediate, 12031-12057 (Repair—Intermediate)
    - Complex, 13100-13153 (Repair—Complex)
  - Local anesthesia included

Nails (11719-11765)

Both toes and fingers

Types of services:
- Trimming, debridement, removal, biopsy, repair

Introduction (11900-11983)

Types of services. Lesion injections, tattooing, tissue expansion, contraceptive insertion/removal, hormone implantation services

Repair (12001-16036)

Repair Factors in Wound Repair

- As types of wounds vary, types of wound repair also vary
- Length, complexity (simple, intermediate, complex), and site

Types of Wound Repair

Simple: Superficial, epidermis, dermis, and subcutaneous tissue

One-layer closure

Intermediate: Layered closure of deeper layers of subcutaneous tissue and superficial fascia with skin closure

Simple closure can be coded as intermediate if extensive debridement required

Complex: Greater than layered

Example: Scar revision, complicated debridement, extensive undermining, stents

Included in Wound Repair Codes

1. Simple ligation of vessels
2. Simple exploration of wound
3. Normal debridement

Grouping of Wound Repair

- Add together lengths by:
  1. **Complexity**
     Simple, intermediate, complex
  2. **Location**
     i.e., face, ears, eyelids, nose, lips

Do Not Group Wound Repairs that Are

- Different complexities
  Example: Simple repair and complex repair
- Different locations
  Example: Simple repairs of scalp (12001) and nose (12011)

Information Needed to Code Graft

1. Type of graft—adjacent, free, flap, etc.
2. Donor site (from)
3. Recipient site (to)
4. Any repair to donor site

Free Skin Graft

15000-15001 preparation of recipient site codes

15050-15261 graft codes

Split graft: Epidermis and some dermis **(Figure 3-7)**

Full-thickness: Epidermis and all dermis

Grafts (15342-15401)

- Bilaminate skin substitute
  Artificial skin
- Allograft: Donor graft
- Xenograft: Nonhuman donor

Flap (15570-15776)

- Some skin left attached to blood supply
  Keeps flap viable
- Donor site may be far from recipient site
- Flaps may be in stages
- Formation of flap (15570-15576)
  Based on location: Trunk, scalp, nose, etc.
- Transfer of flap (15650): Previously placed flap released from donor site
  Also known as walking or walk up of flap

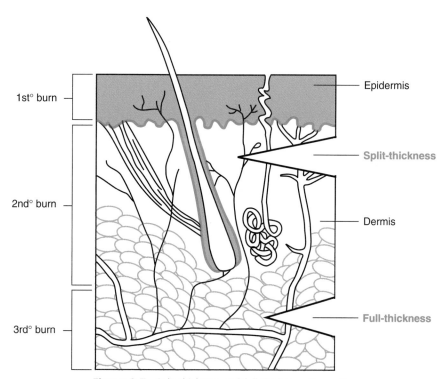

Figure 3-7   Split-thickness and full-thickness skin grafts.

- Muscle, Myocutaneous, or Fasciocutaneous Flaps (15732-15738)
  - Repairs made with
    - Muscle
    - Muscle and skin
    - Fascia and skin
  - Flaps rotated from donor to recipient site
  - Includes closure donor site
  - Codes divided on location, i.e.:
    - Trunk
    - Extremity

Pressure Ulcers (15920-15999)

- Excision and various closures
  Primary, skin flap, muscle, etc.
- Many codes "with ostectomy"
  Bone removal
- Locations
  1. Coccygeal (end of spine)
  2. Sacral (between hips)
  3. Ischial (lower hip)
  4. Trochanteric (outer hip)
- Site prep only 15936 or 15946
  Defect repair or donor site reported separately

Burns (16000-16036)

- Codes for small, medium, and large
- Most calculate percentage of body burn using Rule of Nine for adults (**Figure 3-8**)
  $4\frac{1}{2}$ small
  $4\frac{1}{2}$ to 9 medium
  >9 large
- Lund-Browder for children (**Figure 3-9**)
  - Proportions of children differ from adults
  - Heads are larger
- Often require multiple debridement and redressing
- Based on:
  1. Initial or subsequent service
  2. Size
  3. With or without anesthesia
- Report % of burn and depth

Destruction (17000-17286)

Ablation (destruction) of tissue

- Laser, electrosurgery, cryosurgery, chemosurgery, etc.

Benign/premalignant, or malignant tissue

- Based on location and size

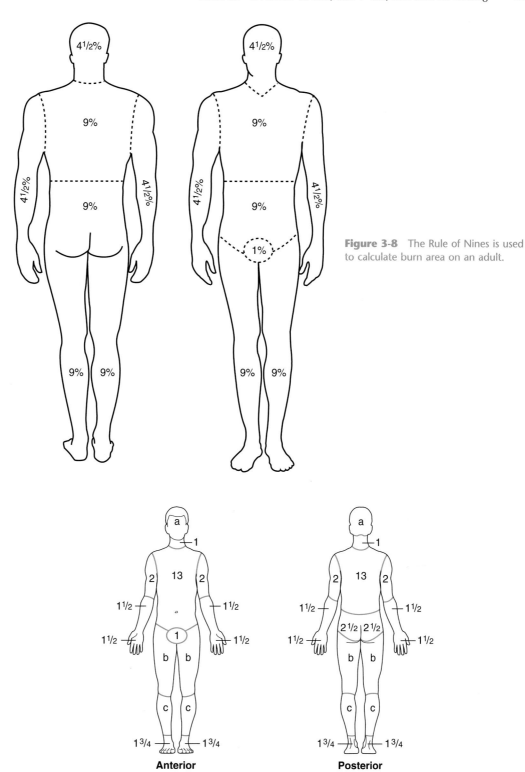

Figure 3-8   The Rule of Nines is used to calculate burn area on an adult.

Anterior   **Posterior**

Relative percentage of body surface areas (% BSA) affected by growth

	0 yr	1 yr	5 yr	10 yr	15 yr
a – ½ of head	9½	8½	6½	5½	4½
b – ½ of 1 thigh	2¾	3¼	4	4¼	4½
c – ½ of lower leg	2½	2½	2¾	3	3¼

Figure 3-9   Lund-Browder chart for estimating the extent of burns on children.

Mohs' Microscope (17304-17310)

- Surgeon acts as pathologist and surgeon
- Removes one layer of lesion at time
- Until no malignant cells remain
- Based on stages stated in report

Other Procedures (17340-17999)

Treatment of acne
- Cryotherapy
- Chemical exfoliation

Electrolysis

Unlisted procedures

Breast Procedures (19000-19499)

Divided based on procedure, i.e.:
- Incision
- Excision
- Repair

Mastectomies based on extent of procedure

Bilateral procedures, use -50

MUSCULOSKELETAL SYSTEM SUBSECTION (20000-29999)

- Subsection divided: Anatomic site, then service (e.g., excision)
- Used extensively by orthopedic surgeons
  *Many codes commonly used by variety of physicians
- Extensive notes
- Most common:
  *Fracture and dislocation treatments
  *"General" subheading
  *Arthroscopic procedures
  *Casting and strapping

Fracture Treatment

Type of treatment depends on type and severity of fracture

Open: Surgically opened to view or remotely opened to place nail across fracture site

Closed: Not surgically opened

Percutaneous: Insertion of devices through skin or a remote site

Traction
- Application of force to align bone
- Force applied by internal device (e.g., wire, pin) inserted into bone (skeletal fixation)
- Application of force by means of adhesion to skin (skin traction)

Manipulation

Use of force to return bone back to normal alignment

Codes often divided based on whether manipulation was or was not used

Dislocation

Bone displaced from normal joint position

Treatment: Return bone to normal joint location

Subheading "General"

Begins "Incision" (20000-20005)

Depth: Difference between Integumentary and Musculoskeletal incision codes

Musculoskeletal used when underlying bone or muscle is involved

Wound Exploration (20100-20103)

Traumatic penetrating wounds

Divided on wound location

Includes:
- Enlargement
- Debridement
- Foreign body(ies) removal
- Ligation
- Repair of tissue and muscle

Excision (20150-20251)

Biopsies for bone and muscle

Divided by:
- Type of biopsy (bone/muscle)
- Depth
- Some by method

Can be percutaneous or excisional

Does not include tumor excision, which is coded separately

Biopsy with excision, only code excision

Introduction and Removal (20500-20694)

Codes for:

1. Injections

2. Aspirations

3. Insertions

4. Applications

5. Removals

6. Adjustments

Therapeutic sinus tract injection procedures:
- Not nasal sinus
- Abscess or cyst with passage (sinus tract) to skin
- Antibiotic injected with use of radiographic guidance

Removal of foreign bodies lodged in muscle or bone

Integumentary removal codes for removal from skin

Injection into tendon, ligament, or ganglion cyst

Arthrocentesis injection "and/or" aspiration of a joint
- Both aspiration and injection reported with one code
- Do not unbundle and report with two codes

Replantation (20802-20838)

Used to report reattachment of amputated limb

Code by body area

Grafts (20900-20938)

Used to report harvesting through separate incision of:

1. Bone
2. Cartilage
3. Fascia lata
4. Tissue

Fascia lata grafts: from lower thigh where fascia is thickest

Some codes include obtaining grafting material (not coded separately)

Other Procedures (20950-20999)

Monitoring muscle fluid pressure (interstitial)
- Pressure increases when blood supply decreases due to increased accumulation of fluids

Bone grafts identified by site taken from (donor site)

Free osseocutaneous flaps: bone grafts
- Taken along with skin and tissue overlying bone

Electrical stimulation
- Used to speed bone healing
- Placement of stimulators externally or internally
- Ultrasound also used externally

External Fixation

Application of device that holds bone in place

Code fracture treatment and external fixation
- Unless treatment and fixation both included in code description

Spinal Instrumentation and Fixation

Spine (Ventral Column), 22100-22855 divided by repair location:

1. Cervical (C1-C7)

   C1 = Atlas

   C2 = Axis

2. Lumbar (L1-L5)

3. Thoracic (T1-T12)

Types of Spinal Instrumentation

Segmental: Devices at each end of repair area + at least 1 other attachment

Nonsegmental: Devices at each end of defect only

Arthrodesis

Fixation of joint

Often performed with other procedure such as fracture repair
- Use -51 on arthrodesis code unless service reported with add-on code

Subsequent Subheadings

After General subheading, divided by anatomic location
- Anatomic subheadings divided by type procedure

Example, subheading "Head" divided by procedure:

1. Incision

2. Excision

3. Introduction or Removal; Repair, Revision, and/or Reconstruction

4. Other Procedures

5. Fracture and/or Dislocation

Casting and Strapping (29000-29799)

Replacement procedure or initial placement to stabilize without additional restorative treatment

Initial fracture treatment includes placement and removal of first cast
- Subsequent cast applications coded separately

Application not coded when part of surgical procedure

Removal bundled into surgical procedure

Supplies reported separately

Subheading Endoscopy/Arthroscopy (29800-29999)

Surgical arthroscopy always includes diagnostic arthroscopy

Codes divided on joint
- Subdivided on procedure

Note: Parenthetical information following codes indicates codes to use if procedure was an open procedure

RESPIRATORY SYSTEM SUBSECTION (30000-32999)

- Anatomic site arrangement:
  Nose
  Larynx

- Further subdivided by procedure:
  Incision
  Excision

Endoscopy

Endoscopy in all subheadings except Nose

Each preceded by "Notes"

Endoscopy Rule One

- Code full extent
  Example: Procedure begins at mouth and ends at bronchial tube
  Bronchial tube = full extent

Endoscopy Rule Two

- Code correct approach
  Example, for removal:
  Interior lung lesion via endoscopy inserted through mouth
  Exterior lung lesion via laparoscope inserted through skin
- Incorrect approach = incorrect code = incorrect reimbursement

Endoscopy Rule Three

- Diagnostic always included in surgical
  Example:
  - Diagnostic bronchial endoscopy begins
  - Identifies foreign body
  - Removed foreign body (surgical endoscopy)

Multiple Procedures

Frequent in respiratory coding
- **Watch for bundled services**

Sequence primary procedure first, no modifier

Sequence secondary procedures next, with -51

Bilateral procedures often performed, use -50

Format for reporting chosen by payer

Example: Nasal lavage
- 31000×2
- 31000 and 31000-50
- 31000-50

Nose (30000-30999)

Used extensively by otorhinolaryngologists (ear, nose, and throat specialists, ENT)

Also used by wide variety of physicians

When approach to nose:
- External approach, use Integumentary System
- Internal approaches, use Respiratory System

Incision (30000-30020)

- Bundled into Incision codes are drain or gauze insertion and removal
- Supplies reported separately

Excision (30100-30160)

- Contains intranasal biopsy codes
- Polyp excision, by complexity
    Excision includes any method of destruction, even laser
    Use -50 (bilateral) for both sides

Introduction (30200-30220)

- Common procedures
    Example: Injections to shrink nasal tissue or displacement therapy (saline flushes) to remove mucus
    Displacement therapy performed through nose

Removal of Foreign Body (30300-30320)

- Divided by if the removal at office or hospital (requires general anesthesia)

Repair (30400-30630)

Many plastic procedures, e.g.:
- Rhinoplasty (reshaping nose internal and/or external)
- Septoplasty (rearrangement of nasal septum)

Destruction (30801-30802)

Use of cauterization or ablation (removing by cutting)

Used for removal of excess nasal mucosa or to reduce turbinate inflammation

Based on intramural or superficial extent of destruction

    Intramural: Deeper mucosa

    Superficial: Outer layer of mucosa

Other Procedures (30901-30999)

- Control of nasal hemorrhage
- Anterior packing for less severe bleeding
- Posterior packing for more severe bleeding

Accessory Sinuses, Incision (31000-31090)

Codes for lavage (washing) of sinuses
- Cannula (hollow tube) placed into sinus
- Saline solution flushed through

Use -50 (bilateral) for both sides

Larynx (31000-31599)

Laryngoscopic Procedures

- Uses terms indirect and direct
  Indirect: Tongue depressor with mirror used to view larynx
  Direct: Endoscopy passed into larynx, physician directly views vocal cords

Excision (31300-31402)

- Laryngotomy: open surgical procedure to expose larynx
  For removal procedure (e.g., tumor)
- May be confused with Trachea/Bronchi codes for tracheostomy
  Used to establish air flow

Introduction (31500-31502)

- Endotracheal intubation, establishment of airway
- Based on planned (ventilation support) or emergency procedure

Repair (31580-31590)

- Several plastic procedures and fracture repairs
- Laryngoplasty procedures based on purpose
- Fracture codes based on whether manipulation used

Trachea and Bronchi (31600-31899)

Incision (31600-31614)

- Most codes: Tracheostomy divided by:
  Planned (ventilation support)
  Emergency
- Divided by type:
  Transtracheal or cricothyroid (position of incision)

Introduction (31700-31730)

- Catheterization
- Instillation
- Injection
- Aspiration
- Trachea tube placement
- Some include inhaled gas as contrast material

Repair (31750-31830)

- Plastic repairs of tracheoplasty and bronchoplasty

Lungs and Pleura (32000-32999)

Incision (31750-31830)

Thoracentesis: Needle inserted into pleural space for aspiration (withdrawal) of fluid

Thoracotomy: Surgical opening of chest to expose to view. Used for:

1. Biopsy

2. Cyst

3. Foreign body removal, or

4. Cardiac massage, etc.

Excision (32310-32540)

- Biopsy codes in both Excision and Incision categories
  Excision biopsy with percutaneous needle
  Incision biopsy with chest open
- Also services of pleurectomy, pneumocentesis, and lung removal
  Segmentectomy: 1 segment
  Lobectomy: 1 lobe
  Bilobectomy: 2 lobes
  Total Pneumonectomy: 1 lung

CARDIOVASCULAR (CV) SYSTEM (33010-37799)

CV coding may require codes for

Radiology: Diagnostic studies

Medicine: Nonsurgical and percutaneous

Surgery: Open and percutaneous

Cardiology Coding Terminology

Invasive: Enters body

Example: Opening chest for removal, i.e., tumor on heart

Both Medicine and Surgery sections contain invasive procedures

Noninvasive: Procedures that do not break skin

Example: Electrocardiogram

Electrophysiology (EP): study of electrical system of heart

Example: Study of irregular heartbeat (arrhythmia)

Nuclear Cardiology: Diagnostic and treatment specialty, uses radioactive substances for cardiac conditions

Example: MRI

Cardiovascular in Surgery Section

Codes for Procedures

Heart/Pericardium (33010-33999)

- Pacemakers, valve disorders

Arteries/Veins (34001-37799)

- Many of same types of procedures but noncoronary procedures

Heart/Pericardium (33010-33999)

Both percutaneous and open surgical

Extensive notes throughout

Frequent changes with medical advances

Examples of categories Heart/Pericardium subheading:
- Pericardium
- Cardiac Tumor
- Pacemaker or Pacing Cardioverter-Defibrillator

Example of services:
- Pericardiocentesis: Percutaneous withdrawal of fluid from pericardial space
- Cardiac Tumor: Open surgical procedure for removal of tumor on heart

Pacemakers and Cardioverter-Defibrillators (33200-33249)

- Devices that assist heart in electrical function
- Divided by where pacer placed, approach, and type of service
- Patient record indicates revision or replacement
- Codes include all services provided within 14 days related to repair, revision, or replacement
- Usual follow-up 90 days (global period)

Placed

Atrium

Ventricle

Both

Biventricular, both ventricles and atrium (uses 3 leads)

Approach

Epicardial: Open procedure to place on heart

Transvenous: Through vein to place in heart

Type of Service

Initial placement or replacement of all or part of device

Number of leads placed is important in code selection

Electrophysiologic Operative Procedures (33250-33261)

- Surgeon repairs defect causing abnormal rhythm
- Chest opened to full view
  Cardiopulmonary (CP) bypass usually used
- Codes based on reason for procedure and if CP bypass used

Patient-Activated Event Recorder (33282-33284)

- Also known as cardiac event recorder or loop recorder
- Internal surgical implantation required
- Divided based on device being implanted or removed

Cardiac Valves (33400-33496)

- Divided by valve:
  1. Aortic
  2. Mitral
  3. Tricuspid
  4. Pulmonary
- Subdivided on if cardiopulmonary bypass was used
- Code descriptions are all similar, requiring careful reading

Coronary Artery Bypass (CAB)

- CAB performed for coronary arteries severely clogged (atherosclerosis)
- Determine what was used in repair:
  Vein (33510-33516)
  Artery (33533-33536)
  Both artery and vein (33517-33523)
- Number of bypass grafts performed
  Example: Three venous grafts

Venous Grafting Only for Coronary Artery Bypass (33510-33516)

- Divided based on number grafts being placed
- Procurement of saphenous vein included in procedure (not coded separately)

Arterial Grafting for Coronary Artery Bypass (33533-33536)

- Divided based on number of grafts
- Obtaining artery for grafting included in codes, except:
  Procuring upper extremity artery (i.e., radial artery), coded separately

  1. Several codes (33542-33545) for myocardial resection and repair of ventricular septal defect

Combined Arterial-Venous Grafting (33517-33523)

- Divided based on number of grafts and if procedure initial or reoperation
- Procuring saphenous vein included
- These codes are never used alone
- Always used with Arterial Grafting codes (33533-33536)
- Arterial-Venous codes report only **venous** graft portion of procedure

Arteries and Veins Subheading (34001-37799)

Only for noncoronary vessels
- Divided based on whether artery or vein used
  Example: Different codes for embolectomy, depending on artery or vein

Catheters placed into vessels for monitoring, removal, repair

Using nonselective or selective catheter placement

Nonselective: Direct placement without further manipulation

Selective: Place and then manipulate into further order(s)

Catheter Placement Example

Nonselective: 36000 Introduction of needle into vein

Selective: 36012 Placement of catheter into second order venous system

Vascular Families Are Like a Tree

- Main branch—first order
- Second-order branch
- Third-order branch
- Brachiocephalic Vascular Family **(Figure 3-10)**
  Report farthest extent of catheter placement in a vascular family

Embolectomy and Thrombectomy (34001-34490)

Embolus: Dislodged thrombus

Thrombus: Mass of material in vessel located in place of formation

Balloon Removal: Threaded into vessel, inflated under mass, pulled out with mass

Venous Reconstruction—CV Repairs (34501-34530)

Types of Repair:

Valve

Vein

Aneurysm

Aneurysm

- Aneurysm: Sac of clotted blood
- Repair by removal or bypass
- Endovascular repair (34800-34832) from inside vessel
- Direct (35001-35162) from outside vessel

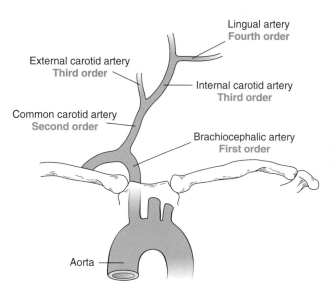

Lingual artery
Fourth order

External carotid artery
Third order

Internal carotid artery
Third order

Common carotid artery
Second order

Brachiocephalic artery
First order

Aorta

Figure 3-10 Brachiocephalic vascular family with first-, second-, third-, and fourth-order vessels.

Endovascular Repair of Abdominal Aortic Aneurysm (34800-34832)

- Extensive notes preceding codes—must reading
- Uses fluoroscopic guidance report Radiology 75952 or 75953
- Includes access, catheter manipulation, balloon angioplasty, site closure
- Other procedures performed at same time, coded separately

Repair Arteriovenous Fistula (35180-35190)

Abnormal passage

Divided based on fistula type:
- Congenital
- Acquired
- Traumatic

Angioplasty and Atherectomy

Transluminal: By way of vessel

Transluminal Angioplasty: Catheter passed into vessel and stretched

Transluminal Atherectomy: Guidewire threaded into vessel and clots destroyed

Noncoronary Bypass Grafts (35500-35671)

- Divided by:
  1. Vein
  2. In Situ Vein (veins repaired in their original place)
  3. Other Than Vein
- Code by type of graft and vessels being used to bypass
    Example: 35506, Bypass graft, with vein; carotid-subclavian
    Graft attached to carotid and to subclavian, bypassing defect of subclavian

Vascular Injection Procedures (36000-36015)

- Divided into:
  1. Intravenous
  2. Intraarterial—Intraaortic
- Used for many procedures
    Example: Injection of opaque substance for venography (radiography of vein)

Cardiovascular in Medicine Section

Services can be:
- Invasive or noninvasive
- Diagnostic or therapeutic
Subheadings:

  Therapeutic Services

  1. Cardiography

  2. Echocardiography

  3. Cardiac Catheterization

4. Intracardiac Electrophysiologic (EP) Procedures

5. Peripheral Arterial Disease Rehabilitation

6. Other Vascular Studies

Therapeutic Services (92950-92998)

Types of services:

1. Cardioversion

2. Infusions

3. Thrombolysis

4. Catheter placement

Many groups of codes divided by:

1. Method (e.g., balloon, blade)

2. Location (e.g., aortic or mitral valve)

3. Number (e.g., single or multiple vessels)

Cardiography (93000-93278)

Types of services:

1. Stress tests

2. Holter monitor

3. Electrocardiogram

Echocardiography (93303-93350)

Noninvasive Diagnostic Procedure: ultrasound detects presence of cardiac or vascular disease

Cardiac Catheterization (93501-93591)

Used to identify valve disorders, abnormal blood flow

Many bundled services in catheterization codes

Examples:

Introduction

Positioning/Repositioning of catheter

Pressure readings inside heart or vessels

Blood samples

Rest/Exercise studies

Final evaluation and report

Three Components of Coding Cardiac Catheterization

- Placement of catheter (93501-93533)
- Injection (93539-93545)
- Imaging supervision, interpretation, and report (93555 or 93556)

Intracoronary Brachytherapy

- New procedure, uses radioactive substances to destroy restenosis of coronary vessel
- Patients have had stent placed in coronary vessel
- Stent "restenosis" (re-formation of plaque)
- Cardiologist: Places guide wire and catheter
- Radiation oncologist: Places radioactive elements

Intracardiac Electrophysiologic Procedures (93600-93662)

Services to diagnose and treat conditions of electrical system of heart

EP System of Heart

Electrical conduction system

Electrical recording codes divided based on location of recording device

Example: Bundle of His or right ventricle

Pacing: Temporary pacing to stabilize beating of heart

Example: Intraventricular or intraarterial pacing

Peripheral Arterial Disease (PAD) Rehabilitation (93668)

Rehabilitation sessions: 45-60 minutes

Use of motorized treadmill/track to build patient's CV endurance

Supervised by exercise physiologist or nurse

Other Vascular Studies (93701-93790)

Category contains codes for services such as:

Plethysmography: Recordings of changes in size of body part when blood passes through it.

Electronic Analysis: Checks electronic function of devices, such as pacemakers

Ambulatory Blood Pressure Monitoring: Outpatient basis over 24-hour period

Thermograms: Visual recordings of temperature body

Cardiovascular in Radiology Section

- Radiology section, Heart (75552-75556) and Aorta/Arteries (75600-75790) subsections
- Prior to 1992, Radiology section contained codes for entire CV procedures
- Major revision to CV radiology codes 1992
- Divided complete procedures into two components: Technical and Professional
  Example: Angiography
     Technical component angiography—remains in Radiology section
     Professional component injection—moved to Surgery section
- Complete angiography requires radiology code and surgery code
- Reflects common practice of cardiologist's performing injection and radiologist's performing angiography

Contrast Material

Often radiologic procedures use contrast material to improve image

Many codes have contrast material bundled into service
- "With contrast" or "with or without contrast"

Only injected contrast qualifies as with contrast

Contrast not included in description, used in procedure, code both contrast material and injection separately

Nonhospital based (not employed by hospital) physician performs procedure in hospital outpatient department use -26 for professional component only

---

A Component Coding Example

Two physicians (cardiologist and radiologist from same facility) perform angiography of 3rd order brachiocephalic artery with contrast
- Cardiologist placing catheter (36217), Surgery section
- Radiologist performs angiography (75658), Radiology section
- Supply of contrast material (99070), Medicine section

HEMIC AND LYMPHATIC SYSTEMS SUBSECTION (38100-38999)

Divisions

1. Spleen
2. General
3. Lymph Nodes and Lymphatic Channels

Spleen Subheading (38100-38200)

Spleen easily ruptured, causes massive hemorrhage

   May require splenectomy

   Splenectomy: total or partial

Often done as part of more major procedure

   Bundled into major procedure

General (38204-38242)

Codes divided on:

Aspiration

Biopsy

Harvesting

Transplantation

Stem Cells

Immature blood cells originating in bone marrow

Used in treatment of leukemia

Types of Stem Cells

Allogenic: Close relative

Autologous: Patient's own

Lymph Nodes and Lymphatic Channels Subheading (38300-38999)

Two types of lymphadenectomies:

Limited: Lymph nodes only

Radical: Lymph nodes, submandibular gland, and surrounding tissue

Often bundled into more major procedure (e.g., prostatectomy)

Do not unbundle and report lymphadenectomy separately

MEDIASTINUM (39000-39499)

- Incision codes for foreign body removal or biopsy
- Excision codes for removal of cyst or tumor

DIAPHRAGM (39501-39599)

Only category: Repair

Most codes hernia or laceration repairs

DIGESTIVE SYSTEM (40490-49999)

Divided by anatomic site from mouth to anus + organs that aid digestive process

Example: Liver and gallbladder

Many bundled procedures

Endoscopy

- Diagnostic procedure always bundled into surgical endoscopic
- Code to furthest extent of procedure

Endoscopy Terminology

Notes define specific terminology
Read notes preceding 45300-45387:
- Proctosigmoidoscopy: Rectum and sigmoid colon (6-25 cm)
- Sigmoidoscopy: Entire rectum, sigmoid colon, and may include part of descending colon (26-60 cm)
- Colonoscopy: Entire colon, rectum to cecum, and may include terminal ileum (greater than 60 cm)

Laparoscopy and Endoscopy

Some subheadings have both laparoscopy (outside) and endoscopy (inside) procedures.

Example: Subheading Esophagus
- Endoscopy views inside
- Laparoscopy inserted through umbilicus, views from outside

Hernia Codes (49491-49611)

Divided by:

1. Type of hernia

    Example: Inguinal, femoral

2. Initial or subsequent repair

3. Age of patient

4. Clinical presentation:

    Strangulated: Blood supply cut off

    Incarcerated: Cannot be returned to cavity (not reducible)

URINARY SYSTEM (50010-53899)

Anatomic division:

- Kidney
- Ureters
- Bladder
- Urethra

Further divided by procedure:

- Incision
- Excision

Kidney Subheading (50010-50590)

Endoscopy codes are for procedure done through previously established stoma or incision

Introduction Category (50390-50398)

- Catheters and injections for radiography
- Aspirations
- Insertion of guide wires
- Tube changes
- Usually reported with radiology component

Ureter Subheading (50600-50980)

Divided on type of procedure:

Incision

Excision

Laparoscopy codes describe surgical procedures

Bladder Subheading (51000-52700)

Many bundled codes
Read all descriptions carefully

Urodynamics (51725-51798)

- Procedures relate to motion and flow of urine
- Used to diagnose urine flow obstructions

- Bundled: All usual, necessary instruments, equipment, supplies, and technical assistance

MALE GENITAL SYSTEM (54000-55899)

1. Penis (most codes)
2. Testes
3. Epididymis
4. Tunica Vaginalis
5. Scrotum
6. Vas Deferens
7. Spermatic Cord
8. Seminal Vesicles
9. Prostate

Biopsy Codes

Located in subheading to which refer

Example: Biopsy codes in subheadings:
- Epididymis (Excision)
- Testis (Excision)

Penis (54000-54450)

Incision codes (54000-54015) differ from Integumentary System codes
- Penis incision codes for deeper structures

Destruction (54050-54065)

- Codes divided on:
  Extent: simple or extensive
  Method of destruction, e.g., chemical, cryosurgery
- Extensive destruction can be by any method

Excision (54100-54164)

- Commonly used codes biopsy and circumcision

Introduction (54200-54250)

- Many procedures for corpora cavernosum (spongy body of penis)
  - Injection procedures for Peyronie disease (toughening of corpora cavernosum)
  - Treatments for erectile dysfunction

Repair (54300-54450)

- Many plastic repairs
- Some repair 1+ stage
  Stage indicated in code description

INTERSEX SURGERY (55970-55980)

There only 2 codes within subsection

1. Male to female

2. Female to male

Complicated procedures completed over extended period of time

Performed by physicians with extensive specialized training

FEMALE GENITAL SYSTEM (56405-58999)

Anatomic division: From vulva to ovaries
* Many bundled services

Vulva, Perineum, & Introitus (56405-56821)

Skene's gland coded with Urinary System, Incision or Excision codes
* Group of small mucous glands, lower end of urethra
  ○ Paraurethral duct

Incision (56405-56441)

I&D of abscess: Vulva, perineal area or Bartholin's gland

Marsupialization:

* Cyst incised
* Drained
* Edges sutured to sides to keep cyst open

Destruction (56501-56515)

* Lesions destroyed by variety of methods
  ○ Destruction = Eradication not excision. Excision is removal
* Divided by simple or complex destruction
  Complexity based on physician's judgment
  Stated in record
* Destruction has no pathology report

Excision (56605-56740)

Biopsy includes:

1. Local anesthetic

2. Biopsy

3. Simple closure

4. Code based number of lesions biopsied

5. Place number of lesions on CMS-1500 in Block 24-G (see **Figure 3-1**)

Vulvectomy: Surgical removal of portion of vulva (56620-56640)
Based on extent and size of area removed

Extent:

1. Simple: Skin and superficial subcutaneous tissues

2. Radical: Skin and deep subcutaneous tissues

Size:

1. Partial: <80%

2. Complete: >80%

Extent and size, indicated in operative report

Repair (56800-56810)

- Many plastic repairs
- Read notes following category
  If repair procedure for wound of genitalia, use Integumentary System code

Endoscopy (56820-56821)

- By means of a colposcopy
  With or without biopsy

Vagina (57000-57421)

Codes divided based on service, e.g., incision, excision

Introduction (57150-57180)

- Includes vaginal irrigation, insertion of devices, diaphragm, cervical caps
- Report device inserted separately
  99070 or HCPCS, such as A4261 (Cervical cap)

Repair (57200-57335)

- For nonobstetric repairs:
  Obstetric repairs, use Maternity Care & Delivery codes

Manipulation (57400-57415)

Dilation: Speculum inserted into vagina and enlarged using dilator

Endoscopy (57420, 57421)

- Colposcopy codes based on purpose
  i.e., biopsy, diagnostic, LEEP
  LEEP uses heated wire to excise; AKA: diathermy

Cervix Uteri (57452-57820)

Cervix uteri, narrow lower end of uterus. Services include excision, manipulation, repair

Excision (57500-57556)

Conization codes

Conization: Removal of cone of tissue from cervix

LEEP technology can be used for conizations

Corpus Uteri (58100-58579)

Many complex procedures
- Often very similar wording in code descriptions
- Requires careful reading

Excision (58100-58294)

- Dilation & curettage (D&C, 58120) of uterus
    After dilation, curette scrapes uterus
- Do not report postpartum hemorrhage service with 58120
    Use 59160—Maternity & Delivery code
- Many hysterectomy codes
    Based on approach (vaginal, abdominal) and extent (uterus, fallopian tubes, etc.)
- Often secondary procedures performed with hysterectomy
- Do not code secondary, related minor procedures separately

Introduction (58300-58353)

- Common procedures
    e.g., insertion of an IUD
- Report supply of device separately
- Specialized services
    e.g., artificial insemination procedures
- Used to report physician component of service
- Component coding:
    Necessary with catheter procedures for hysterosonography
    Notes following codes indicate radiology guidance component codes

Oviduct/Ovary (58600-58770)

Oviduct: Fallopian tube
Incision category contains tubal ligations
- When during same hospitalization as delivery, ligation not coded separately

Laparoscopy (58660-58679)

- Through abdominal wall
- Based on purpose of procedure
    e.g., lysis, lesion removal
- Caution: If only diagnostic laparoscopy:
    Do not use Female Genital System codes
    Use 49320, Digestive System

Ovary (58800-58960)

Two categories only: Incision and Excision

Incision: Primarily for drainage of cysts and abscesses
* Divided on surgical approach

Excision: Biopsy, wedge resection, and oophorectomy

In Vitro Fertilization (58970-58999)

Specialized codes used by physicians trained in fertilization procedures
* Codes divided by type of procedure and method used

MATERNITY CARE & DELIVERY SUBSECTION (59000-59899)

Divided by service:
* Antepartum
* Delivery
* Postpartum
* Abortion

Gestation

Fetal gestation: Approximately 266 days (40 weeks)

EDD: Estimated Date of Delivery
* 280 days from last menstrual period (LMP)

Trimesters

First, LMP to Week 12

Second, Weeks 13-27

Third, Week 28-EDD

Global Package and Delivery

Uncomplicated maternity care includes:

1. Antepartum care = Before
2. Delivery
3. Postpartum care = After

Antepartum Care Includes

1. Initial and subsequent H&P
2. Blood pressures
3. Weight
4. Routine urinalysis
5. Fetal heart tones
6. Monthly visits to 28 weeks
7. Twice a month visits weeks 29 to 36
8. Weekly visits from week 37 to delivery

> - Services not related to antepartum care are reported separately
>   - i.e., pregnant female with complaint of suspicious mole on left shoulder
>   - Visits OB/GYN physician, who provides antepartum care
>   - Service regarding mole not antepartum care
>   - Listed in notes preceding 59000

Delivery Includes

1. Admission to hospital with admitting H&P

2. Management of uncomplicated labor

3. Vaginal or cesarean section delivery

- Complications coded separately
- Listed in notes preceding 59000

Postpartum Care Includes

Normal follow-up care for 6 weeks after delivery:
- i.e., hospital visits, office visits
- Listed in notes preceding 59000

Antepartum (59990-59051)

Amniocentesis: Insertion of needle into pregnant uterus, withdraws fluid (59000)

Ultrasound guidance with this service (76946)

Component coding often part of services in subheading

Fetal services: Include stress tests, blood sampling, and monitoring

Excision (59100-59160)

Postpartum curettage: removes remaining pieces of placenta or clotted blood (59160)

Nonobstetric curettage: 58120 (Corpus Uteri, Excision)

Introduction (59200)

Insertion of cervical dilator: Used to prepare cervix for an abortive procedure or delivery

Cervical ripening agents may be introduced to prepare cervix
- Is a separate procedure and not reported when part of more major procedure

Repair (59300-59350)

Only for repairs during pregnancy

Repairs done during delivery or after pregnancy

Routine Global Obstetric Care

59400, Vaginal delivery

59510, Cesarean delivery

59610, Vaginal delivery after previous cesarean delivery (VBAC)

59618, Cesarean delivery following attempted vaginal delivery after previous cesarean delivery

Episiotomies and Use of Forceps

Included in delivery

Not reported separately

Physician Provides Only Portion of Global Routine Care, Delivery

59409, Vaginal delivery only

59514, Cesarean delivery only

59612, Vaginal delivery only, after previous cesarean delivery

59620, Cesarean delivery only, following attempted vaginal delivery after previous cesarean delivery

Delivery of Twins

Payers differ on reporting format
- -22 (Unusual Procedural Services)
- -51 (Multiple Procedures)

Abortion Services (59812-59857)

Spontaneous: Happens naturally

Incomplete: Requires medical intervention

Missed: Fetus dies naturally during first half of pregnancy

Septic: Missed abortion with infection

Medical intervention:
- Dilation & curettage or evacuation (suction removal)
- Intraamniotic injections (saline or urea)
- Vaginal suppositories (prostaglandin)

ENDOCRINE SYSTEM SUBSECTION (60000-60599)

9 glands in endocrine system, only 4 included in subsection:

1. Thyroid
2. Parathyroid
3. Thymus
4. Adrenal

Pituitary & Pineal: Nervous System subsection

Pancreas: Digestive System

Ovaries and Testes: Respective genital systems
   Divided into 2 subheadings:

Thyroid Gland

Parathyroid, Thymus, Adrenal Glands, & Carotid Body

Carotid Body: Refers to area adjacent to carotid artery
Can be site of tumors

Thyroid Gland, Excision Category (60001-60281)

Code descriptions often refer to:
- **Partial or subtotal:** Something less than total
- **Total:** All

NERVOUS SYSTEM SUBSECTION (61000-64999)

Divided anatomically:
- Skull, Meninges, and Brain
- Spine and Spinal Cord
- Extracranial Nerves, Peripheral Nerves, and Autonomic Nervous System

Skull, Meninges, and Brain Subheading (61000-62258)

Categories:

- Injection, Drainage, or Aspiration
- Twist Drills, Burr Hole(s), or Trephine

Conditions that Require Openings into Brain to:

1. Relieve pressure

2. Insert monitoring devices

3. Place tubing

4. Inject contrast material

Craniotomy or Craniotomy Category:

- Removal of portion of skull, usually as operative site
- Codes divided by site and condition for which procedure is performed

Surgery at Skull Base Category

Skull base: Area at base of cranium
- Lesion removal from this area very complex

Extensive category notes

Surgery at Skull Base Terminology

- Approach procedure used to gain exposure of lesion
- Definitive procedure what is done to lesion
- Repair/reconstruction procedure reported separately only if extensive repair

Surgery of Skull Base (61580-61616)

- Approach procedure and definitive procedure coded separately
  Example: Removal of an intradural lesion using middle cranial fossa approach
  - 61590 approach procedure, middle cranial fossa and
  - 61608 definitive procedure of intradural resection of lesion

Cerebrospinal Fluid Shunt (CSF) Shunt Category (62180-62258)

- Used to drain fluid
- Codes describe placement of:
  1. Devices
  2. Repair
  3. Replacement
  4. Removal of shunting devices

Spine and Spinal Cord Subheading (62263-63746)

Codes divided on condition and approach

Often used are:
- Unilateral or bilateral procedures (-50)
- Multiple procedures (-51)

EYE AND OCULAR ADNEXA SUBSECTION (65091-68899)

Terminology extremely important
- Code descriptions often vary only slightly

Codes divided anatomically, e.g.:
- Eyeball
- Conjunctiva

Some codes specifically for patients previously operated on
Much bundling:
  Example: Subheading Posterior Segment, Prophylaxis category notes indicate:
  - "The following descriptors intended to include (67141-67145) sessions in defined treatment period."

AUDITORY SYSTEM SUBSECTION (69000-69990)

Codes divided on:

1. External Ear

2. Middle Ear

3. Internal Ear

Further divisions on procedure:

1. Incision

2. Excision

3. Removal

4. Repair

RADIOLOGY SECTION (70010-79999)

> **Radiology:** Branch of medicine that uses radiant energy to diagnose and treat patients
>
> **Specialist in radiology:** Radiologist (doctor of medicine)

Four Radiology Subsections

>   1. Diagnostic Radiology
>   2. Diagnostic Ultrasound
>   3. Radiation Oncology
>   4. Nuclear Medicine

Procedures

> Fluoroscopy views inside of body, projects onto television screen
>
> Live images by which physician can view function and structure of organ
>
>   **Example:** 71034, chest x-ray with fluoroscopy

Magnetic Resonance Imaging

> MRI uses magnetic energy to view soft tissue structures
>
>   **Example:** 72148 an MRI of spinal canal

Tomography or CT

> Tomography used to view single plane of body
>
>   **Example:** 70450 tomographic scan of head or brain

Planes of Body (Figure 3-11)

Position and Projection

> Position way in which patient placed
>
> Projection path x-ray beam travels

Component Coding

>   **Three component terms:**
>   1. Professional
>   2. Technical
>   3. Global

Professional Component

> Physician portion of service, includes:
>
> Supervision of technician
>
> Interpretation of results, including written report

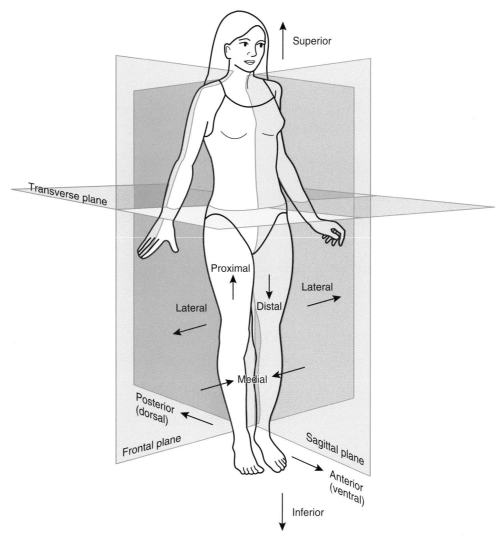

Figure 3-11 Planes of the body.

Technical Component

- Technologist's services
- Equipment, film, and supplies

Global Procedure

Both professional and technical portions of radiology service

Component Modifiers

If only professional component of radiology service provided: -26 to code

If only technical component provided: -TC to code
- -TC HCPCS modifier used with CPT and HCPCS codes

If both professional and technical components of radiology service provided (global): No modifier

Example: Chest x-Ray

- Professional component: 71030-26 (Supervision and final report)
- Technical component: 71030-TC (Technician, supplies, equipment)
- Global procedure: 71030

Third-party payers usually reimburse:

- 40% professional component
- 60% technical component
- 100% global procedure

Contrast Material

Statement "with contrast" implies injection service included in code.

Oral or rectal contrast does not qualify for "with contrast"

Notes indicate codes for components

> **Example:** 75801, lymphangiography; see 38790 (Injection procedure)

Interventional Radiologist

Combination radiologist and surgeon

Provides total procedure for cystography with contrast

- Report 74430, x-ray portion
- 51600 for injection procedure
- Plus code for supply of contrast material (e.g., 99070)

Overview of Radiology Subsections

1. Diagnostic Radiology
2. Diagnostic Ultrasound
3. Radiation Oncology
4. Nuclear Medicine

DIAGNOSTIC RADIOLOGY (70010-76499)

Most standard radiographic procedures

Codes often divided on whether contrast material used

Codes further divided on number of views

Used to:

- Diagnose disease
- Monitor disease process—progression or remission
- Therapeutic procedures

Diagnostic Procedures Include:

- X-ray
- Computerized axial tomography (CAT or CT scan)
- Magnetic resonance imaging (MRI)
- Angiography

Computerized Axial Tomography

- X-ray image taken in sections
- Computer reconstructs and enhances image

Magnetic Resonance Imaging

- Uses magnetic fields to produce an image displayed on computer screen
- Codes of same area (e.g., spine) divided on whether or not contrast material used

Angiography

- Used to view vessel obstructions
- Dye injected into vessel
- Radiologist uses angiography to diagnose vascular conditions
    Examples:
    Malformations
    Strokes
    Myocardial infarctions

Remember
- If fewer than total number of views specified in code provided: Use -52, Reduced Service

---

DIAGNOSTIC ULTRASOUND (76506-76999)

Uses high-frequency sound waves to image anatomic structures

Nine subheadings of Diagnostic Ultrasound

Primarily based on anatomy

Ultrasound Modes and Scans

- A-mode
- M-mode
- B-scan
- Real-time scan

A-Mode

A = Amplitude

Technique used to map structure outline

Displays one-dimensional image

M-Mode

M = Motion

Technique used to display movement of structure

Displays one-dimensional image

B-Scan

B = Brightness

Technique used to display movement of tissues and organs

Known as gray scale ultrasound

Displays two-dimensional image

Real-Time Scan

Technique used to display both structure and motion of organ and tissues

Displays two-dimensional image

Extent of Study

Codes often divided on extent of study

Example: Extent of scan as follows

Complete: Scans entire body

Limited: Scans part of body, i.e., one organ

Follow-up/repeat: Limited study of part body that was scanned previously

Three Locations for Ultrasound Services

76506-76886: Radiology codes for diagnostic ultrasound services

93875-93990: Medicine codes for vascular studies

93303-93350: Medicine codes for echocardiography

RADIATION ONCOLOGY (77261-77799)

Therapeutic use of radiation

Codes both professional and technical services

Subheading divided based on treatment

Initial consultation, prior to decision to treat, reported with E/M consultation code

Outpatient: 99241-99245

Inpatient: 99251-99255

Clinical Treatment Planning—Professional Component (77261-77299)

Includes:
- Interpretation of special testing
- Tumor localization
- Determination of treatment volume
- Choice of treatment method
- Determination of number of treatment ports
- Selection of treatment devices
- Other necessary procedures

Clinical Treatment Planning Consists of

1. Planning

2. Simulation

Three Levels of Planning

1. **Simple:** One treatment area, one port or one set of parallel ports

2. **Intermediate:** Three or more ports, two separate treatment areas, multiple blocking

3. **Complex:** Complex blocking, custom shielding blocks, tangential ports, special wedges, 3+ treatment areas, special beams

Simulation

- Determining placement of treatment areas/ports for radiation treatment
- Does not include administration of radiation

Three Levels of Simulation

1. **Simple:** 1 treatment area with 1 port or pair of ports

2. **Intermediate:** 3+ ports, 2 separate treatment areas, multiple blocking

3. **Complex:** Tangential ports, 3+ treatment areas, complex blocking

Medical Radiation, Physics, Dosimetry, Treatment Devices, and Special Services

Decision making services of physicians

- Treatment types
- Dose calculation and placement (dosimetry)
- Development of treatment device

Radiation Treatment Delivery (77401-77418)

Technical component of actual delivery of radiation

Information Needed to Code Radiation Treatment Delivery

Amount of radiation delivered

Number of

1. Areas treated (single, two, three or more)

2. Ports involved (single, three or more, tangential)

3. Blocks used (none, multiple, custom)

Reporting Clinical Treatment Management

Professional (physician) portion of services, including:
- Review port films
- Review dosimetry, dose delivery, treatment parameters
- Treatment setup
- Patient examination for medical E/M

Clinical Brachytherapy (77750-77799)

Placement of radioactive material into or around site of tumor:
- Intracavitary (within body cavity)
- Interstitial (within tissues)

Source

Radioactive element delivers radiation dose over time
Examples: Seeds, ribbons, or capsules
Ribbons: Seeds embedded on tape
- Tape cut to desired length controls amount radiation and inserted into tissue

Clinical Brachytherapy Codes Divided Based on

Number of sources applied:

1. Simple 1-4

2. Intermediate 5-10

3. Complex 11+

NUCLEAR MEDICINE (78000-79999)

Placement of radioactive material into body and measurement of emissions

Used for both diagnosis and treatment

Codes divided primarily on organ system

Except "Therapeutic," which is for radiopharmaceutical therapies

PATHOLOGY AND LABORATORY SECTION (80048-89356)

Includes:

Organ or Disease Panels

Drug Testing

Therapeutic Drug Assays

Evocative/Suppression Testing

Consultation (Clinical Pathology)

Urinalysis

Chemistry

Molecular Diagnostics

Infectious Agent Antibodies

Microbiology Infectious Agent Detection

Anatomic Pathology

Cytopathology

Cytogenetic Studies

Surgical Pathology

Pathology and Laboratory

Codes for laboratory test only

Specimen collection coded separately

Example: Venous blood draw reported 36415 (Surgery section)

Facility Indicators

Allow additional tests without physician written order

Example: Urinalysis positive for bacteria, built-in indicator for culture

Pathology/Laboratory Caution

Report 2nd or subsequent tests without -51, multiple procedures

Organ or Disease-Oriented Panels (80048-80076)

Groups of tests often ordered together

Examples:
- Basic Metabolic Panel
- General Health Panel
- Electrolyte Panel

Rules of Panels

- All tests must have been conducted
- Do not use -52, Reduced Service
- Additional tests, over those in panel are reported separately
- If all tests in panel not done
  1. List each test separately
  2. Do not use panel code

Drug Testing (80100-80103)

Identifies presence or absence of drug—qualitative analysis

Confirmation conducted to double check results of positive drug test (80102)

Chromatography procedure in which multiple drugs identified
- Some machines identify all drugs present in 1 procedure
- Others require 2+ procedures to identify 2+ drugs

Code the number of procedures, not number of drugs tested for

Example:
- 2 procedures to identify 3 drugs = 80100 × 2
- 1 procedure to identify 3 drugs = 80100

Does not identify amount of drug present
- Only presence or absence

Report the presence and amount (quantitative)
- Therapeutic Drug Assays (80150-80299) or
- Chemistry (82000-84999)

Therapeutic Drug Assays (80150-80299)

Material examined can be from any source

Drugs listed by generic names

Example: amitriptyline generic name for brand name Elavil

Evocation/Suppression Testing (80400-80440)

Measures stimulating (evocative) or suppressing agents

Codes report only technical component of service

Additional services reported:
- Supplies and/or drugs used in testing (99070 or HCPCS code)

Physician administered agent
- Infusion or injection code (90780 and 90781)

E/M code reported for physician monitoring of test

Consultations (Clinical Pathology) (80500-80502)

At request of physician

Additional information about specimen

Consultant prepares written report

Levels

Limited without review of medical record

Comprehensive with review of medical record

More Consultation Codes (88321-88332)

Surgical Pathology

Used when pathologist either
- Reviews slides, material, or reports
- Provides consultation during surgery

Reported on number of specimens

Urinalysis (81000-81099)

Tests on Urine

1. Method of test
   - e.g., tablet, reagent, or dipstick
2. Reason for test
   - e.g., pregnancy
3. Constituents being tested for
   - e.g., bilirubin, glucose

Equipment Used

- Automated or nonautomated

Chemistry (82000-84999)

Specific tests on any bodily substances:
- Urine
- Blood

- Breath
- Feces
- Sputum

Most are for quantitative (presence of) screenings only

4 codes report qualitative (amount of) screenings (80100-80103)

Samples from different sources, reported separately, e.g., blood, feces

Samples taken different times of day reported separately

Hematology and Coagulation (85002-85999)

Laboratory procedures on blood

Example:
- Complete blood count (CBC)
- White blood cell count (WBC)

Codes divided based on method of
- Blood draw
- Test being conducted

Immunology (86000-86849)

Identifying immune system conditions caused by antibodies and antigens

Example: Hepatitis C antibody screening

Transfusion Medicine (86850-86999)

Blood bank codes

Tests performed on blood or blood products

Do NOT identify supply of blood, but:
- Collection
- Processing
- Typing

Microbiology (87001-87999)

Study of Microorganisms

Identification of organism

Sensitivities of organism to antibiotics

> **Microbiology Caution:** Many code descriptions similar to those in Immunology (86000-86849)
> - Difference is technique used

Anatomic Pathology (88000-88099)

Postmortem examinations
- Autopsies

Reports only physician service

Codes divided on extent of exam

> **Example:** With or without central nervous system

Cytopathology (88104-88199)

Identifies cellular changes

Common laboratory procedures, e.g., Pap smear

Codes divided on

1. Type of procedure
2. Technique used

Cytogenetic Studies (88230-88299)

Branch of genetics concerned with cellular abnormalities and pathologic conditions

> **Example:** Chromosomes

Surgical Pathology (88300-88399)

Pathology Terminology

Specimen sample of tissue of suspect area
- Basis of reporting is specimen

Block frozen piece of specimen

Section is a slice of frozen block

Evaluation of Specimens to Determine Disease Pathology

- All tissue removed during procedures undergoes pathology evaluation
- Operative report usually coded after pathology report received
- Pathology reports usually coded with operative report
- Unit of measure (88300-88309), specimen
  2 anus tags, each examined, 88304 × 2
  1 anus tag examined in 2 different areas of tag, 88304

Types of Pathologic Examination
Microscopic: With microscope

Gross: Without microscope
- 88300, only gross exam code
- Other codes are gross and microscopic

Six Levels of Surgical Pathology

- Based on specimen examined, i.e., breast, prostate, lung, and reason for evaluation, i.e., radical procedure for suspected carcinoma
- Levels divided on complexity of examination
  Example:
  88305, Colon, Biopsy

88307, Colon, Segmental Resection, Other than for Tumor

88309, Colon, Total Resection

Not Included in Codes 88300-88309

Any special services necessary during specimen examination

Example: Special stains

Additional services reported separately (88311-88399)

MEDICINE SECTION (90281-99600)

Most procedures noninvasive (not entering body)

Contains invasive procedures

Example: 92973, Percutaneous thrombectomy

Numerous notes throughout

Many specialized tests

Example: Audiology and biofeedback

Immunizations

Often used

Two types immunizations
* Active and passive

Active—Bacteria or Virus

Bacteria that cause disease made nontoxic (toxoid)
* Injected to build immunity

Small dose active virus injected (vaccine)
* Injected to build immunity

Example: Poliovirus

Passive Immunization

Does not cause immune response

Contains antibodies against certain diseases—immune globulins

Immune Globulins (90281-90399)

Identifies immune globulin product

Example: Botulism antitoxin

Report administration separately

Immune Globulins Codes Divided By:

Type

e.g., rabies, hepatitis B

Method

e.g., intramuscular, intravenous, subcutaneous

Dose

e.g., full dose, minidose

Immunization Administration (90471-90474)

Administration (giving substance) of substance
* Reported with substance given

Methods of Administration

1. Percutaneous
2. Intradermal
3. Subcutaneous
4. Intramuscular
5. Jet
6. Intranasal
7. Oral

Report Administration for Each Dose—Single or Combination

Example: Patient receives 3 separate injections:
* 90471 administration tetanus
* 90472 administration rubella
* 90472 administration diphtheria

OR depending on payer:
* 90471 administration tetanus
* 90472 × 2 administration rubella and diphtheria

Vaccines, Toxoids (90476-90749)

Many codes age specific

Example: 90658, influenza vaccine, for ages 3 and over

Codes for products for single diseases

Example: 90703, tetanus

Codes for combination diseases

Example: 90701, diphtheria, tetanus, and DTP

Some vaccines given on schedule

Example: 90633, 2-dose hepatitis A vaccine
* 1st dose 1st visit
* 2nd dose 2nd visit

Remember
Do not use modifier -51 with Vaccine/Toxoid codes
Rather, depending on payer:
* List each code multiple times or
* Use times (×) symbol and indicate number

Important Reporting Rule

If vaccine administered during an office visit that was not for vaccine
- Report E/M service (with modifier -25) + Vaccine

Office visit for vaccine only, code only vaccine, NO E/M service

Routine Vaccinations

Influenza

Substance (vaccine) 90657-90665

Administration
- G0008 HCPCS
- 90471/90472

Pneumococcal

Substance (vaccine) 90732

Administration
- G0009 HCPCS
- 90471/90472 administration

Therapeutic or Diagnostic Infusions (90780-90781)

Infusion: Therapeutic procedure to introduce fluid into body

Example: Fluid into vein for patient rehydration

Codes represent infusion service only
- Report substance infused separately

Psychiatry (90801-90802)

Psychiatric treatment at same time as E/M service, report
- Psychiatric treatment + E/M service

Time major billing factor
- Codes divided on time
- Record indicates session time

Many services provided in partial hospital settings
- Patient in hospital during day, return to home for evenings and weekends

Biofeedback (90901-90911)

Used to help patients gain control over body processes

Example: Elevated BP or manage chronic pain

Patient training in biofeedback by professional

Continues on own

Services often part psychophysiologic (mind/body) therapy

Dialysis (90918-90999)

Cleanses blood

1. Temporary (non-ESRD)
2. Permanent (ESRD)

Two parts to report ESRD dialysis services:

- Physician service + hemodialysis procedure

ESRD Physician Services (90918-90925)
Include:

1. Establishment dialyzing cycle

2. Physician services

3. E/M outpatient dialysis visits

4. Telephone calls

5. Patient management during dialysis

Reported for month: 90918-90921

- Less than full month of service 90922-90925 per day
- Codes divided on age

Hemodialysis Service (90935-90940)

Hemodialysis is the procedure
- Used for ESRD and non-ESRD

Billed per day for inpatients receiving ESRD

Includes all physician E/M services related to procedure
- Use modifier -25 if separate E/M service provided

Miscellaneous Dialysis Procedures (90945-90999)

- Describes other dialysis procedures
  Example: Peritoneal dialysis in which toxins are passively absorbed into dialysis fluid

Peritoneal Dialysis (90989-90993)

- Services billed on per day basis for inpatient ESRD patients
- Patients can receive training in self-dialysis
  Codes divided by complete or partial training program

Gastroenterology (91000-91299)

For tests and treatments of esophagus, stomach, and intestine

Codes usually reported with E/M or consultation service code

   Caution: Many bundled services

Ophthalmology (92002-92499)

Contains E/M codes

Definitions for new and established patients same as for E/M section

Codes are for bilateral services
- If only one eye, use modifier -52 (reduced service)

Special Ophthalmologic Services (92502-92700)

For special evaluations of visual system

Goes beyond those usually provided in evaluation

May be reported in addition to basic visual service

Special Otorhinolaryngologic Services (92502-92700)

Special treatments and diagnostic services

> **Example:** Nasal function tests (rhinomanometry) or audiometric tests

All hearing tests bilateral unless indicated one ear in description

Noninvasive Vascular Diagnostic Studies (93875-93990)

Vascular codes for procedures on noncoronary veins and arteries
Includes:

1. Patient care

2. Supervision and interpretation (S&I)

3. Copy of results

Pulmonary (94010-94799)

For therapies and diagnostic tests

Includes procedure and interpretation of test results
- Additional E/M service reported separately

Allergy and Clinical Immunology (95004-95199)

Divided into two suheadings:

1. Allergy Testing (95004-95078)

2. Allergen Immunotherapy (95115-95199)

Allergy Testing (95004-95078)

- Sensitivity testing using various types of tests
   Example: Percutaneous, intracutaneous, inhalation
- Tests use numerous substances
   Example: Extracts, venoms, biologics, and foods
- Type and number of tests based on physician's judgment

Coding Allergy Testing

Medical record will indicate
- Number tests
- Type test
- Method testing

Allergen Immunotherapy (95115-95199)

- Codes divided into three types services:

    1. Injection only

    2. Prescription and injection

    3. Provision antigen (substance) only

- Physician service bundled into immunotherapy codes
  If separate E/M service provided, report separately

Neurology and Neuromuscular Procedures (95805-96004)

Contains codes to report tests, such as:

- Sleep tests
- Muscle tests (electromyography)
- Range-of-motion measurements
- Electroencephalogram (EEG)

Many bundled services

Services usually provided in addition to E/M service

Central Nervous System (CNS) Assessments/Tests (96105-96117)

Used to report:

- Psychological tests
- Speech/Language assessments
- Developmental progress assessments
- Thinking/Reasoning examinations
  Codes based on per hour basis
- Except for basic developmental testing
  Includes written report of results

Chemotherapy Administration (96400-96549)

Represents only preparation and administration chemotherapy
- If separate E/M service provided, report E/M code + -25
Chemical can be administered (injected) into

    1. Lesion

    2. Vein

    3. Tissue

    4. Muscle

    5. Artery

    6. Cavity

    7. Nerve

Intravenously injected chemicals two methods of delivery of chemical

    1. IV push quickly puts into vein

    2. IV infusion delivers over longer period time

Codes often divided on time the injection procedure takes

    Example: 96410 chemotherapy administration, intravenous push, up to hour

Chemical agent (substance) reported separately using 96545 or HCPCS J code

Special supplies (e.g., special needles) reported separately using 99070 or HCPCS code

Report any intraarterial catheter placement with 36620-36640

Injections with chemotherapy
- Report separately any analgesic or antiemetic (for vomiting)
- Before or after chemotherapy

Photodynamic Therapy (96567-96571)

Used in addition to bronchoscopy or endoscopy codes

Injected agent remains in cancerous cells longer than normal cells
- After agent dissipates from normal cells, patient exposed to laser light
- Agent absorbs light
- Light produces oxygen and cancer cell destroyed

Special Dermatological Procedures (96900-96999)

Usually specialized procedures provided on consultation basis
- Separate E/M consultation code would then be appropriate

Treatment of skin conditions:

Actinotherapy—with ultraviolet light

Photochemotherapy—with light-sensitive chemicals and light rays

Physical Medicine & Rehabilitation (97001-97799)

Used by physicians and therapists to report services for variety of services

Treatments

- Traction
- Electrical stimulation (used to help heal fractures)

Patient Training

- Gait training
- Functional activities

Codes often have time components

> **Example:** 97504 reports orthotics fitting and training, per 15 minutes

Active Wound Care Management (97601-97602)

Debridement

- Selective only necrotic (dead) tissue removed
- Nonselective healthy tissue removed along with necrotic tissue

Each code for ongoing care reported on per session basis

Osteopathic and Chiropractic Services (98925-98943)

Both inpatient and outpatient settings

Physician services bundled into codes

Codes divided by body area

Special Services, Procedures, and Reports (99000-99091)

Handling and conveyance laboratory specimens
- 99000-99022

Postoperative follow-up visits included in surgical package
- 99024

Office visits after posted hours or in locations other than office
- 99050-99056

Supplies and materials
- 99070

Hospital mandated on call services
- 99026-99027

HCPCS CODING

Developed by Centers for Medicare & Medicaid Services, CMS
- Formerly HCFA

HCPCS developed, 1983

CPT did not contain all codes necessary for Medicare services reporting

One of Two Levels of Codes

1. Level I, CPT

2. Level II, HCPCS, also known as national codes

Phased Out Level III, Local Codes

Developed by Medicare carriers for use at local level

Varied by locale

Discontinued October 2002
- Some codes incorporated into HCPCS

Level II, National Codes

Codes for wide variety providers
- Physicians
- Dentists
- Orthodontists

Codes for wide variety services
- Specific drugs
- Durable medical equipment (DME)
- Ambulance services

Format

Begins with letter, followed by 4 digits

Example: E0608, apnea monitor

Each letter represents group codes

Example: "J" codes used to report drugs

Temporary Codes

Certain letters indicate temporary codes

Example: K0459, heavy-duty wheeled walker
- K codes are temporary codes

HCPCS Index

Directs coder to specific codes

Do not code directly from index

Reference main portion of text before assigning code

Alphabetical order

Ambulance Modifiers

Origin and destination used in combination:
- 1st letter origin
- 2nd letter destination

Example:
- -R = Residence
- -H = Hospital
- -RH origin (1st letter) residence and destination (2nd letter) hospital

PET Modifiers

Positron Emission Tomography: Noninvasive imaging procedure

Assesses metabolic organ activity
- PET scan modifiers 1 letter
  - Used in combination to indicate scan results:
    - 1st current results
    - 2nd previous results

N = Negative

E = Equivocal (means "same")

P = Positive, not suggestive extensive ischemia

S = Positive and suggestive extensive ischemia (>20% left ventricle)

Example: -EP
- E = current scan
- P = previous scan

Table of Drugs

Listed by generic name, not brand name

Often used to when reporting immunizations or injections

ICD-9-CM

Introduction

Morbidity (Illness)

Mortality (death)

CM = Clinical Modification

Provides continuity of data

WHO's ICD-9 used globally

1977: US develops ICD-9 version
- Has more code subsets
- Data collapse back to ICD-9 for uniformity of data

Medicare

- Medicare Catastrophic Act of 1988
  Required use of ICD-9-CM codes for outpatient claims
- Act abolished but codes still used

Uses of ICD-9-CM

- Some payers reimburse hospital based on patient's diagnosis
- Facilities track patient use through codes
- Fiscal entities track health care costs
- Research
  Health care quality
  Future needs
  Newer cancer center built if patient use warrants

Predict health care trends
Plan for future health care needs

✱ ICD-9-CM on Insurance Forms

p. 238
copy
from
new
book

- Diagnoses establish medical necessity
- Services and diagnoses must correlate
- CMS-1500 in Block 21 and 24E **(Figure 3-12)**
  Office visit: croup, 464.4, Block 21, 1; 1 placed in Block 24E, Line 1

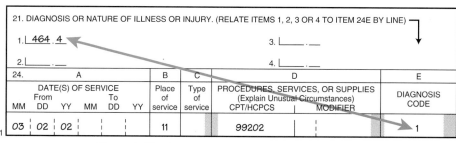

Figure 3-12 Diagnosis code and service must correlate.

> **Ethics**
> Documentation must support diagnosis
> **Example:**
>   Services provided
>   Diagnosis justifies services
> If in doubt, check it out; don't make assumptions
> **Your Job:** Translate documentation into ICD-9-CM codes

Format of ICD-9-CM

Volume 1, Diseases, Tabular List

Volume 2, Diseases, Alphabetic Index

Volume 3, Procedures, Tabular List + Alphabetic Index

Volume 1, Diseases, Tabular List

- Contains code numbers
- 001.0-999.9 Diagnosis codes describe condition
- V & E codes = supplemental information

Volume 2, Diseases, Alphabetic Index

Volume 3
· Index + Tabular List used for
Procedures + therapists

- Appears first in book
- Refers coder to code numbers in Volume 1
- Never code directly from Index!

· Inpatient settings
· Procedures + therapists

ICD-9-CM Conventions

Symbols, abbreviations, punctuation, and notations
NEC: not elsewhere classifiable
- No more specific code exists
NOS: not otherwise specified
- Unspecified in documentation

[ ] BRACKETS

Enclose synonyms, alternative wording, or explanatory phrases

Helpful, additional information

Can affect code

Found only in Tabular List (001.0-999.9)

( ) PARENTHESES

Contain nonessential modifiers
- Take them or leave them

Found in Tabular List and Index

Do not affect code

COLON & BRACE

: **Colon:** Tabular List, completes statement with one or more modifiers

} **Brace:** Tabular List, modifying statements to left of brace

New Book Copy Bottom of Page p. 238   Figure 3-4

LOZENGE, SECTION MARK, & BOLD TYPE

□ **Lozenge:** Can indicates codes unique to ICD-9-CM

§ **Section:** Can be footnote indicator

Bold type: Codes and code titles in Tabular List, Volume 1

ITALICIZED TYPE

All excludes notes

Codes NOT used as principal diagnosis

SLANTED BRACKETS [ ]

Enclose manifestations of underlying condition

Code underlying condition first

INCLUDES, EXCLUDES, USE ADDITIONAL CODE

Includes notes: In chapter, section, or category

Excludes notes: Conditions are coded elsewhere

Use Additional Code: Assignment of other code(s) is necessary

AND/WITH

And: means and/or

With: one condition with (in addition to) another condition

CODE, IF APPLICABLE, ANY CAUSAL CONDITION FIRST:

May be principal diagnosis if no causal condition applicable or known

Example, 707.10, Ulcer of lower limb, except decubitus; states:
  • Chronic venous hypertension with ulcer (459.31)

If ulcer caused by chronic venous hypertension:

   First: 459.31 chronic venous hypertension

   Second: 707.10 ulcer of lower limb

Volume 2, Alphabetic Index

Nonessential Modifiers: have no effect on code selection

Enclosed in parentheses

Clarify diagnosis

   Example: Ileus (adynamic) (bowel) . . .

Terms

Main terms (bold typeface)
• Subterms
• Indented 2 spaces to right
• Not bold

Cross References

- Directs you: *see, see* also
- "*see*" directs you to specific term
  - **Example,** Panotitis—"*see*" Otitis media
- "*see* also" directs you to another term for more information
  - **Example,** Perivaginitis (*see* also Vesiculitis)
- "*see* category" Volume 1, Tabular List, specific information about use of code
  - **Example,** Mesencephalitis (*see* also Encephalitis) 323.9; late effect—*see* category 326

Notes

- Define terms
- Give further coding instructions
  - **Example:** Index: "Melanoma"
  - Note: "Except where otherwise indicated . . ."
- Mandatory fifth digits also appear as notes (one reason to never code from Index)

Eponyms

- Disease or syndromes named for person
  - **Example:** Arnold-Chiari (see also Spina bifida)

Etiology and Manifestation of Disease

Etiology = cause of disease

Manifestation = symptom

Combination codes = etiology and manifestation in one code

Neoplasm

- In Volume 2, Index, locate Neoplasm Table under "Ns"

Sections

Section 1, Index to Diseases

Section 2, Table of Drugs and Chemicals

Section 3, Index to External Causes of Injuries and Poisonings (E Codes)

Section 1, Index to Diseases

- Largest part of Volume 2—Index
- First step in coding, locate main term in Index
- Subterms indented two spaces to right
- May have more than one subterm

Section 2, Table of Drugs and Chemicals

- Drug name placed alphabetically on left under heading "Substance" **(Figure 3-13)**
- First column: "Poisoning" code for substance involved
- E codes identify how poisoning occurred

Example: if Alkaline antiseptic solution poisoning occurred by accident, E858.7
*Accidental poisoning by alkaline antiseptic solution: 976.6 (substance) and E858.7 (how it occurred)
*Code any resulting condition (i.e., coma)

Headings

Accident: Unintentional

Therapeutic: Correct dosage, correctly administered with adverse effects

Suicide attempt: Self-inflicted

Assault: intentionally inflicted by another person

Undetermined: Unknown cause

Section 3, E Codes

- Alphabetic Index to External Causes of Injuries and Poisonings
- Provides additional information
- Never principal (inpatient) or primary (outpatient) diagnosis
- Separate Index to External Causes
   Alphabetical, main terms in bold
   Subterms are indented 2 spaces to right under main term

Volume 1, Tabular List

Two Major Divisions:

1. Classification of Diseases and Injuries (codes 001.0-999.9)

2. Supplementary Classification (V codes and E codes)

a word of Caution alphabetic Index
" Some words in Index do not appear in Tabular - Saves space
• Exact word may not be in code Tabular description
But found in alphabetic Index .
That is why you must locate term in Index , then locate Tabular

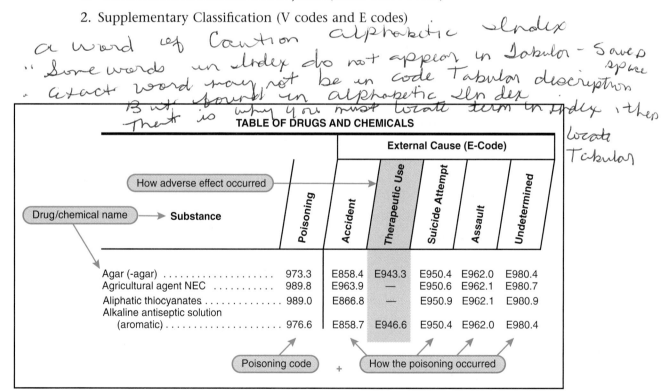

TABLE OF DRUGS AND CHEMICALS

Drug/chemical name → Substance	Poisoning	External Cause (E-Code)				
		Accident	Therapeutic Use	Suicide Attempt	Assault	Undetermined
Agar (-agar)	973.3	E858.4	E943.3	E950.4	E962.0	E980.4
Agricultural agent NEC	989.8	E963.9	—	E950.6	E962.1	E980.7
Aliphatic thiocyanates	989.0	E866.8	—	E950.9	E962.1	E980.9
Alkaline antiseptic solution (aromatic)	976.6	E858.7	E946.6	E950.4	E962.0	E980.4

How adverse effect occurred

Poisoning code + How the poisoning occurred

Figure 3-13   Section 2, Table of Drugs and Chemicals. *(From International Classification of Diseases, 9th Revision. U.S. Department of Health and Human Services, Public Health Service, Center for Medicare and Medicaid Services.)*

Classification of Diseases and Injuries

- Main portion of ICD-9-CM
- Codes from 001.0-999.9
- Most chapters are body systems
   Example:
   Digestive System
   Respiratory System

Divisions of Classification of Diseases and Injuries

Chapters: 1 through 17

Section: A group of related conditions

Category: Represents single disease/condition

Subcategory: More specific

Subclassification: Most specific

Remember
Assign to highest level of specify, based on documentation
If 4-digit code exists, do not report 3-digit code
If 5-digit code exists, do not report 4-digit code

Appendices in Volume 1

There are five appendices in official ICD-9-CM

Private publishers may have more

Appendix A, Morphology of Neoplasms

- Used in conjunction with codes from Chapter 2, Neoplasm
   Inpatient setting: Cancer registries and claim forms
   Not used by outpatient coders
- Begins with M followed by 5 digits:
   M8400/0, Sweat gland adenoma
   First four digits: Histologic type of neoplasm
   Fifth digit: Behavior (i.e., 0 = benign)

Appendix B, Glossary of Mental Disorders

- Contains psychiatric terms that appear in Chapter 5, Mental Disorders
- Listed in alphabetical order
- Valuable tool for cross referencing psychiatric conditions
- *Deleted in 2005*

Appendix C, Drugs

- American Hospital Formulary Service (AHFS) publishes list of all drugs
- Tracks drugs nationally, used by pharmacists, not outpatient coders
- Each drug coded with up to 5-digit code (e.g., 8:12.04)

- AHFS listing correlated with ICD-9-CM Table of Drugs and Chemicals
- New drugs not identified by name
  Rather listed under heading "Drug" in Table of Drugs and Chemicals
  Example, 84:04.04 antibiotic

Appendix D, Industrial Accidents

- Three-digit codes that identify occupational hazards
- Not placed on insurance or billing form
- Used by state and federal organizations (OSHA) to summarize industrial accident data, not used by outpatient coders

Appendix E, Three-Digit Categories

- Presented by chapter
- Categories are labeled 1 through 17
- Provides quick overview of ICD-9-CM contents

USING ICD-9-CM

Guidelines developed by Cooperating Parties
- AHA
- AHIMA
- CMS
- NCHS

General Guidelines

Appendix A of this text contains Official Guidelines for Coding and Reporting

Inpatient coders use Sections I-III

Outpatient coders primarily use Section I and IV, however

Diagnostic Coding and Reporting Guidelines do NOT cover all situations;
  - Outpatient coders also use many Section II and III guidelines

Steps to Diagnosis Coding

Identify MAIN term(s) in diagnosis

Locate MAIN term(s) in Index

Review subterms

Follow cross-reference instructions (e.g., *see, see also*)

Verify code(s) in Tabular

  1. Read Tabular notes

  2. Code to highest specificity

  3. Never code from index!

[handwritten margin notes:]

Copy from New Book
p. 244, 245
Volume 3 Procedures
90% of codes refer
the surgical procedures
10% refer to diagnostic
& therapeutic procedures
Volume 3. Table of Contents
Tabular List
Alphabetic Index
Volume 3 - Bundling

Guidelines for following labels

(1) indicates inpatient setting guidelines
(0) indicates outpatient setting guidelines
(1/0) guidelines apply to both inpt. &
outpt. settings
You have type up to code both inp
& outpt. facility services on the
cert specation examination.

Guideline Section I, B, 3, Level of Specificity in Coding

Assign diagnosis (dx) to highest level of specificity

Do NOT use 3-digit code if there is 4th

Do NOT use 4-digit code if there is 5th

Section I, 10B and 10,3, Acute and Chronic Conditions

Exists alone or together

May be separate or combination codes

If two codes, code acute first

Example, acute and chronic pancreatitis

When two separate codes exist, code:
- Acute cystitis 595.0
- Chronic cystitis 595.2

Handwritten: Section I, A, 2 other (NEC) or Unspecified (NOS) (1/0)
NEC - Not Elsewhere Classifiable — More specific code does not exist.
NOS = Not otherwise specified (Means "Unspecified") available information NOT Specific enough — use only if more specific code NOT available

Combination code: Both acute and chronic condition
- Diarrhea (acute) (chronic) 787.91, Acute and subacute bacterial endocarditis 421.0
- Otitis acute and subacute 382.9

Handwritten: Uncertain Conditions (1)
If diagnosis at time of discharge States:
probable
suspected
likely
questionable
possible
rule out
Code condition as if condition existed, until proven otherwise.
Example: Cough & fever probably pneumonia. Code pneumonia, do not code cough & fever. Outpt. Code cough & fever, do not code pneumonia

Section I, 11A, Combination Code

Always use combination code if one exists

Example, encephalomyelitis (dx) due to rubella (manifestation), 056.01

Section I, B, 9, Multiple Diagnosis Coding

Etiology (cause)

Manifestation (symptom)
- Slanted brackets [ ]
  Example: Retinopathy, diabetic 250.5 [362.01]
  ○ Must check Tabular notes to assign correct 5th digit for diabetes
  ○ Tabular: 362.0, Diabetic retinopathy, instructs to "Code first diabetes 250.5"

Handwritten: New Book 247

Selection of Primary Diagnosis

Condition for encounter

Documented

That condition that is responsible for services provided

Also list co-existing conditions

Diagnosis and procedure MUST correlate

Medical necessity established

No correlation = no reimbursement

Section I, C17, Codes in Brackets

- Never sequence as principal dx
- Always sequence in order listed in Index
  Example:
  - Index lists: Diabetes, gangrene 250.7 *[785.4]*
  - 785.4 = gangrene
  - Tabular, 785.4 indicates "Code first any associated underlying condition: diabetes (250.7X) . . ."
  - Code first diabetes, then gangrene
  - 250.7X = diabetes (X = 5th digit)
  - 785.4 = gangrene

Section II, B, Two or More Interrelated Conditions

- When two or more interrelated conditions exist and either could be principal dx, either may be sequenced first
  Example: Patient with mitral valve stenosis and coronary artery disease (two interrelated conditions)
  - Either can be principal dx and sequenced first
  - Resource intensiveness affects choice

V Codes

Located after 999.9 in Tabular

Two digits before decimal (e.g., V10.10)

Index for V codes Alphabetic Index to Diseases

Main terms: contraception, counseling, dialysis, status, examination

Not sick BUT receives health care (e.g., vaccination)

Services for known disease/injury (e.g., chemotherapy)

A circumstance/problem that influences patient's health BUT NOT current illness/injury

Examples: Organ transplant status

Birth status and outcome of delivery (newborn)

Special Note About "History of"
Index to Disease, MAIN term "History"
Entries between "family" and "visual loss V19.0" = "family history of"
Entries before "family" and after "visual loss V19.0" = "personal history of"

Section I, 12, Late Effects

Late effect residual of (remaining from) previous illness/injury, e.g., burn that leaves scar

Residual coded first (scar)

Cause (burn) coded second

Diagnostic Coding and Reporting Guidelines

Physician's office

Hospital-based outpatient services

Part of Official Guidelines for Coding and Reporting, Section IV

Guideline A

- The term *first-listed diagnosis* is used rather than *principal diagnosis*

Guideline B

- Use codes 001.0 through V83.89 to code dx, symptoms, conditions, problems, complaints, or other reason(s) for visit

Guideline C

- Documentation should describe patient's condition, using terminology that includes specific diagnoses as well as symptoms, problems, or reasons for encounter

Guideline D

- Selection of codes 001.0 through 999.9 (Chapters 1-17) will frequently be used to describe reason for encounter

Guideline E

- Codes that describe symptoms and signs, as opposed to diagnoses, acceptable for reporting purposes when an established dx has NOT been confirmed by physician

Guideline F

- V codes deal with encounters for circumstances other than disease or injury

  Example: Well-baby checkup (V20.2)

Guideline G

- Codes have either three, four, or five digits
- 4th and/or 5th digit codes provide greater specificity
- Three-digit code used ONLY if it is 4th or 5th digit
- Where 4th and/or 5th digits provided, must be assigned
- Diagnoses NOT coded to full digits available invalid

Guideline H

- List first code for dx, condition, problem, or other reason for encounter/visit shown in medical record to be chiefly responsible for services provided
- List additional codes that describe any coexisting conditions

Guideline I

- Do NOT code diagnoses documented as probable, suspected, questionable, ruled out, or working diagnoses
- Rather, code condition(s) to highest degree of certainty for that encounter/visit, such as symptoms, signs, abnormal test results, or other reason for visit
  Example: Cough and fever, probably pneumonia
  Code as cough (786.2) and fever (780.6) [in this order]

Guideline J

- Chronic diseases treated on an ongoing basis may be coded and reported as many times as patient receives treatment and care for condition(s)

Guideline K

- Code all documented conditions that coexist at time of visit, that require or affect patient care, treatment, or management
- Do NOT code conditions previously treated, no longer existing
- "History of" codes (V10-V19) may be used as secondary codes if:
- Impacts current care or treatment

Guideline L & M

- For patients receiving diagnostic or therapeutic services ONLY
- Sequence first:

    Diagnosis,

    Condition,

    Problem, or

    Other reason shown in medical record to be chiefly responsible for encounter
- Codes for other diagnoses (e.g., chronic conditions)

    May be sequenced as secondary diagnoses
- **Exception:**

    Patients receiving chemotherapy (V58.1), radiation therapy (V58.0), or rehabilitation (code depends on type):

    V code 1^{st,} dx or problem for which service being performed 2nd

Guideline N

- For patients receiving preoperative evaluations ONLY:

    Code from category V72.8 (Other specified examinations)

    Assign secondary code for reason for surgery

    Code also any findings related to preoperative evaluation

Guideline O

- Code dx which required surgery
- And op dx different

    Code op dx

Guideline P

- Code routine prenatal visits with no complications:

    V22.0 (Supervision of normal 1st pregnancy)

    V22.1 (Supervision of other normal pregnancy)

    DO NOT use these codes with pregnancy complication codes

ICD-9-CM, Chapter 1, Infectious and Parasitic Diseases

Divided based on etiology (cause of disease)

Many Combination Codes

> **Example:** 112 candidiasis infection of mouth

Reports both organism and condition

Multiple Codes

> Sequencing must be considered
> UTI due to *Escherichia coli*
> - 599.0 (UTI) etiology
> - 041.4 (*E. coli*) organism [in this order]

Section I, C1, Human Immunodeficiency Virus

> Code HIV or HIV-related illness ONLY if stated as <u>confirmed</u> in diagnostic statement
> - 042 HIV or HIV-related illness
> - V08 Asymptomatic HIV or HIV-related illness
> - 795.71 Nonspecific HIV and infants with inconclusive HIV tests

Previously Diagnosed HIV-Related Illness
> - Code prior dx HIV-related disease 042 (HIV)
> - NEVER assign these patients to:
> V08 (Asymptomatic) or
> 795.71 (Nonspecific serologic evidence of HIV)

HIV Sequencing
> - Sequence first that reason most responsible for encounter
> - Followed by secondary dx that affects encounter or patient care

HIV and Pregnancy
> - This an exception to HIV sequencing
> - During pregnancy, childbirth, or puerperium, code:
> 647.8X (Other specified infections and parasitic diseases),
> followed by 042 (HIV)
> - Asymptomatic HIV during pregnancy, childbirth, or puerperium:
> 647.8X (Other specified infections and parasitic diseases) and
> V08 (Asymptomatic HIV infection status)

Inconclusive Laboratory Test for HIV
> - 795.71 (Inconclusive serologic test for HIV)

HIV Screening
> - Code V73.89 (Screening for other specified viral disease)
> Patient in high-risk group for HIV
> V69.8 (Other problems related to lifestyle)
> - Patients returning for HIV screening results = V65.44 (HIV counseling)

Caution
Incorrectly applying these HIV coding rules can cause patient hardship
- Insurance claims for patients with HIV usually need patient's written agreement to disclosure

---

ICD-9-CM, Chapter 2, Neoplasms

Two steps for coding neoplasms:

Index:

1. Locate histologic type of neoplasm (e.g., sarcoma, melanoma)
   - Review all instructions

2. Locate code identified by body site
   - Usually in Neoplasm Table in Index under "N"

Treatment directed at malignancy: Neoplasm is principal dx
   Except for chemotherapy or radiotherapy:
   - Therapy (treatment) followed by neoplasm code
     Chemotherapy: V58.1
     Radiotherapy: V58.0
Surgical removal of neoplasm and subsequent chemotherapy or radiotherapy:
- Code malignancy as principal dx
Surgery to determine extent of malignancy:
- Code malignancy as principal dx
  V10, "Personal history of malignant neoplasm" if

1. Neoplasm was previously destroyed

2. No longer being treated

If patient receives treatment for secondary neoplasm (metastasis):

1. Secondary neoplasm is principal dx

2. Even though primary is known

Patient treated for anemia or dehydration due to neoplasm or therapy code:
- Anemia or dehydration followed by neoplasm
Patient admitted to repair complication of surgery for an intestinal malignancy:
- Complication principal dx
  Complication is reason for encounter
  Malignancy secondary dx

V Codes and Neoplasms

Patient receiving chemotherapy or radiotherapy post-op removal of neoplasm:

Code: Therapy followed by active neoplasm

Do NOT report H/O (history of) neoplasm

ICD-9-CM, Chapter 3, Endocrine, Nutritional, and Metabolic Diseases and Immunity Disorders

Disorders of Other Endocrine Glands

- Diabetes Mellitus 250 coded frequently
  Subterms often have 2 codes
  Example:
  1. Diabetic iritis 250.5X for diabetes (etiology)
  2. *[364.42]* for iritis (manifestation)

- 5th digit indicates type of diabetes
  1. Adult or juvenile
  2. 2 type II (non-insulin-dependent)
  3. 3 type I (insulin-dependent)

Other Metabolic and Immunity Disorders Section

- Disorders such as gout and dehydration
- Disorders often have many names
  Example: 242.0X Toxic diffuse goiter also known as:
  1. Basedow's disease
  2. Graves' disease
  3. Primary thyroid hyperplasia

ICD-9-CM, Chapter 4, Diseases of Blood and Blood-Forming Organs

Short chapter with 10 sections

Includes anemia, blood disorders, coagulation defects

Often used code, anemia

Many different types of anemia:
- Hereditary hemolytic (282)
- Iron deficiency (280)
- Acquired hemolytic (283)
- Aplastic (284)
- Unspecified (285)

Multiple coding often necessary

Identify underlying disease condition

ICD-9-CM, Chapter 5, Mental Disorders

Includes codes for:

1. Personality disorders
2. Stress disorders
3. Neuroses
4. Psychoses
5. Sexual deviation/dysfunction, etc.

5th digit = status of episode

Example: 304.2, cocaine dependence is assigned the following 5th digits:
- 0 unspecified (episode)
- 1 continuous
- 2 episodic
- 3 in remission

ICD-9-CM, Chapter 6, Diseases of Nervous System and Sense Organs

Central Nervous System

Peripheral Nervous System

Disorders of Eye

Diseases of Ear

ICD-9-CM, Chapter 7, Diseases of Circulatory System

Three types of hypertension:

1. Malignant accelerated, severe, poor prognosis

2. Benign continuous, mild (BP elevated) controllable

3. Unspecified NOT indicated as either malignant or benign

Hypertension (401-405)

Hypertension, Essential, or NOS

- Assign hypertension (arterial, essential, primary, systemic, NOS) to 401
- 4th digit to indicates type

Hypertension with Heart Disease

402 Category:

Certain heart conditions when stated "due to hypertension" or implied ("hypertensive")

Add 4th digit for type

Use additional code to specify type of heart failure

Hypertensive Renal Disease with Chronic Renal Failure

- Cause-and-effect relationship assumed in chronic renal failure with hypertension
- Category 403, Hypertensive renal disease, used when following present:
  Chronic renal failure (585)
  Renal failure, unspecified (586)
  Renal sclerosis, unspecified (587)

Hypertensive Heart and Renal Disease

- Assign 404 when both hypertensive renal disease and hypertensive heart disease stated
- Assume cause-and-effect relationship
- Assign 5th digit for mention of renal and/or congestive heart failure
  Use additional code to specify type of heart failure

Hypertensive Cerebrovascular Disease

Code:
- Cerebrovascular disease (430-438)
- Type of hypertension (401-405)

Hypertensive Retinopathy

Code:
- Hypertensive retinopathy
- Type of hypertension (401-405)

Hypertension, Secondary

Hypertension caused by an underlying condition
   Code:
- Underlying condition
- Type of hypertension (401-405)

Hypertension, Transient

- Transient hypertension: Temporary elevated BP
- NOT assign 401-405 Hypertensive Disease
  Hypertension dx NOT established
  Use:
  796.2, Elevated blood pressure or
  642.3X, Transient hypertension of pregnancy

Hypertension, Controlled

- Hypertension controlled by therapy:
  Assign code from 401-405

Hypertension, Uncontrolled

- Untreated or uncontrolled hypertension
  Assign code from 401-405

Elevated Blood Pressure

- Elevated blood pressure coded 796.2
  Elevated BP reading without hypertension is dx
  Hypertension NOT stated, NOT coded to 401

ICD-9-CM, Chapter 8, Diseases of Respiratory System

> "Use additional code to identify infectious organism"
> Some codes indicate specific organism

Acute Respiratory Infection Section

Frequently used codes, such as:
- Common cold (460, acute nasopharyngitis)
- Sore throat (462, acute pharyngitis)
- Acute tonsillitis (463)
- Bronchitis (490-491)
- Acute upper respiratory infection (465, URI)
- Influenza (487, flu)

ICD-9-CM, Chapter 9, Diseases of Digestive System

Mouth to anus + accessory organs

Extensive subcategories
- 574 Cholelithiasis (10 subcategories)
- Each has 5th digit subclassification

Commonly used codes:

Ulcers (531-534)

Gastric (531)

Duodenal (532)

Peptic (533)

Gastrojejunal (534)

Hernias (550-553)

ICD-9-CM, Chapter 10, Diseases of Genitourinary System

Commonly used codes:

Urinary tract infection (599.0)

Inflammation of prostate (601.X)

Disorders of menstruation (625-627)

ICD-9-CM, Chapter 11, Complications of Pregnancy, Childbirth, and Puerperium

Extensive multiple coding with many 5th digit assignments and notes

Admission for pregnancy, complication
- Obstetric complication = primary dx

General Rules

- Not all encounters are pregnancy related
  Example, pregnant woman, broken ankle (medial malleolus, open)
  Broken ankle (824.1)
  V22.2 Pregnant state incidental

Complications of Pregnancy, Childbirth, and Puerperium

- Chapter 11 codes (630-677)
- Only used on mother's medical record
- Not on newborn medical record

Selection of Primary Diagnosis

- Routine prenatal visits no complications:
  V22.0, Supervision, normal **first** pregnancy or
  V22.1, Supervision, **other** normal pregnancy
- Prenatal outpatient visits for high-risk pregnancies:
  V23, Supervision of high-risk pregnancy

5th Digit

- All categories EXCEPT 650 (Normal delivery)
- Requires 5th digit for:
  Antepartum
  Postpartum, or
  If delivery has occurred
- Appropriate 5th digit listed under each code
    Example: 640.0, Threatened abortion
      0 unspecified episode
      1 delivered with or without complication
      3 antepartum condition or complication
- Note that NOT all 5th digits are applicable (cannot assign 2 or 4)

Postpartum Period

- After delivery + 6 weeks

Abortions

- Codes 634-637 require 5th digits:
  0 unspecified
  1 incomplete (POC, product of conception) NOT expelled
  2 complete, all (POC) expelled prior to care

Abortions With Liveborn Fetus

- Attempted abortion results in liveborn fetus:
  644.21 (Early onset of delivery) appropriately
  Use V27 (Outcome of delivery)
  Attempted abortion code also assigned

ICD-9-CM, Chapter 12, Diseases of Skin and Subcutaneous Tissue

Skin

1. Epidermis
2. Dermis
3. Subcutaneous tissue
4. Infectious Skin/Subcutaneous Tissue
5. Scar tissue

Accessory Organs

1. Sweat glands
2. Sebaceous glands
3. Nails
4. Hair and hair follicles
5. Other

Multiple Codes Often Necessary

Example, cellulitis due to Staph

1. Cellulitis 682
2. Staph 041

ICD-9-CM, Chapter 13, Diseases of Musculoskeletal System and Connective Tissue

Bone

Bursa

Cartilage

Fascia

Ligaments

Muscle

Synovia

Tendons

Chapter 13 Sections

Extensive notes and 5th digits
- Arthropathies (joint disease) and Related Disorders
- Dorsopathies (curvature of spine)
- Rheumatism, Excluding back
- Osteopathies, Chondropathies, and Acquired Musculoskeletal Deformities

ICD-9-CM, Chapters 14 and 15

Congenital Anomalies (abnormality at birth)

Conditions Originating in Perinatal Period
- Perinatal period through 28th day following birth
- Codes can be used after 28th day if documented that condition originated during perinatal period

ICD-9-CM, Chapter 16, Symptoms, Signs, and Ill-Defined Conditions

Do NOT code a sign or symptom if:
- Definitive dx made (symptoms are part of disease)

Only used if no specific dx made

ICD-9-CM, Chapter 17 Injury and Poisoning

Section Examples

Fractures

Dislocations

Sprains and Strains

Intracranial Injury

Internal Injury

Crushing Injury

Foreign Body

Burns

Late Effects

Poisoning

E Codes

Provides supplemental information

Never principal dx

Identify:

1. Cause of an injury or poisoning

2. Intent (unintentional or intentional)

3. Place it occurred

General E Code Guidelines

- Use with any code in Volume 1
- Initial encounter
  Use E code
- Subsequent encounter
  Use late effects E codes

Intent

- Unknown, Undetermined (E980-E989)
- Unspecified, Undetermined (E980-E989)
- Questionable, Undetermined (E980-E989)

Table of Drugs and Chemicals

- Alphabetic listing with codes (see **Figure 3-13**)
- Do NOT code directly from Table
- Always reference Tabular

Two or More Substances Involved

- If two or more substances involved code:
  Each unless combination code exists
- Code substance more closely related to principal dx, and
  Include one code from each category (cause, intent, place)
- Interaction of a drug(s) and alcohol
  Using poisoning and E codes for both

Unknown or Suspected Intent

- Unknown
- Unspecified
- Questionable

Undetermined Cause

- Intent known, cause unknown, use:
  E928.9, Unspecified accident
  E958.9, Suicide and self-inflicted injury by unspecified means
  E968.9, Assault by unspecified means

Late Effects of External Cause

- Should be used with late effect of a previous injury/poisoning
- Should NOT be used with related current injury code

Multiple Injuries and Burns

- Sequence most severe injury first (physician determined)

Current Burns

- Sequence highest degree burn first
- Current burns (940-948) classified by
  Depth (severity)
  Extent (% body surface)
  Site
  And if necessary, agent

Depth of burn:

  1st degree: erythema

  2nd degree: blistering

  3rd degree: full-thickness involvement

Burns classified

- According to extent body surface involved
- Burn site NOT specified
- Additional data required

Category 948

- 4th digits = % body surface involved
- 5th digits = % body surface involved in 3rd-degree burns
- Rule of Nines applies

Burn example:

Third-degree burn of abdomen, 10%, and second-degree burn of thigh (5%):

  942.33 Burn, abdomen, third degree

  945.26 Burn, thigh, second degree

948.11, 15% burn area

E924.0, Burn by hot liquid

Coding for Multiple Injuries

- Separate code for each injury
- Most serious injury first

Vessel and Nerve Damage

- Code primary injury first
  Use additional code if minor nerve damage
- Primary injury = nerve damage
  Code nerve damage first

Multiple Fractures

- Same coding principles as multiple injuries
- Code multiple fractures, by site
- Sequenced by severity

Fractures

- Not indicated as closed or open = closed
- Same bone fractured AND dislocated
  Code Fx ONLY (highest level of injury)

UNIT IV

Coding Challenge

EXAMINATIONS

You have three opportunities to practice taking an examination:
- Practice Examination (before study)
- Practice Examination (after study)
- Final Examination (at the end of your complete program of study)

You should have a current edition of the following texts:
- ICD-9-CM (International Classification of Diseases, 9th Edition, Clinical Modification)
- HCPCS (Health Care Common Procedural Coding System)
- CPT (Current Procedural Terminology)

No other reference material is allowed for the Practice Examination or Final Examination.
- For the Practice Examination, you will need a computer that can use a CD-ROM.
- For the Final Examination, you will not need a computer; rather, you will need paper, pencils, erasers, and the three coding references listed above (ICD-9-CM, HCPCS, CPT).
- Each organization's certification examination has different scoring requirements, but as you take these examinations, you should strive for an 80% to 90% on the second Practice Examination and 70% as a minimum on the Final Examination.

PRACTICE EXAMINATIONS

The Practice Examination contains 150 questions and is located on the **CD-ROM.** Take this examination before you begin your studies and then immediately on completion of your study. The software on the CD will automatically grade your first attempt at the examination and will store the results for comparison to the second time you take this examination. Ideally, you should complete the examination in one sitting (5 hours, or 300 minutes); if time does not allow, spread the examination times over several periods. There are no time extensions in the real certification examination setting, and learning how to judge the amount of time you have to spend on each question is an important part of this learning experience to prepare you for the real certification experience. There are rationales for each question in the Practice Examination, but do not read the rationales after the first Practice Examination; rather, wait until after you have taken the examination again before reviewing the rationales. The purpose of the Practice Examination is only to assess your beginning level of knowledge and skill—your starting place.

After your studies, take the same Practice Examination again. The software will display the results of the second examination and will compare these scores with the scores from the first examination to illustrate the improvements you have achieved. Keep track of your time; again you have 5 hours (300 minutes) to complete the examination. Study the questions for which you did not choose the correct response. Did you misread the question, did you not know the material well enough to answer correctly, or did you run out of time? Knowing why you missed a question is an important step to improve your skill level.

FINAL EXAMINATION

If you scored well on all areas of the Practice Examination (80%–90%), you are ready to move on to the Final Examination, which is a paper and pencil examination. The real certification is a paper and pencil examination. The time for the Final Examination is 5 hours (300 minutes). There is an answer sheet on which to place your answers; it is located directly before the Final Examination. Remove the answer sheet from the text, and use a no. 2 pencil to enter your answer for each of the 150 questions. If you change an answer, erase the previous entry completely. When you have finished the examination, review the score sheet to ensure that there are no stray pencil marks.

You will need to calculate your percent on each of the three sections in the Final Examination. Each section contains 50 questions. You should strive for a minimum of 70% on each section to consider the Final Examination successful. After you have taken the examination and checked your answers in the Answers to Final section of this text, count the number of incorrect responses per section. Each question is worth 2% (50 questions per section, divided by 100 the total percent = 2% per question). Take the number of incorrect questions times 2 (i.e., Section 1, if you got three questions incorrect, the calculation is $3 \times 2 = 6$) and subtract the resulting number from 100 (100 minus 6 = 94%) to calculate your percent. Calculate your percentage score for each of the three sections. These three scores represent your Final Examination score. Each of the three scores must be at a minimum of 70% to be considered a passing grade. If you did not attain a 70% on each section, you should develop a plan to restudy those particular areas where the examination indicates you are having difficulties. You can take the Final Examination again for practice after your additional study.

ANSWER SHEET

SECTION 1

Medical term
1. Ⓐ Ⓑ Ⓒ Ⓓ
2. Ⓐ Ⓑ Ⓒ Ⓓ
3. Ⓐ Ⓑ Ⓒ Ⓓ
4. Ⓐ Ⓑ Ⓒ Ⓓ
5. Ⓐ Ⓑ Ⓒ Ⓓ
6. Ⓐ Ⓑ Ⓒ Ⓓ
7. Ⓐ Ⓑ Ⓒ Ⓓ
8. Ⓐ Ⓑ Ⓒ Ⓓ
9. Ⓐ Ⓑ Ⓒ Ⓓ
10. Ⓐ Ⓑ Ⓒ Ⓓ

Anatomy
11. Ⓐ Ⓑ Ⓒ Ⓓ
12. Ⓐ Ⓑ Ⓒ Ⓓ
13. Ⓐ Ⓑ Ⓒ Ⓓ
14. Ⓐ Ⓑ Ⓒ Ⓓ
15. Ⓐ Ⓑ Ⓒ Ⓓ
16. Ⓐ Ⓑ Ⓒ Ⓓ
17. Ⓐ Ⓑ Ⓒ Ⓓ
18. Ⓐ Ⓑ Ⓒ Ⓓ
19. Ⓐ Ⓑ Ⓒ Ⓓ
20. Ⓐ Ⓑ Ⓒ Ⓓ

ICD-9-CM
21. Ⓐ Ⓑ Ⓒ Ⓓ
22. Ⓐ Ⓑ Ⓒ Ⓓ
23. Ⓐ Ⓑ Ⓒ Ⓓ
24. Ⓐ Ⓑ Ⓒ Ⓓ
25. Ⓐ Ⓑ Ⓒ Ⓓ
26. Ⓐ Ⓑ Ⓒ Ⓓ
27. Ⓐ Ⓑ Ⓒ Ⓓ
28. Ⓐ Ⓑ Ⓒ Ⓓ
29. Ⓐ Ⓑ Ⓒ Ⓓ
30. Ⓐ Ⓑ Ⓒ Ⓓ

HCPCS
31. Ⓐ Ⓑ Ⓒ Ⓓ
32. Ⓐ Ⓑ Ⓒ Ⓓ
33. Ⓐ Ⓑ Ⓒ Ⓓ
34. Ⓐ Ⓑ Ⓒ Ⓓ
35. Ⓐ Ⓑ Ⓒ Ⓓ

Concepts of coding
36. Ⓐ Ⓑ Ⓒ Ⓓ
37. Ⓐ Ⓑ Ⓒ Ⓓ
38. Ⓐ Ⓑ Ⓒ Ⓓ
39. Ⓐ Ⓑ Ⓒ Ⓓ
40. Ⓐ Ⓑ Ⓒ Ⓓ

E/M
41. Ⓐ Ⓑ Ⓒ Ⓓ
42. Ⓐ Ⓑ Ⓒ Ⓓ
43. Ⓐ Ⓑ Ⓒ Ⓓ
44. Ⓐ Ⓑ Ⓒ Ⓓ
45. Ⓐ Ⓑ Ⓒ Ⓓ
46. Ⓐ Ⓑ Ⓒ Ⓓ
47. Ⓐ Ⓑ Ⓒ Ⓓ
48. Ⓐ Ⓑ Ⓒ Ⓓ
49. Ⓐ Ⓑ Ⓒ Ⓓ
50. Ⓐ Ⓑ Ⓒ Ⓓ

SECTION 2

Anesthesia
51. Ⓐ Ⓑ Ⓒ Ⓓ
52. Ⓐ Ⓑ Ⓒ Ⓓ
53. Ⓐ Ⓑ Ⓒ Ⓓ
54. Ⓐ Ⓑ Ⓒ Ⓓ
55. Ⓐ Ⓑ Ⓒ Ⓓ
56. Ⓐ Ⓑ Ⓒ Ⓓ
57. Ⓐ Ⓑ Ⓒ Ⓓ
58. Ⓐ Ⓑ Ⓒ Ⓓ
59. Ⓐ Ⓑ Ⓒ Ⓓ
60. Ⓐ Ⓑ Ⓒ Ⓓ

10,000
61. Ⓐ Ⓑ Ⓒ Ⓓ
62. Ⓐ Ⓑ Ⓒ Ⓓ
63. Ⓐ Ⓑ Ⓒ Ⓓ
64. Ⓐ Ⓑ Ⓒ Ⓓ
65. Ⓐ Ⓑ Ⓒ Ⓓ
66. Ⓐ Ⓑ Ⓒ Ⓓ
67. Ⓐ Ⓑ Ⓒ Ⓓ
68. Ⓐ Ⓑ Ⓒ Ⓓ
69. Ⓐ Ⓑ Ⓒ Ⓓ
70. Ⓐ Ⓑ Ⓒ Ⓓ

20,000
71. Ⓐ Ⓑ Ⓒ Ⓓ
72. Ⓐ Ⓑ Ⓒ Ⓓ
73. Ⓐ Ⓑ Ⓒ Ⓓ
74. Ⓐ Ⓑ Ⓒ Ⓓ
75. Ⓐ Ⓑ Ⓒ Ⓓ
76. Ⓐ Ⓑ Ⓒ Ⓓ
77. Ⓐ Ⓑ Ⓒ Ⓓ
78. Ⓐ Ⓑ Ⓒ Ⓓ
79. Ⓐ Ⓑ Ⓒ Ⓓ
80. Ⓐ Ⓑ Ⓒ Ⓓ

30,000
81. Ⓐ Ⓑ Ⓒ Ⓓ
82. Ⓐ Ⓑ Ⓒ Ⓓ
83. Ⓐ Ⓑ Ⓒ Ⓓ
84. Ⓐ Ⓑ Ⓒ Ⓓ
85. Ⓐ Ⓑ Ⓒ Ⓓ
86. Ⓐ Ⓑ Ⓒ Ⓓ
87. Ⓐ Ⓑ Ⓒ Ⓓ
88. Ⓐ Ⓑ Ⓒ Ⓓ
89. Ⓐ Ⓑ Ⓒ Ⓓ
90. Ⓐ Ⓑ Ⓒ Ⓓ

40,000
91. Ⓐ Ⓑ Ⓒ Ⓓ
92. Ⓐ Ⓑ Ⓒ Ⓓ
93. Ⓐ Ⓑ Ⓒ Ⓓ
94. Ⓐ Ⓑ Ⓒ Ⓓ
95. Ⓐ Ⓑ Ⓒ Ⓓ
96. Ⓐ Ⓑ Ⓒ Ⓓ
97. Ⓐ Ⓑ Ⓒ Ⓓ
98. Ⓐ Ⓑ Ⓒ Ⓓ
99. Ⓐ Ⓑ Ⓒ Ⓓ
100. Ⓐ Ⓑ Ⓒ Ⓓ

SECTION 3

50,000
101. Ⓐ Ⓑ Ⓒ Ⓓ
102. Ⓐ Ⓑ Ⓒ Ⓓ
103. Ⓐ Ⓑ Ⓒ Ⓓ
104. Ⓐ Ⓑ Ⓒ Ⓓ
105. Ⓐ Ⓑ Ⓒ Ⓓ
106. Ⓐ Ⓑ Ⓒ Ⓓ
107. Ⓐ Ⓑ Ⓒ Ⓓ
108. Ⓐ Ⓑ Ⓒ Ⓓ
109. Ⓐ Ⓑ Ⓒ Ⓓ
110. Ⓐ Ⓑ Ⓒ Ⓓ

60,000
111. Ⓐ Ⓑ Ⓒ Ⓓ
112. Ⓐ Ⓑ Ⓒ Ⓓ
113. Ⓐ Ⓑ Ⓒ Ⓓ
114. Ⓐ Ⓑ Ⓒ Ⓓ
115. Ⓐ Ⓑ Ⓒ Ⓓ
116. Ⓐ Ⓑ Ⓒ Ⓓ
117. Ⓐ Ⓑ Ⓒ Ⓓ
118. Ⓐ Ⓑ Ⓒ Ⓓ
119. Ⓐ Ⓑ Ⓒ Ⓓ
120. Ⓐ Ⓑ Ⓒ Ⓓ

70,000
121. Ⓐ Ⓑ Ⓒ Ⓓ
122. Ⓐ Ⓑ Ⓒ Ⓓ
123. Ⓐ Ⓑ Ⓒ Ⓓ
124. Ⓐ Ⓑ Ⓒ Ⓓ
125. Ⓐ Ⓑ Ⓒ Ⓓ
126. Ⓐ Ⓑ Ⓒ Ⓓ
127. Ⓐ Ⓑ Ⓒ Ⓓ
128. Ⓐ Ⓑ Ⓒ Ⓓ
129. Ⓐ Ⓑ Ⓒ Ⓓ
130. Ⓐ Ⓑ Ⓒ Ⓓ

80,000
131. Ⓐ Ⓑ Ⓒ Ⓓ
132. Ⓐ Ⓑ Ⓒ Ⓓ
133. Ⓐ Ⓑ Ⓒ Ⓓ
134. Ⓐ Ⓑ Ⓒ Ⓓ
135. Ⓐ Ⓑ Ⓒ Ⓓ
136. Ⓐ Ⓑ Ⓒ Ⓓ
137. Ⓐ Ⓑ Ⓒ Ⓓ
138. Ⓐ Ⓑ Ⓒ Ⓓ
139. Ⓐ Ⓑ Ⓒ Ⓓ
140. Ⓐ Ⓑ Ⓒ Ⓓ

90,000
141. Ⓐ Ⓑ Ⓒ Ⓓ
142. Ⓐ Ⓑ Ⓒ Ⓓ
143. Ⓐ Ⓑ Ⓒ Ⓓ
144. Ⓐ Ⓑ Ⓒ Ⓓ
145. Ⓐ Ⓑ Ⓒ Ⓓ
146. Ⓐ Ⓑ Ⓒ Ⓓ
147. Ⓐ Ⓑ Ⓒ Ⓓ
148. Ⓐ Ⓑ Ⓒ Ⓓ
149. Ⓐ Ⓑ Ⓒ Ⓓ
150. Ⓐ Ⓑ Ⓒ Ⓓ

FINAL EXAMINATION

SECTION 1

Questions 1-50

Medical Terminology

1. The cup-shaped depression on the hip joint that receives the head of the femur is the:
   A. acetabulum
   B. calcaneus
   C. trochlea
   D. medial malleolus

2. The lower third of the small intestine is the:
   A. jejunum
   B. tenue
   C. ileum
   D. duodenum

3. This term means to divert or make an artificial passage:
   A. burr
   B. occipital
   C. shunt
   D. catheter

4. This term means to identify the presence of and the amount of:
   A. qualitative
   B. definitive
   C. authoritative
   D. quantitative

5. The term that means the expansion of:
   A. dilation
   B. curettage
   C. tocolysis
   D. manipulation

6. This term means the outermost covering of the eyeball:
   A. sclerae
   B. lacrimal
   C. ciliary
   D. chorea

7. This term means the soft tissue around the nail border:
   A. sebaceous
   B. dermis
   C. lunula
   D. perionychium

8. This term means to turn downward:
   A. flexion
   B. adduction
   C. circumduction
   D. pronation

9. This combining form means artery:
   A. angi/o
   B. aort/o
   C. arteri/o
   D. atri/o

10. This abbreviation means that the neonate has a lower than normal weight:
    A. VLBW
    B. LNBW
    C. BWLN
    D. LBWV

Anatomy

11. This gland is located at the base of the brain in a depression in the skull:
    A. thymus
    B. hypothalamus
    C. pituitary
    D. pineal

12. Which of the following is not a part of the kidney?
    A. cortex
    B. trigone
    C. medulla
    D. pyramids

13. Which of the following is NOT a lymph organ?
    A. spleen
    B. bone marrow
    C. tonsils
    D. adrenal

14. This is nature's pacemaker:
    A. atrioventricular node
    B. bundle of His
    C. septum
    D. sinoatrial node

15. This is divided into the medulla oblongata, pons, and midbrain:
    A. brainstem
    B. diencephalon
    C. cerebellum
    D. cerebrum

16. This is located in the middle ear:
    A. vestibule
    B. cochlea
    C. auricle
    D. stapes

17. This is located in the pharynx and contains the adenoids:
    A. oropharynx
    B. laryngopharynx
    C. nasopharynx
    D. sphenoidal

18. This is another name for the bulbourethral gland:
    A. tunica albuginea
    B. seminal vesicles
    C. prostate
    D. Cowper's

19. The approximate number of days of gestation of the fetus:
    A. 240
    B. 255
    C. 266
    D. 277

20. This is the makeup of the liquid part of the blood (plasma):
    A. 90% water, 2% protein, 8% other
    B. 95% water, 3% protein, 2% other
    C. 91% water, 1% protein, 2% other
    D. 88% water, 5% protein, 6% other

ICD-9-CM

21. A patient is diagnosed with bilateral otitis media:
    A. 382.9
    B. 382.4
    C. 381.6
    D. 382.02

22. A patient is diagnosed with bacterial endocarditis due to AIDS:
    A. 421.0, 042
    B. 042, 421.9
    C. 421.1, 042
    D. 042, 421.0

23. HOLTER REPORT

    LOCATION: Outpatient, Clinic

    INDICATION: Patient with atrial fibrillation on Lanoxin. Patient with known cardiomyopathy

    BASELINE DATA: An 86-year-old man with congestive heart failure on Elavil, Vasotec, Lanoxin, and Lasix. The patient was monitored for the 24 hours in which the analysis was performed.

    INTERPRETATION:

    1. The predominant rhythm is atrial fibrillation. The average ventricular rate is 74 beats per minute, minimum 49 beats per minute, and maximum 114 beats per minute.

    2. A total of 4,948 ventricular ectopic beats were detected. There were four forms. There were 146 couplets with one triplet and five runs of bigeminy. There were two runs of ventricular tachycardia, the longest for 5 beats at a rate of 150 beats per minute. There was no ventricular fibrillation.

    3. There were no prolonged pauses.

CONCLUSION:

1. Predominant rhythm is atrial fibrillation with well-controlled ventricular rate.

2. There are no prolonged pauses.

3. Asymptomatic, nonsustained, ventricular tachycardia.

A. 427.3, 425.4
B. 425.4, 427.3
C. 427.31, 425.4
D. 427.32, 425.4

24. A 51-year-old male patient had surgery to remove two separate carbuncles of the left axilla. Pathology report indicated staphylococcal infection.
    A. 680.3, 041.10
    B. 680.9, 041.09
    C. 680.3, 041.19
    D. 680.9, 041.09

25. The discharge diagnoses for a patient who was admitted for dyspnea were as follows: pneumonia, *Klebsiella pneumoniae,* COPD with emphysema, multifocal atrial tachycardia, middle dementia.
    A. 482, 492.8, 427.5, 294.8
    B. 486, 492.8, 427.89, 294.8
    C. 486, 492.0, 427.89, 294.11
    D. 482.0, 492.8, 427.89, 294.8

26. A patient with spinal stenosis of cervical disk C4-5 and C5-6 with intervertebral disk displacement had a cervical diskectomy, corpectomy, allograft from C4 to C6, and placement of arthrodesis (a 34-mm plate from C4 to C6)
    A. 722.90
    B. 723.0, 722.1
    C. 723.0, 722.0
    D. 723.1, 722.51

27. A patient presents for an influenza vaccination and pneumococcal vaccination.
    A. V04.8, V03.89
    B. V04.7, V03.82
    C. V04.81, V03.82
    D. V04.7, V03.2

28. A patient with a family history of malignant neoplasm of the breast receives a screening mammography, bilaterally (76092).
    A. V76.11
    B. V76.11, V16.3
    C. V16.3
    D. V10.3, V76.11

29. A patient with unstable angina, hypertension, diabetes with hypoglycemia, and a history of myocardial infarction is admitted for cardiac catheterization.
    A. 413.9, 401.9, 250.80, 412
    B. 411.1, 401.9, 250.80, 412
    C. 411.1, 401.1, 250.80, 412
    D. 411.1, 401.9, 250.00, 410.9

30. A 4-year-old patient is seen by the physician in the outpatient clinic setting for chronic lymphoid leukemia that is currently in remission.
   A. 204.11
   B. 204.21
   C. 203.11
   D. 204.81

HCPCS

31. All third-party payers require the use of HCPCS codes when submitting for service provided to any patient.
   A. True
   B. False

32. A 62-year-old male Medicare patient presents for a digital rectal examination and a total prostate-specific antigen test (PSA).
   A. G0102
   B. G0103
   C. G0102, G0107
   D. G0102, G0103

33. An 82-year-old female Medicare patient has a single-energy x-ray absorptiometry (SEXA) bone density study of two sites of the wrist.
   A. 76071
   B. 76075
   C. G0130
   D. 76070

34. A 72-year-old male Medicare patient receives 30 minutes of individual diabetes outpatient self-management training session.
   A. G0109
   B. G0176
   C. 99213
   D. G0108

35. A Medicare patient presents for an influenza vaccination and pneumococcal vaccination.
   A. G0008
   B. G0009
   C. G0008, G0009
   D. G0010, G0008

Concepts of Coding

36. The term OIG stands for the Office of the:
   A. Information Group
   B. Insurance Group
   C. Inspector General
   D. Insurance General

37. This part of Medicare is the non-hospital portion:
   A. Part A
   B. Part B
   C. Part C
   D. Part D

38. This is the group to which the CMS delegates the daily operation of the Medicare and Medicare programs:
    A. FI
    B. OG
    C. PRO
    D. HEW

39. This physician receives reimbursements for Medicare directly from the fiscal intermediary:
    A. PIB
    B. PRA
    C. PAR
    D. PEER

40. Which of the following is NOT true about the Outpatient Prospective Payment System?
    A. Known as the APC
    B. Was implemented in 2000
    C. Payment rates for each APC are published in the *Federal Register*
    D. Is applicable to non-Medicare and Medicare patients

Evaluation and Management

41. A second opinion is requested by a 90-year-old patient whose ophthalmologist recently diagnosed the patient with bilateral senile cataracts. Her regular ophthalmologist has recommended surgical removal of the cataracts and implantation of lens. The patient presents to the clinic stating that she is concerned about the necessity of the procedure at this time. During the detailed history, the patient states that she has had decreasing vision over the last year or two, but has always had excellent vision. She cannot recall any eye trauma in the past. The physician conducted a detailed visual examination and confirmed the diagnosis of the patient's ophthalmologist. The medical decision making was of low complexity.
    A. 99263
    B. 92002
    C. 99243
    D. 99273

42. The attending physician requests a confirmatory consultation from an interventional radiologist for a second opinion about a 63-year-old male with abnormal areas within the liver. The recommendation for a CT-guided biopsy is requested, which the attending has recommended be performed. During the comprehensive history, the patient reported right upper-quadrant pain. His liver enzymes were elevated. Previous CT study revealed multiple low attenuation areas within the liver (infection versus tumor). The laboratory studies were creatine, 0.9; hemoglobin, 9.5; PT and PTT, 13.0/31.5 with an INR of 1.2. The comprehensive physical examination showed that the lungs were clear to auscultation and the heart had regular rate and rhythm. The mental status was oriented times three. Temperature, intermittent low-grade fever, up to 101°F, usually occurred at night. The CT-guided biopsy was considered appropriate for this patient. The medical decision making was of high complexity.
    A. 99245
    B. 99255
    C. 99275
    D. 99274

43. A cardiology consultation is requested for a 71-year-old inpatient for recent onset of dyspnea on exertion and chest pain. The comprehensive history reveals that the patient cannot walk three blocks without exhibiting retrosternal squeezing sensation with shortness of breath. She relates that she had the first episode 3 months ago, which she attributed to indigestion. Her medical history is negative for stroke, tuberculosis, cancer, or rheumatic fever but includes seborrheic keratosis and benign positional vertigo. She has no known allergies. A comprehensive physical examination reveals a pleasant, elderly female in no apparent distress. She has a blood pressure of 150/70 with a heart rate of 76. Weight is 131 pounds, and she is 5 foot 4 inches. Head and neck reveal JBP less than 5 cm. Normal carotid volume and upstroke without bruit. Chest examination shows clear to auscultation with no rales, crackles, crepitations, or wheezing. Cardiovascular examination reveals a normal PMI without RV lift. Normal S1 and S2 with an S3, without murmur, are noted. The medical decision making complexity is high based on the various diagnosis options.
    A. 99275
    B. 99245
    C. 99255
    D. 99274

44. A new patient presents to the emergency department with an ankle sprain received when he fell while roller blading. The patient is in apparent pain, and the ankle has begun to swell. He is unable to flex the ankle. The patient reports that he did strike his head on the sidewalk as a result of the fall. The physician completes an expanded problem-focused history and examination. The medical decision making complexity is low.
    A. 99232
    B. 99282
    C. 99202
    D. 99284

45. A 89-year-old female patient is admitted to the skilled nursing facility after being seen in the office earlier today. The daughter brought the patient to the office. As a part of the detailed history, conducted with the patient's daughter, it is found that the patient was diagnosed with dementia last year. The patient was moved to this city from Anytown so that the daughter could care for her mother. The patient is noncontributory, and the physician relies on medical record documentation brought in by the daughter from her mother's previous physician. Of late, the patient has become more and more withdrawn and noncommunicative. She has wandered away from the daughter's home twice in the last week and on the last occasion was found walking on the street. After a comprehensive examination, it was decided that the patient would be admitted to the nursing facility today. The physician spent 45 minutes with the patient and in preparation of the medical documentation for admittance to the nursing facility. The level of medical decision making was of high complexity.
    A. 99313
    B. 99323
    C. 99302
    D. 99301

46. The physician provides a service to a new patient in a custodial care center. The patient is a paraplegic who has pneumonia of moderate severity. The physician performed an expanded problem-focused history and examination. The examination focused on the respiratory and cardiovascular systems, based on the patient's current complaint and past history of tachycardia. The medical decision making was of moderate complexity.
    A. 99332
    B. 99322
    C. 99342
    D. 99312

47. A 66-year-old male presents for a complete physical. There are no new complaints since my previous examination on 06/09 of last year. The patient spends 6 hours a week golfing and reports a brisk and active retirement. He does not smoke and has only an occasional glass of wine. He sleeps well but has been having nocturia times three. On physical examination, the patient is a well-developed, well-nourished male. The physician continues and provides a complete examination of the patient lasting 45 minutes.
    A. 99387
    B. 99403
    C. 99450
    D. 99397

48. A new patient is seen in the office with complains of a fever, chills, and difficulty breathing. The patient states that he has not been well for several weeks now and has progressively gotten weaker. He has not been able to work for the past week and before that was frequently absent from work over the course of 2 weeks. He is uncertain how long fever has been present but believes that it has been approximately 4 days. He does not have a thermometer at home and does not know what his temperature has been. He has been sleeping in a living room recliner because when he lies down, he has increased difficulty breathing. The detailed history and examination centered around the respiratory and cardiovascular systems. The upper respiratory findings included conjunctival injection, nasal discharge, and pharyngeal erythema. A rapid test pack was used to diagnosis the viral infection. Chest x-ray showed patchy bilateral infiltrates. The physician diagnosed the patient with influenza A. The medical decision making complexity was low.
    A. 99203
    B. 99213
    C. 99205
    D. 99215

49. A new patient is admitted to the observation unit of the local hospital after a 10-foot fall from a ladder. The patient struck his head on the side of the garage as he fell into a hedge that somewhat broke his fall. He has significant bruising on the left side of his body and complains of a 5/10 pain under his left arm. A series of x-rays have been ordered in addition to an MRI. The physician completed a comprehensive history and physical examination. It was decided to admit the patient to observation based on some evidence that he may have hit the left side of his head during the fall. The medical decision making is moderately complex.
    A. 99222
    B. 99219
    C. 99235
    D. 99220

50. An established patient is admitted to the hospital by his attending physician after a car accident in which the patient hit the steering wheel of the automobile with significant enough force to fold the wheel backwards. The patient complains of significant pain in the right shoulder. After a detailed history and physical examination, the physician believed the patient may have sustained a right rotator cuff injury. The medical decision was straightforward in complexity.
   A. 99283
   B. 99263
   C. 99221
   D. 99253

SECTION 2

Questions 51-100

Anesthesia

51. If the anesthesia service was provided to a patient who had mild systemic disease, what would the physical status modifier be?
   A. P1
   B. P2
   C. P3
   D. P4

52. The qualifying circumstances code indicates a 72-year-old female:
   A. 99100
   B. 99116
   C. 99135
   D. 99140

53. This type of sedation decreases the level of the patient's alertness but allows the patient to cooperate during the procedure:
   A. topical
   B. local
   C. regional
   D. conscious

54. The national unit values for anesthesia services are listed in this publication:
   A. BVR by AS
   B. RVG by ASA
   C. ASA by RVG
   D. RVP by ASA

55. When reporting anesthesia services performed for two procedures performed on the same patient during the same operative procedure, you would do the following to calculate the unit value of the services:
   A. Add the units of the two procedures together.
   B. Subtract the procedure with the lowest unit value from the procedure with the highest unit value.
   C. Report only the units for the lowest unit value procedure.
   D. Report only the units for the highest unit value procedure.

56. Anesthesia provided for an anterior cervical diskectomy with decompression of a single interspace of the spinal cord and nerve roots and including osteophytectomy (63075).
    A. 00620
    B. 00630
    C. 00600
    D. 00640

57. A 16-year-old female patient has a left thyroid mass, which is removed by total thyroidectomy. The anesthesia service would be reported with the following:
    A. 00320
    B. 00322
    C. 00326
    D. 00300

58. General anesthesia for a limited ophthalmological examination and evaluation with the manipulation of the globe for range of motion (92019) using an ophthalmoscope:
    A. 00145
    B. 00140
    C. 00148
    D. 00147

59. The following indicates anesthesia for a procedure on the lower posterior abdominal wall for a patient with severe hypertension:
    A. 00820-P3
    B. 00820-P2
    C. 00800-P3
    D. 00800-P2

60. What combination of CPT code and modifier would you use to report anesthesia services for a patient who is 87 years of age and is not expected to survive without the surgical procedure being performed and for which anesthesia is being provided?
    A. 99116, P4
    B. 99100, P4
    C. 99100, P5
    D. 99140, P6

Integumentary

61. A 24-year-old female is seen in the office for a single subcutaneous cyst that needs to be incised and drained:
    A. 10061
    B. 10080
    C. 10060
    D. 11400

62. A 10-year-old boy presents for injuries caused by falling off his bike. All wounds were superficial. He has a 2-cm wound to his nose and a 1-cm wound to his cheek. He also has a 2.5-cm wound to his elbow. All injuries were simple repair by means of suture.
    A. 12011, 12001
    B. 12013, 12001
    C. 12013, 12002
    D. 12011, 12002

63. Dr. Smith performed a bilateral radical mastectomy, including the pectoral muscles and axillary lymph nodes, on a 63-year-old female with breast cancer:
   A. 19200, 174.9
   B. 19220-50, 174.9
   C. 19200-50, 174.9
   D. 19240-50, 174.9

64. What code(s) would you use to report chemosurgery, Mohs' micrographic technique, with six specimens of fresh tissue, first stage?
   A. 17304-51
   B. 17310-51
   C. 17304, 17307
   D. 17304, 17310

65. A 40-year-old male is in for layered closure of wounds due to a motor vehicle accident. The patient sustained injuries to the forehead, 1.5 cm, and a 1-cm wound to the eyebrow when his head hit the steering wheel. Code the service code only.
   A. 12011
   B. 12051
   C. 13131
   D. 12001

66. Which code would the surgeon use to report the shaving of an epidermal lesion of the arm when a lesion diameter is greater than 2.0 cm?
   A. 11402
   B. 11200
   C. 11303
   D. 11602

67. A 73-year-old male is admitted by Dr. Smith for an excision of a nail and nail matrix, complete, for permanent removal with amputation of a tuft of distal phalanx. A 2.0-cm single pinch skin graft was needed to cover the tip of the digit.
   A. 11752
   B. 11750
   C. 11750, 15050
   D. 11752, 15050

68. What code would you use for an initial large debridement of both arms resulting from burns, without general anesthesia?
   A. 16010
   B. 16025
   C. 16030-50
   D. 16030

69. Donna, a 41-year-old female, presents for biopsies of both breasts. Dr. Smith will be doing the biopsies using fine-needle aspiration with imaging guidance:
   A. 19102-50
   B. 10022-50
   C. 10021
   D. 19103-50

70. Katie is seen in the clinic by Dr. Smith for several scars on her face caused by acne. Dr. Smith decides to do an epidermal chemical peel of the face.
    A. 15780
    B. 15781
    C. 15789
    D. 15788

Musculoskeletal System

71. Richard, a 34-year-old male, fell from a 4-foot scaffolding and hit his heel on the bottom rung of the support, fracturing his calcaneus in several locations. The orthopedic surgeon manipulated the bone pieces back into position and secured the fracture sites by means of percutaneous fixation.
    A. 28415
    B. 28405
    C. 28406
    D. 28456

72. Sammy, a 5-year-old male, tumbled down the stairs at daycare, striking and fracturing his coccygeal bone. The physician manually manipulated the bone into proper alignment and told Sammy's mother to have the child sit on a rubber ring to alleviate the pain.
    A. 27510
    B. 28445
    C. 27202
    D. 27200

73. Alice, a 42-year-old female, is a carpenter at the local college. While on a ladder repairing a window frame, the weld on the rung of the metal ladder loosened, and she fell backwards a distance of 8 feet. She landed on her left hip, resulting in a dislocation. With the patient under general anesthesia, the Allis maneuver is used to repair an anterior dislocation of the right hip. The pelvis is stabilized and pressure applied to the thigh to reduce the hip and bring it into proper alignment.
    A. 27250
    B. 27252
    C. 27253
    D. 27254

74. A 13-year-old female sustained multiple tibial tuberosity fractures of the left knee while playing soccer at her local track meet. The physician extended the left leg and manipulated several fragments back into place. The knee was then aspirated. A long-leg knee brace was then placed on the knee.
    A. 27334
    B. 27550
    C. 27538
    D. 27330

75. Under general anesthesia, 5-year-old Michael's tarsal dislocation was reduced by means of manipulation. Two-view intraoperative x-rays demonstrated that the tarsus was in correct alignment, and a short leg cast was then applied. Code only the reduction service.
    A. 28545, 29405
    B. 28545, 29405, 73620
    C. 28540, 73620
    D. 28545

76. Dr. Clark applied a cranial halo to Gordon to stabilize the cervical spine in preparation for x-rays and subsequent surgery. The scalp was sterilized and local anesthesia injected over the pin insertion sites. Posterior and anterior cranial pins are inserted and the halo device attached.
    A. 20664
    B. 20661, 90782
    C. 20661
    D. 20664, 90782

77. Samantha was playing in the back yard when her brother fired a pellet gun at her leg at close range. The pellet penetrated the skin and lodged in the muscle underlying the area. The physician removed the pellet without complication or incident.
    A. 20520
    B. 20525
    C. 10120
    D. 10121

78. Kevin comes in with a deep hematoma on his shoulder that he has had for some time. After an exam was performed of the shoulder area, the physician decides that the hematoma needs to be incised and drained.
    A. 23030
    B. 10140
    C. 10060
    D. 10160

79. Marsha is admitted to same-day surgery after having an abnormal shoulder x-ray in the clinic yesterday. The physician decides to do a diagnostic arthroscopy.
    A. 29806
    B. 29805
    C. 23066
    D. 23100

80. Cole comes into the orthopedic department today with his mother after falling from the top bunk bed where he and his brother were wrestling. Cole is having pain in his left lower leg and is unable to bear weight on it. Cole was taken to the x-ray department. After the physician talked with the radiologist regarding the diagnosis of sprained ankle, the physician decides to apply a walking short leg cast from just below his knee to his toes.
    A. 29405, 845.00, E884.4
    B. 29515, 845.00, E888.9
    C. 29355, 959.7, E884.4
    D. 29425, 845.00, E884.4

10,000 Respiratory System, Cardiovascular System, Mediastinum, and Diaphragm

81. PREOPERATIVE DIAGNOSIS: Deviated septum

    PROCEDURE PERFORMED:

    1. Septoplasty

    2. Resection of turbinates

    The patient was taken to the operating room and placed under general anesthesia. The fracture of the turbinates was first performed to do the septoplasty. Once this was done, the septoplasty was completed and the turbinates were placed back in their

original position. The patient was taken to recovery in satisfactory condition. Code the procedure(s) and the diagnosis:
A. 30520, 30130, 470
B. 30520, 30130-51, 470
C. 30520, 30140-51, 478.1
D. 30520, 30140-52, 470

82. The patient is seen in the clinic for chronic sinusitis. The physician decides to schedule an endoscopic sinus surgery for the next day. The patient arrives to same-day surgery, and the physician performs an endoscopic ethmoidectomy total with an endoscopic maxillary antrostomy with removal of maxillary tissue. Code the procedure(s) and diagnosis.
A. 31254, 31256-51, 473.9
B. 31255, 31267-51, 461.9
C. 31255, 31267-51, 473.9
D. 31200, 31225-51, 473.9

83. Faye, an 88-year-old female, is taken to same-day surgery for a possible small chicken bone stuck in her larynx. The physician does a direct laryngoscopy to check the larynx. On inspection, a small bone fragment is seen obstructing the larynx. The physician using an operating microscope removes the bone fragment. The patient is sent home in satisfactory condition.
A. 31526, 933.1, E915
B. 31531, 933.1, E912
C. 31530, 935.0, E912
D. 31511, 933.1, E912

84. OPERATIVE REPORT

PREOPERATIVE DIAGNOSIS: Ventilator dependency, aspiration pneumonia

PROCEDURE PERFORMED: Tracheostomy

DESCRIPTION OF PROCEDURE: After consent was obtained, the patient was taken to the operating room and placed on the operating room table in the supine position. After an adequate level of general endotracheal anesthesia was obtained, the patient was positioned for tracheostomy. The patient's neck was prepped with Betadine and then draped in a sterile manner. A curvilinear incision was marked approximately a finger breadth above the sternal notch in any area just below the cricoid cartilage. This area was then infiltrated with 1% Xylocaine with 1:100,000 units of epinephrine. After several minutes, sharp dissection was carried down through the skin and subcutaneous tissue. The subcutaneous fat was removed down to the strap muscles. Strap muscles were divided in the midline and retracted laterally. The cricoid cartilage was then identified. The thyroid gland was divided in the midline with the Bovie, and then the two lobes were retracted laterally, exposing the anterior wall of the trachea. The space between the second and third tracheal rings was then identified. This was infiltrated with local solution. A cut was then made through the anterior wall. The endotracheal tube was then advanced superiorly. An inferior cut into the third tracheal ring was then done to make a flap. This was secured to the skin with 4-0 Vicryl suture. A no. 6 Shiley cuffed tracheotomy tube was then placed and secured to the skin with ties as well as the tracheostomy strap. The patient tolerated the procedure well and was taken to the critical care unit in stable condition. Report the procedure(s) and diagnosis:
A. 94656, 60220, 31600-51, 507.0
B. 31500, 31600-51
C. 31600, 507.0
D. 94656, 31502-51, 31600-51, 518.81, 507.0

85. Carl, a 58-year-old male, is taken to the operating room to remove his permanent pacemaker after successfully getting his heart back to normal sinus rhythm.
    A. 33236
    B. 33238
    C. 33243
    D. 33233

86. This 70-year-old male is admitted for coronary ASHD. A prior cardiac catheterization showed numerous native vessels to be 70% to 100% blocked. The patient was taken to the operating room. After opening the chest and separating the rib cage, a coronary artery bypass was performed using five venous grafts and four coronary arterial grafts. Code the graft procedure(s) and the diagnosis:
    A. 33536, 33517-51, 414.9
    B. 33533, 33522, 414.05
    C. 33536, 33522, 414.01
    D. 33514, 414

87. What code(s) would be used to report an arterial catheterization?
    A. 36600
    B. 36620, 36625
    C. 36620
    D. 36640

88. This patient is taken to the operating room for a ruptured spleen. Repair of the ruptured spleen with a partial splenectomy is done.
    A. 38101-58, 38115-51-58, 289.59
    B. 38115, 289.59
    C. 38120, 865.04
    D. 38129, 865.14

89. This 60-year-old female was seen previously for a laparoscopic biopsy of her cervical lymph nodes. The biopsy came back showing abnormal cells. The decision was made to do a lymphadenectomy. The patient was brought to the operating room and put under general anesthesia. After completing a radical neck dissection, the lymph nodes were excised. The patient was returned to recovery in satisfactory condition. Code the lymphadenectomy only.
    A. 38720, 38570-51
    B. 38720, 38500-51
    C. 38571
    D. 38724

90. Connie is brought to the operating room for a diaphragmatic hernia. Transthoracic repair will be done to fix the hernia.
    A. 39520
    B. 39503
    C. 39530
    D. 39540

40,000 Digestive System

91. OPERATIVE REPORT

    PROCEDURE: Excision of parotid tumor or gland or both

    Once the patient was successfully under general anesthetic, Dr. Green, assisted by Dr. Smith, opened the area in which the parotid gland is located. After carefully

inspecting the gland, the decision was made to excise the total gland because of the size of the tumor (5.0 cm). With careful dissection and preservation of the facial nerve, the parotid gland was removed. The wound was cleaned and closed, and the patient was brought to recovery in satisfactory condition. Report only Dr. Smith's service.
A. 42410-80, 11041, 142.0
B. 42426-62, 210.2
C. 42420-80, 239.0
D. 11426, 239.0

92. A 9-year-old boy is in for a tonsillectomy because of chronic tonsillitis and possible adenoidectomy. On inspection of the adenoids, they were found not to be inflamed; then we did a tonsillectomy only. Code the tonsillectomy only:
A. 42820, 474.10
B. 42825, 474.00
C. 42830, 42825-51, 474.10
D. 42826, 42835-51, 474.02

93. What code would you use to report a rigid proctosigmoidoscopy with guide wire?
A. 52260
B. 45386
C. 45339
D. 45303

94. A 62-year-old female presents to Acute Surgical Care for a sigmoidoscopy. The physician inserts a flexible scope into the patient's rectum and determines the rectum is clear of any polyps. The scope is advanced to the sigmoid colon, and a total of three polyps are found. Using the snare technique, the polyps are removed. The remainder of the colon is free of polyps. The flexible scope is withdrawn.
A. 45383, 211.3
B. 44110, 153.9
C. 45338, 211.3
D. 44111, 153.3

95. This patient is in for multiple external hemorrhoids. After inspection of the hemorrhoids, the physician decides to excise all the hemorrhoids.
A. 46250, 455.3
B. 46615, 455.0
C. 46255, 455.3
D. 46083, 455.5

96. OPERATIVE REPORT

PREOPERATIVE DIAGNOSIS: Barrett's esophagus with severe dysplasia, possible carcinoma

POSTOPERATIVE DIAGNOSIS: Same

PROCEDURE PERFORMED: Exploratory laparotomy, biopsy of liver lesion, immobilization of stomach with pyloroplasty and placement of feeding tube

OPERATIVE NOTE: With the patient under general anesthesia, the abdomen was prepped and draped in a sterile manner. Midline incision was made from the xiphoid to below the pubis. Sharp dissection was carried down into the peritoneal cavity, and hemostasis was maintained with electrocautery. We began by exploring the abdominal cavity. The liver was carefully palpated. The area that had been identified on CT was at the very apex of the right lobe of the liver. We could feel this area, and it did not have a thickened feel to it but was more consistent with an area of hemangioma.

There was a small secondary lesion on the undersurface of the right lobe. A biopsy was taken, and it did return a diagnosis of hemangioma. The rest of the liver appeared normal, and in my opinion we did not need to proceed with anything further. We thus began with mobilization of the stomach, taking down the greater curvature vessels, preserving the gastroepiploica. We carried our dissection all the way up into the hiatal hernia, preserving the blood supply to the spleen and not injuring it. We were then able to detach the left gastric artery such that the stomach was tethered on its other vasculature but appeared completely viable. All these vessels were taken down with clamps and ligatures of 2-0 silk. We then circumferentially went around the esophagus and carried our dissection all the back toward the pylorus. We then had the entire stomach freed up from the pylorus all the way up to the diaphragm. The stomach appeared viable with reasonable circulation. A Heineke-Mikulicz pyloroplasty then was performed to open the pylorus in one direction and close it in another using interrupted 3-0 silk sutures to complete the pyloroplasty. With this accomplished, we then picked up the jejunum approximated 40 or 50 cm beyond the ligament of Treitz and placed a red rubber feeding tube using a Witzel technique; this was a number 18-2. This was attached to the skin and brought out through a separate stab incision. The abdominal cavity was then checked for hemostasis, and everything appeared to be intact. We then closed the incision using running 0 loop nylon. We closed the skin with staples. A sterile dressing was applied. Code the biopsy of the liver lesion and pyloroplasty only.
A. 49000, 43830-51, 47000-51, 228.00, 150.9
B. 43800, 47001-51, 150.9
C. 43800, 47001
D. 43800, 47001-51

97. OPERATIVE REPORT

PREOPERATIVE DIAGNOSIS: Upper gastrointestinal bleeding

POSTOPERATIVE DIAGNOSIS: Multiple serpiginous ulcers in the gastric antrum and body, not bleeding

FINDINGS: The video therapeutic double-channel endoscope was passed without difficulty into the oropharynx. The gastroesophageal junction was seen at 42 cm. Inspection of the esophagus revealed no erythema, ulceration, exudates, stricture, or other mucosal abnormalities. The stomach proper was entered. The endoscope was advanced to the second duodenum. Inspection of the second duodenum, first duodenum, duodenal bulb, and pylorus revealed no abnormalities. Retroflexion revealed no lesion along the cardia or lesser curvature. Inspection of the antrum, body, and fundus of the stomach revealed no abnormality except there were multiple serpiginous ulcerations in the gastric antrum and body. They were not bleeding. They had no recent stigmata of bleeding. Photographs and biopsies were obtained. The patient tolerated the procedure well.
A. 43258, 531.9
B. 43234, 531.30
C. 43239, 531.90
D. 43239, 532.9

98. How would you code an excision of a ruptured appendix with generalized peritonitis?
    A. 44970
    B. 44950
    C. 44960
    D. 44960-22

99. Kevin is admitted to same-day surgery today for a laparoscopic cholecystectomy.
    A. 47600
    B. 47562, 47550
    C. 47560
    D. 47562

100. INDICATION: Sean is a 2-year-old boy who was born with a cleft lip.

    PROCEDURE: This 2-year-old male was taken to the operating room for plastic repair of a unilateral cleft lip.
    A. 40701-52, 749.10
    B. 40700, 749.10
    C. 30460, 749.20
    D. 40525, 749.20

SECTION 3

Questions 101-150

50,000

101. OPERATIVE REPORT

    DIAGNOSIS: Acute renal insufficiency

    PROCEDURE: Renal biopsy

    The patient was taken to the operating room for a percutaneous needle biopsy of the right and left kidneys.
    A. 49000-50
    B. 50555-50
    C. 50542-LT, 50542-RT
    D. 50200-50

102. What code(s) would you use to report a biopsy of the bladder?
    A. 52354
    B. 52204
    C. 52224
    D. 52250

103. OPERATIVE REPORT

    DIAGNOSIS: Large bladder neck obstruction

    PROCEDURE PERFORMED: Cystoscopy and transurethral resection of the prostate

    The patient is a 78-year-old male with obstructive symptoms and subsequent urinary retention. The patient underwent the usual spinal anesthetic, was put in the dorsolithotomy position, prepped, and draped in the usual fashion. Cystoscopic visualization showed a marked high-riding bladder. Median lobe enlargement was such that it was difficult even to get the cystoscope over. Inside the bladder, marked trabeculation was noted. No stones were present.

    The urethra was well lubricated and dilated. The resectoscopic sheath was passed with the aid of obturator with some difficulty because of the median lobe. TURP of the median lobe was performed, getting several big loops of tissue, which helped to improve visualization. Anterior resection of the roof was carried out from the bladder neck. Bladder-wall resection was taken from 10 to 8 o'clock. This eliminated the rest

of the median lobe tissue as well. The patient tolerated the procedure well. Code the procedure(s) performed and the diagnosis.
A. 52450, 52001-51, 596.0
B. 52450, 52001-51, 753.6
C. 52450, 52000-59, 596.0
D. 52450, 52000, 753.6

104. What code(s) would you use to code reconstruction of the penis for straightening of chordee?
A. 54435
B. 54328
C. 54360
D. 54300

105. Clamp circumcision of a newborn:
A. 54160
B. 54150
C. 54152
D. 54161

106. Jim is a 42-year-old male in for a bilateral vasectomy that will include three postoperative semen examinations:
A. 52347 × 3
B. 52648
C. 55250
D. 55250 × 3

107. Patient is seen for a Bartholin's gland abscess. The physician incised and drained the abscess.
A. 56420
B. 50600
C. 53060
D. 56405

108. This 21-year-old female is seen at the clinic today for a colposcopy. The physician will take multiple biopsies of the cervix.
A. 56821
B. 57421
C. 57455
D. 57456

109. Sarah is a 37-year-old female diagnosed with an ectopic pregnancy. The patient was taken to the operating room for treatment of a tubal ectopic pregnancy, abdominal approach.
A. 59130
B. 59150
C. 59120
D. 59121

110. What code(s) do you use to report a cesarean delivery including the postpartum care?
A. 58611, 59430
B. 59400
C. 59515
D. 59622

60,000

111. OPERATIVE REPORT

    DIAGNOSIS: Malignant tumor, thyroid

    PROCEDURE: Thyroidectomy, total

    The patient was prepped and draped. The neck area was opened. With careful radical dissection of the neck completed, one could visualize the size of the tumor. The decision was made to do a total thyroidectomy. Note: The pathology report later indicated that the tumor was malignant.
    A. 60240, 193
    B. 60271, 193
    C. 60220, 164.0
    D. 60254, 193

112. What code(s) would you use to report burr hole(s) to drain an abscess of the brain?
    A. 61253
    B. 61150
    C. 61156
    D. 61151

113. This patient was brought to the operating room to repair an aneurysm of the intracranial artery by balloon catheter:
    A. 61698
    B. 61697
    C. 61710
    D. 61700

114. OPERATIVE REPORT

    PREOPERATIVE DIAGNOSIS: Obstructed ventriculoperitoneal shunt

    PROCEDURE PERFORMED: Revision of shunt. Replacement of ventricular valve and peritoneal end. Entire shunt replacement.

    PROCEDURE: Under general anesthesia, the patient's head, neck, and abdomen were prepped and draped in the usual manner. An incision was made over the previous site where the shunt had been inserted in the posterior right occipital area. This shunt was found to be nonfunctioning and was removed. The problem was that we could not get the ventricular catheter out without probably producing bleeding, so it was left inside. The peritoneal end of the shunt was then pulled out through the same incision. Having done this, I placed a new ventricular catheter into the ventricle. I then attached this to a medium pressure bulb valve and secured this with 3-0 silk to the subcutaneous tissue. We then went to the abdomen and made an incision below the previous site, and we were able to trocar the peritoneal end of the shunt by making a stab wound in the neck and then connecting it up to the shunt. This was then connected to the shunt. Pumping on the shunt, we got fluid coming out the other end. I then inserted this end of the shunt into the abdomen by dividing the rectus fascia, splitting the muscle, and dividing the peritoneum and placing the shunt into the abdomen. One 2-0 chromic suture was used around the peritoneum. The wound was then closed with 2-0 Vicryl, 2-0 plain in the subcutaneous tissue, and surgical staples on the skin. The stab wound on the neck was closed with surgical staples. The head wound was closed with 2-0 Vicryl on the galea and surgical staples on the skin. A dressing was applied. The patient was discharged to the recovery room.
    A. 63740, 996.2
    B. 62256, 996.59
    C. 62160, 996.2
    D. 62230, 996.2

115. OPERATIVE REPORT

DIAGNOSIS: Herniated disk

PROCEDURE: Hemilaminectomy L4-5 and L5-S1

The patient was taken to the operating room prepped and draped in the usual fashion. Once the lower back area was opened, after decompression of the nerve roots, the interspace at L4-5 disk was excised. Next the interspace at L5-S1 disk was excised. The patient tolerated the procedure well.
A. 63045, 63048, 722.2
B. 63040, 63043, 839.00
C. 63030, 63035, 722.10
D. 63040, 63043, 722.10

116. Delores, a 67-year-old female, is seen today for destruction of a lesion of her cornea. The lesion is removed by thermocauterization.
A. 65400
B. 65450
C. 65435
D. 65410

117. What code(s) would you use to code the removal of a foreign body embedded in the eyelid?
A. 67830
B. 67413
C. 67801
D. 67938

118. Kristie is a 14-year-old female with a diagnosis of chronic otitis media. The patient was taken to same-day surgery and placed under general anesthesia. Dr. White performed a bilateral tympanostomy with the insertion of ventilating tubes. The patient tolerated the procedure well.
A. 69421-50, 69433-51, 382.1
B. 69420-50, 382.4
C. 69436-50, 382.9
D. 69436-50, 382.02

119. Kristie, a 15-year-old female, is seen today for removal of bilateral ventilating tubes that Dr. White inserted 1 year ago.
A. 69205-50
B. 69424-79
C. 69424-50
D. 69424-50-78

120. What code would you use for a revision mastoidectomy resulting in a radical mastoidectomy?
A. 69502
B. 69511
C. 69602
D. 69603

70,000 Radiology

121. A 62-year-old male comes into the clinic complaining of shortness of breath. The physician orders a chest x-ray, frontal and lateral.
    A. 71015, 786.09
    B. 71020, 786.05
    C. 71035, 786.9
    D. 71020 × 2, 786.05

122. A patient is in for an MRI (magnetic resonance imaging) of the pelvis with contrast material(s):
    A. 72125
    B. 72198
    C. 72196
    D. 72159

123. What code(s) would you use for an endoscopic catheterization of the biliary ductal system for the professional radiology component only?
    A. 43271, 74328
    B. 74328-26
    C. 74300-26
    D. 74330-26

124. Jennifer is a 29-year-old pregnant female in for a follow-up ultrasound with image documentation of the uterus.
    A. 74740
    B. 76816
    C. 74710
    D. 76856

125. What codes would you use for complex brachytherapy isodose calculation for a patient with prostate cancer?
    A. 77776, 184
    B. 77300, 185
    C. 77327-22, 186
    D. 77328, 185

126. Therapeutic radiology treatment planning is the "prescription" for a patient who will start radiation therapy for a cancerous neoplasm of the adrenal gland. What code would you use for a complex treatment planning?
    A. 60540
    B. 77315
    C. 77263
    D. 77401

127. Because of the number of headaches this 50-year-old female had been experiencing, her physician ordered a CT of her head, without contrast materials.
    A. 70450
    B. 70460
    C. 70470
    D. 70496

128. A patient presents to the clinic for a barium enema that was ordered by his physician. Once the patient drinks the barium, the patient will be taken to radiology for a colon x-ray, including KUB.
   A. 74000
   B. 74241
   C. 74270
   D. 74247

129. Margie is a 62-year-old female in to see her primary physician with complaints of chest pain and shortness of breath. She has been experiencing these symptoms on and off for the last 2 months. Her primary physician refers Margie to a cardiologist to consult her about her symptoms.

   Dr. Tom, a cardiologist, consults Margie for chest pain and shortness of breath. He performs a comprehensive history and exam, the medical decision making of moderate complexity. Dr. Tom calls the hospital to set up a tomographic chemical stress test (myocardial perfusion imaging single study at rest). When the test is completed, he will interpret the results. Code the consult, the supervision and interpretation of the stress test, the diagnosis(s), and the radiologist's part of the stress test:
   A. 99244-57, 93016, 93018, 78464-26, 786.50, 786
   B. 99243, 78460, 786.50, 786.05
   C. 99244, 78461-76, 78480-26, 786, 786.05
   D. 99244-25, 93016, 93018, 78464-26, 786.50, 786.05

130. Tina is a patient who suffers from lower back pain. Her physician has ordered an x-ray of her lumbar spine, four views.
   A. 72110, 724.2
   B. 72074, 724.5
   C. 72110, 307.89
   D. 72080, 721.42

80,000 Pathology and Laboratory

131. A patient presents to the laboratory at the clinic for the following tests: thyroid stimulating hormone, comprehensive metabolic panel, and an automated hemogram with manual differential WBC count (CBC). How would you code this lab?
   A. 84443, 80053, 85027, 85007
   B. 80050
   C. 84443
   D. 84445, 80051, 85025

132. An 80-year-old female patient presented to the laboratory for a lipid panel that includes measurement of total serum cholesterol, lipoprotein (direct measurement, HDL), and triglycerides.
   A. 82465, 83718, 84478
   B. 82465-52, 83718, 84478
   C. 80061-52
   D. 80061

133. Philip has end-stage renal failure and comes to the clinic lab today for his monthly urinalysis (qualitative, microscopic only).
   A. 81015, 586
   B. 81001, 584.9
   C. 81015, 585
   D. 81003, 585

134. This 33-year-old male has been suffering from chronic fatigue. His physician has ordered a TSH:
    A. 80418, 780.71
    B. 80438, 780.79
    C. 80440, 780.71
    D. 84443, 780.79

135. Surgical pathology, gross examination, or microscopic examination is most often required when a sample of an organ, tissue, or body fluid is taken from the body. What code(s) would you use to report biopsy of the colon, hematoma, pancreas, and a tumor of the testis?
    A. 88304, 88304, 88309, 88309
    B. 88305, 88303, 88307, 88309
    C. 88305, 88304, 88307, 88309
    D. 88307, 88304, 88309, 88309

136. A patient presents to the clinic laboratory for a prothrombin time measurement because of his use of long-term use of Coumadin.
    A. 85210, V58.62
    B. 85610, V58.61
    C. 85230, V58
    D. 85210, V58.61

137. The patient presented to the laboratory at the clinic for the following blood tests ordered by her physician: albumin (serum), bilirubin (total), and BUN (quantitative):
    A. 82044, 82248, 84520
    B. 82040, 82252, 84525
    C. 82040, 82247, 84520
    D. 82044, 82247, 84540

138. A 70-year-old male who suffers from atrial fibrillation has been on long-term use of digoxin. He comes into the lab today to have a quantitative drug assay performed for digoxin:
    A. 80100
    B. 80102
    C. 80299
    D. 80162

139. This 68-year-old female suffers from chronic liver disease and needs a hepatic function panel performed every 6 months. Tests include total bilirubin (82247), direct bilirubin (82248), total protein (84155), alanine aminotransferases [ALT and SGPT] (84460), aspartate aminotransferases [AST and SGOT] (84450), and what other lab tests?
    A. 80061, 83718
    B. 82040, 82247
    C. 84295, 84450
    D. 82040, 84075

140. Edgar is status post kidney transplant and comes into the clinic lab for a follow-up creatinine clearance:
    A. 82540, V42.0
    B. 82575, V42.0
    C. 82565, 586
    D. 82570, 585

90,000 Medicine

141. An elderly male comes in for his flu (split virus, IM) and pneumonia (23-valent, IM) vaccines. Code only the immunization administration and diagnoses for the vaccines:
A. 90471, 90659, 90472, 90732, V04.8, V03.82
B. 90471 × 2, 90658, 90732, V04.8
C. 90471, 90472, V04.8, V03.82
D. 90658, 90732, V05.8, V04.8

142. Code the substance of DTP given intramuscularly:
A. 90700, 90471
B. 90702
C. 90701, 90471
D. 90701

143. Katie is a 9-year-old female who comes into the clinic to have her first ophthalmological exam. The exam was intermediate.
A. 99203
B. 92002
C. 92002, 99203
D. 92004

144. Katie is back for a 2-year follow-up comprehensive ophthalmological exam. The physician gives her contact lenses. She is to follow-up in 1 week to see how her contacts are working for her. Code the exam and the supply of contact lenses.
A. 92014, 92391
B. 92391
C. 92014, 92396
D. 92014, 92393

145. This 70-year-old male is taken to the emergency room with severe chest pain. The physician provided an expanded problem-focused history and examination. While the physician is examining the patient, his pressures drop and he goes into cardiac arrest. Cardiopulmonary resuscitation is given to the patient, and his pressure returns to normal; he is transferred to the intensive care unit in critical condition. Code the cardiopulmonary resuscitation and the diagnosis. The medical decision making complexity was of low complexity.
A. 99282, 92950, 427.5
B. 99238, 92970, 427.5
C. 92950, 427.5
D. 92960, 427.5

146. The patient is taken to the operating room for insertion of a Swan-Ganz catheter. The physician inserts the catheter for monitoring cardiac output measurements and blood gases.
A. 36013, 93503
B. 36013
C. 93508
D. 93503

147. Dr. Green orders a sleep study for Dan, a 51-year-old male who has been diagnosed with obstructive sleep apnea. The sleep study will be done with c-pap (continuous positive airway pressure).
A. 95806, 786.03
B. 95807, 780.53
C. 95811, 780.57
D. 95806, 780.57

148. Ann is a 58-year-old female with end-stage renal failure. She receives dialysis Tuesdays, Thursdays, and Saturdays each week. Code a full month of dialysis for the month of December.
    A. 90918, 593.9
    B. 90921, 585
    C. 90921-52, 585
    D. 90935, 586

149. OPERATIVE REPORT

    PROCEDURE PERFORMED: Primary stenting of 70% proximal posterior descending artery stenosis.

    INDICATIONS: Atherosclerotic heart disease.

    DESCRIPTION OF PROCEDURE: Please see the computer report. Please note that a 2.5 × 13 mm pixel stent was deployed.

    COMPLICATIONS: None

    RESULTS: Successful primary stenting of 70% proximal posterior descending artery stenosis with no residual stenosis at the end of the procedure.
    A. 92980-RC, 92981, 414.01
    B. 92982-RC, 414.9
    C. 92980-RC, 413.9
    D. 92980-RC, 414.01

150. Dr. Barrette is a neurosurgeon who has taken Betty, a 42-year-old female, with a diagnosis of carotid stenosis, to the operating room to perform a thromboendarterectomy, unilateral. During the surgery, the patient is monitored by electroencephalogram (EEG). Code the monitoring only:
    A. 35301, 95955, 433.10
    B. 35301-50, 433.30
    C. 95955, 433.10
    D. 95955

ANSWERS WITH RATIONALES FOR FINAL EXAMINATION

SECTION 1

Questions 1-50

Medical Terminology

1. The cup-shaped depression on the hip joint that receives the head of the femur is the:
   A. acetabulum
   B. calcaneus
   C. trochlea
   D. medial malleolus

Correct Answer: A. ***Acetabulum is the cup-shaped depression on the hip joint that receives the head of the femur.***
   Rationale: B. *Calcaneus, also known as the heel bone, is located at the back of the tarsus.*
   C. *Trochlea is located at the distal end of the humerus.*
   D. *Medial malleolus is located at the distal end of the tibia.*

2. The lower third of the small intestine is the:
   A. jejunum
   B. tenue
   C. ileum
   D. duodenum

Correct Answer: C. ***The ileum is the term for the lower third of the small intestine.***
   Rationale: A. *Jejunum is the second portion of the small intestine.*
   B. *Tenue is a term that means the small intestine.*
   D. *Duodenum the first portion of the small intestine.*

3. This term means to divert or make an artificial passage:
   A. burr
   B. occipital
   C. shunt
   D. catheter

Correct Answer: C. ***The term shunt means to divert or make an artificial passage.***
   Rationale: A. *Burr is a circular hole that is drilled into the skull by means of a drill.*
   B. *Occipital refers to the posterior cranial area, the occipital bone, or the occipital lobe of the brain.*
   D. *Catheter is a tube that is inserted into the body.*

4. This term means to identify the presence of and the amount of:
   A. qualitative
   B. definitive
   C. authoritative
   D. quantitative

Correct Answer: D.   ***Quantitative means to identify the presence of and the amount of.***
Rationale: A.   *Qualitative only identifies the presence of.*
B.   *Definitive means clear and final, without questions.*
C.   *Authoritative means the one who knows best.*

5. The term that means the expansion of:
   A. dilation
   B. curettage
   C. tocolysis
   D. manipulation

Correct Answer: A.   ***Dilation is the act of expanding or enlarging.***
Rationale: B.   *Curettage is scrapping of a cavity.*
C.   *Tocolysis is repression of uterine contractions.*
D.   *Manipulation is maneuvering.*

6. This term means the outermost covering of the eyeball:
   A. sclerae
   B. lacrimal
   C. ciliary
   D. chorea

Correct Answer: A.   ***Sclerae is the outermost covering of the eyeball.***
Rationale: B.   *The lacrimal is related to the tears, such as the lacrimal sac.*
C.   *Ciliary refers to the eyelash or other cilia, such as ciliary muscle or ciliary nerve.*
D.   *Chorea is an involuntary jerky movement.*

7. This term means the soft tissue around the nail border:
   A. sebaceous
   B. dermis
   C. lunula
   D. perionychium

Correct Answer: D.   ***Perionychium means the soft tissue around the nail border.***
Rationale: A.   *Sebaceous refers to the oil-secreting gland.*
B.   *Dermis is the middle layer of the skin, also known as true skin or corium.*
C.   *Lunula is the white half-moon at the base of the nail plate.*

8. This term means to turn downward:
   A. flexion
   B. adduction
   C. circumduction
   D. pronation

Correct Answer: D.   ***Pronation means to turn downward.***
Rationale: A.   *Flexion is to bend.*
B.   *Adduction is to move toward the median plane of the body.*
C.   *Circumduction is to make a circular motion.*

9. This combining form means artery:
   A. angi/o
   B. aort/o
   C. arteri/o
   D. atri/o

Correct Answer: C.   ***Arteri/o is the combining form that means artery.***
   Rationale: A.   *Angi/o means vessel.*
   B.   *Aort/o means aorta.*
   D.   *Atri/o means atrium.*

10. This abbreviation means that the neonate has a lower than normal weight:
    A. VLBW
    B. LNBW
    C. BWLN
    D. LBWV

Correct Answer: A.   ***VLBW means very low birth weight.***
   Rationale: A, B, C.   *These are not authentic abbreviations.*

Anatomy

11. This gland is located at the base of the brain in a depression in the skull:
    A. thymus
    B. hypothalamus
    C. pituitary
    D. pineal

Correct Answer: C.   ***This is the gland that is located at the base of the brain in a depression in the skull.***
   Rationale: A.   *The thymus is located behind the sternum.*
   B.   *The hypothalamus is located below the thalamus.*
   D.   *The pineal is located behind the hypothalamus.*

12. Which of the following is not a part of the kidney?
    A. cortex
    B. trigone
    C. medulla
    D. pyramids

Correct Answer: B.   ***The trigone is the triangular area at the base of the bladder.***
   Rationale: A.   *The cortex is the outer layer of the kidney.*
   C.   *The medulla is the inner portion of the kidney.*
   D.   *The pyramids are the divisions of the medulla.*

13. Which of the following is NOT a lymph organ?
    A. spleen
    B. bone marrow
    C. tonsils
    D. adrenal

Correct Answer: D.   ***The adrenal is an endocrine gland.***
   Rationale: A, B, and C are all lymph organs.

14. This is nature's pacemaker:
    A. atrioventricular node
    B. bundle of His
    C. septum
    D. sinoatrial node

Correct Answer: D.   ***The sinoatrial node is nature's pacemaker.***
    Rationale: A.   *The atrioventricular node is located on the interatrial septum and sends impulses to the bundle of His.*
        B.   *The bundle of His is divided into the right and left bundle branches.*
        C.   *The septum is the division of the upper right and left chambers of the heart.*

15. This is divided into the medulla oblongata, pons, and midbrain:
    A. brainstem
    B. diencephalon
    C. cerebellum
    D. cerebrum

Correct Answer: A.   ***The brainstem is divided into the medulla oblongata, pons, and midbrain.***
    Rationale: B.   *The diencephalon is where the hypothalamus and thalamus are located.*
        C.   *The cerebellum controls muscle contractions.*
        D.   *The cerebrum is the largest part of the brain and controls mental processes.*

16. This is located in the middle ear:
    A. vestibule
    B. cochlea
    C. auricle
    D. stapes

Correct Answer: D.   ***The stapes is a bone located in the middle ear.***
    Rationale: A.   *The vestibule is located in the inner ear.*
        B.   *The cochlea is located in the inner ear.*
        C.   *The auricle is the external ear, also known as the pinna.*

17. This is located in the pharynx and contains the adenoids:
    A. oropharynx
    B. laryngopharynx
    C. nasopharynx
    D. sphenoidal

Correct Answer: C.   ***The nasopharynx is located in the pharynx and contains the adenoids.***
    Rationale: A.   *The oropharynx contains the tonsils and is located in the pharynx.*
        B.   *The laryngopharynx leads to the trachea and esophagus and is also located in the pharynx.*
        D.   *The sphenoidal is a sinus.*

18. This is another name for the bulbourethral gland:
    A. tunica albuginea
    B. seminal vesicles
    C. prostate
    D. Cowper's

Correct Answer: D.   ***The Cowper's gland is also known as the bulbourethral gland.***
  Rationale: A. *The tunica albuginea is the covering of the testes.*
     B. *The seminal vesicles produce most of the seminal fluid.*
     C. *The prostate is a gland that produces some of the seminal fluid and activates the sperm.*

19. The approximate number of days of gestation of the fetus:
    A. 240
    B. 255
    C. 266
    D. 277

Correct Answer: C.   ***266 is the approximate number of days of gestation of the fetus.***
  Rationale: A, B, and D are not the correct number of gestational days for a fetus.

20. This is the makeup of the liquid part of the blood (plasma):
    A. 90% water, 2% protein, 8% other
    B. 95% water, 3% protein, 2% other
    C. 91% water, 1% protein, 2% other
    D. 88% water, 5% protein, 6% other

Correct Answer: C.   ***The makeup of the liquid part of the blood (plasma) is 91% water, 1% protein, and 2% other.***
  Rationale: A, B, and D are not the correct makeup of the liquid part of the blood (plasma).

ICD-9-CM

21. A patient is diagnosed with bilateral otitis media:
    A. 382.9
    B. 382.4
    C. 381.6
    D. 382.02

Correct Answer: A.   ***382.9, unspecified otitis media, is the correct diagnosis code because there is no indication of any particular type of otitis media.***
  Rationale: B. *382.4 is not correct because the term suppurative or purulent was not mentioned in the diagnosis statement.*
     C. *381.6 is not correct because this code describes obstruction of the eustachian tube and also requires a 5th digit.*
     D. *382.02 is not correct because this code is used to identify acute suppurative otitis media when another condition (i.e., influenza or scarlet fever) is the primary condition and the otitis media is a secondary condition.*

22. A patient is diagnosed with bacterial endocarditis due to AIDS:
    A. 421.0, 042
    B. 042, 421.9
    C. 421.1, 042
    D. 042, 421.0

Correct Answer: D.   *This correctly identifies AIDS with 042 and bacterial endocarditis with 421.0. The AIDS code is sequenced first.*

Rationale: *A.*   *042, the code for AIDS, should be sequenced first, not second; 421.0 identifies bacterial endocarditis.*

             B.   *421.9 identifies acute unspecified endocarditis as the cause, whereas the question identified bacterial endocarditis.*

             C.   *The code for AIDS should be sequenced first, not second; 421.1 identifies infective endocarditis.*

23. HOLTER REPORT

LOCATION: Outpatient, Clinic

INDICATION: Patient with atrial fibrillation on Lanoxin. Patient with known cardiomyopathy

BASELINE DATA: An 86-year-old man with congestive heart failure on Elavil, Vasotec, Lanoxin, and Lasix. The patient was monitored for the 24 hours in which the analysis was performed.

INTERPRETATION:

1. The predominant rhythm is atrial fibrillation. The average ventricular rate is 74 beats per minute, minimum 49 beats per minute, and maximum 114 beats per minute.

2. A total of 4,948 ventricular ectopic beats were detected. There were four forms. There were 146 couplets with one triplet and five runs of bigeminy. There were two runs of ventricular tachycardia, the longest for 5 beats at a rate of 150 beats per minute. There was no ventricular fibrillation.

3. There were no prolonged pauses.

CONCLUSION:

4. Predominant rhythm is atrial fibrillation with well-controlled ventricular rate.

5. There are no prolonged pauses.

6. Asymptomatic, nonsustained, ventricular tachycardia.
    A. 427.3, 425.4
    B. 425.4, 427.3
    C. 427.31, 425.4
    D. 427.32, 425.4

Correct Answer: C.   *The report states two diagnoses for the patient in the Indications section of the report—atrial fibrillation (427.31) and cardiomyopathy (425.4). The codes are placed in the order the diagnoses statements are stated on the report.*

Rationale: *A.*   *427.3 is atrial fibrillation and flutter, but because a five-digit code is available, you must assign that code rather than the four-digit 427.3. 425.4 is correct to report the cardiomyopathy.*

             B.   *425.4 is correct but should be the second-listed code rather than the first listed; also, 427.3 is the four-digit code, not the five-digit code.*

             D.   *427.32 is for atrial flutter, not atrial fibrillation.*

24. A 51-year-old male patient had surgery to remove two separate carbuncles of the left
    axilla. Pathology report indicated staphylococcal infection.
    A. 680.3, 041.10
    B. 680.9, 041.09
    C. 680.3, 041.19
    D. 680.9, 041.09

Correct Answer: A.   *The carbuncle is listed first using 680.3, and the cause of the
                          infection (staphylococcal, unspecified, 041.10) is listed second.*

Rationale: B.   *041.09 is the code used to report streptococcus, not staphylococcal; 680.9 is
                  for a site that is not specified.*

         C.   *041.19 is used to report other staphylococcus, which means other than
                staphylococcus not specified and not S. aureus. 680.3 is correct for the
                carbuncle.*

         D.   *041.09 is used to report other staphylococcus, but again, 680.9 is for a site
                that is not specified.*

25. The discharge diagnoses for a patient who was admitted for dyspnea were as follows:
    pneumonia, *Klebsiella pneumoniae*, COPD with emphysema, multifocal atrial
    tachycardia, middle dementia.
    A. 482, 492.8, 427.5, 294.8
    B. 486, 492.8, 427.89, 294.8
    C. 486, 492.0, 427.89, 294.11
    D. 482.0, 492.8, 427.89, 294.8

Correct Answer: D.   *482.0 (bacterial pneumonia), 492.8 (emphysema), 427.89
                          (tachycardia), and 294.8 (dementia) correctly identifies the
                          diagnoses stated in the question and are in the order stated.*

Rationale: A.   *482 is not a valid code because when there is a four-digit code available to
                  report pneumonia due to K. pneumoniae, that four-digit code must be used.
                  427.5 indicates cardiac arrest, which was not indicated for this patient.*

         B.   *486 is listed in the Index as the code to reference for pneumonia, but in
                referencing the Tabular, you will find that this code is for pneumonia when
                the organism is unspecified and because the organism was known to be K.
                pneumoniae. The remaining codes in this choice are correct.*

         C.   *As in choice B, 486 is used to report pneumonia when the organism is
                unspecified; because the organism was known to be K. pneumoniae, the
                unspecified organism code would not be correct. 492.0 is to report an
                emphysematous bleb, which was not indicated in this case. 427.89 is correct
                to identify the tachycardia. 294.11 identifies dementia that is classified
                elsewhere with behavioral disturbances, and behavior disturbances were not
                indicated.*

26. A patient with spinal stenosis of cervical disk C4-5 and C5-6 with intervertebral disk
    displacement had a cervical diskectomy, corpectomy, allograft from C4 to C6, and
    placement of arthrodesis (a 34-mm plate from C4 to C6).
    A. 722.90
    B. 723.0, 722.1
    C. 723.0, 722.0
    D. 723.1, 722.51

Correct Answer: C. ***723.0 describes the spinal stenosis, and 722.0 describes displacement of the cervical intervertebral disk.***

Rationale: A. *722.90 is used to report unspecified disk disorders, and the disk disorder was specified as spinal stenosis. Further, there is no code to report the displacement of the cervical intervertebral disk.*

B. *723.0 is correct for the spinal stenosis; however, 722.1 is used to report displacement of a thoracic or lumbar intervertebral disk, not a cervical disk and 722.1 requires a 5th digit.*

D. *723.1 is used to report pain in the neck (cervicalgia), and 722.51 is used to report degeneration of the thoracic or thoracolumbar intervertebral disk.*

27. A patient presents for an influenza vaccination and pneumococcal vaccination.
    A. V04.8, V03.89
    B. V04.7, V03.82
    C. V04.81, V03.82
    D. V04.7, V03.2

Correct Answer: C. ***V04.81 (influenza vaccination) and V03.82 (pneumococcal vaccination) correctly describe the reason for the services provided to this patient***

Rationale: A. *V04.8 in correctly reports influenza vaccination as the fifth digit 1 is missing. V03.89 is for a vaccination against a bacterial disease not specified; in the question pneumococcal was specified.*

B. *V04.7 is for a common cold vaccination, and V03.82 is correct for the pneumococcal vaccination.*

D. *V04.7 is again for the common cold, and V03.2 is for tuberculosis.*

28. A patient with a family history of malignant neoplasm of the breast receives a screening mammography, bilaterally (76092).
    A. V76.11
    B. V76.11, V16.3
    C. V16.3
    D. V10.3, V76.11

Correct Answer: B. ***V76.11 describes the screening mammography for high-risk patients, and V16.3 reports the family history of the malignant neoplasm of the breast.***

Rationale: A. *V76.11 reports only the screening mammography for high-risk patients, but this patient also has a family history of malignant neoplasm, which must also be reported.*

C. *V16.3 reports only the family history of malignant neoplasm of the breast and does not report the current screening mammography.*

D. *V10.3 reports a personal history of malignant neoplasm of the breast, and this patient has a family history only. V76.11 is correct for the screening mammography, but it should be the first-listed code.*

29. A patient with unstable angina, hypertension, diabetes with hypoglycemia, and a history of myocardial infarction is admitted for cardiac catheterization.
    A. 413.9, 401.9, 250.80, 412
    B. 411.1, 401.9, 250.80, 412
    C. 411.1, 401.1, 250.80, 412
    D. 411.1, 401.9, 250.00, 410.9

Correct Answer: B. *411.1, unstable angina; the includes the note under 411.1, Intermediate coronary syndrome, and indicates "Unstable angina," which is the condition stated for this patient; 401.9 is hypertension that is unspecified as to malignant or benign, which is the case for this patient; 250.80, diabetes with hypoglycemia; 412, history of myocardial infarction.*

Rationale: A. *413.9 is listed first in the Index, but that is for other or unspecified angina pectoris. The remaining codes are correct.*

C. *411.1 is correct for unstable angina, but 401.1 is for malignant hypertension, which was not specified. The remaining codes are correct.*

D. *250.00 is for diabetes without mention of complication, but the diabetes specified in the statement is diabetic hypoglycemia. 410.9 is for a current myocardial infarction, not a history of myocardial infarction. 410.9 also requires a 5th digit. The remaining codes are correct.*

30. A 4-year-old patient is seen by the physician in the outpatient clinic setting for chronic lymphoid leukemia that is currently in remission.
    A. 204.11
    B. 204.21
    C. 203.11
    D. 204.81

Correct Answer: A. *204.11 reports chronic lymphoid leukemia.*

Rationale: B. *204.21 is used to report subacute lymphoid leukemia in remission.*

C. *203.11 is used to report plasma cell leukemia in remission.*

D. *204.81 is used to report other lymphoid leukemia in remission.*

HCPCS

31. All third-party payers require the use of HCPCS codes when submitting for service provided to any patient.
    A. True
    B. False

Correct Answer: B. *This statement is false because the government payment programs require the use of HCPCS codes, such as Medicare and Medicaid.*

Rationale: A. *Other payers may or may not require the use of the HCPCS codes; it is up to each individual payer to state how providers are to submit for payment for services.*

32. A 62-year-old male Medicare patient presents for a digital rectal examination and a total prostate-specific antigen test (PSA).
    A. G0102
    B. G0103
    C. G0102, G0107
    D. G0102, G0103

Correct Answer: **D.** *G0102 reports the digital rectal examination; G0103 reports the PSA.*

    Rationale: A.   *G0102 is for only the digital rectal examination and does not include the PSA.*

             B.   *G0103 is for only the PSA and does not include the digital rectal examination.*

             C.   *G0102 is for a digital rectal examination, but G0107 is for colorectal cancer screening, not PSA.*

33. An 82-year-old female Medicare patient has a single energy x-ray absorptiometry (SEXA) bone density study of two sites of the wrist.
    A. 76071
    B. 76075
    C. G0130
    D. 76070

Correct Answer: **C.** *G0130 reports a single energy x-ray absorptiometry (SEXA) bone density study of one or more sites of the appendicular skeleton.*

    Rationale: A.   *76071 is for a computerized tomography bone mineral density study, not a SEXA.*

             B.   *Because this is a Medicare patient, the use of the HCPCS code for the SEXA is appropriate, not 76075, which is a DEXA (dual energy x-ray absorptiometry) bone density study of the axial skeleton, which would be used to report hips, pelvis, spine, and so on, not the appendicular skeleton that includes radius, wrist, heel, and so on.*

             D.   *76070 is for a computerized tomography bone mineral density study of the axial skeleton, which would be used to report hips, pelvis, spine, and so on, not the appendicular skeleton that includes radius, wrist, heel, and so on.*

34. A 72-year-old male Medicare patient receives 30 minutes of individual diabetes outpatient self-management training session.
    A. G0109
    B. G0176
    C. 99213
    D. G0108

Correct Answer: **D.** *G0108 reports a diabetic patient receiving self-management training for 30 minutes.*

    Rationale: A.   *G0109 is used to report group sessions of outpatient training.*

             B.   *G0176 is used to report activity therapy, such as music and dance.*

             C.   *99213 is an office visit for an established patient, not a training service.*

35. A Medicare patient presents for an influenza vaccination and pneumococcal vaccination.
    A. G0008
    B. G0009
    C. G0008, G0009
    D. G0010, G0008

Correct Answer: C. **G0008 reports the administration of the influenza vaccination, and G0009 reports the administration of the pneumococcal vaccination.**

    Rationale: A.   *G0008 is used to report the influenza virus vaccination, but this patient also had a pneumococcal vaccination.*

           B.   *G0009 is used to report the pneumococcal vaccination, but this patient also had an influenza virus vaccination.*

           D.   *G0010 is used to report administration of hepatitis B vaccine, but G0008 is correct for the influenza virus vaccination.*

Concepts of Coding

36. The term OIG stands for the Office of the:
    A. Information Group
    B. Insurance Group
    C. Inspector General
    D. Insurance General

Correct Answer: C. **The term OIG stands for the Office of the Inspector General and is part of the Department of Health and Human Services. The OIG is responsible for monitoring and investigating fraud and abuse of the government health care systems.**

    Rationale: A, B, and D are not legitimate terms that relate to the OIG.

37. This part of Medicare is the non-hospital portion:
    A. Part A
    B. Part B
    C. Part C
    D. Part D

Correct Answer: B. **Part B is the non-hospital portion of Medicare.**

    Rationale: A.   *Part A is the hospital insurance.*

           C.   *Part C is Medicare + Choice.*

           D.   *There is no Part D of Medicare.*

38. This is the group to which the CMS delegates the daily operation of the Medicare and Medicare programs:
    A. FI
    B. OG
    C. PRO
    D. HEW

Correct Answer: A. **FI means fiscal intermediaries.**

    Rationale: B.   *There is no OG.*

           C.   *PRO is the Peer Review Organization used to review the use of the DRG system within the hospital setting.*

           D.   *HEW is Health, Education and Welfare.*

39. This physician receives reimbursements for Medicare directly from the fiscal intermediary:
    A. PIB
    B. PRA
    C. PAR
    D. PEER

Correct Answer: C.   **PAR is the Participating Provider; reimbursement is sent directly from the FI to the provider. Non-PAR provider reimbursements are sent to the patient, who must then pay the provider.**

Rationale: A, B, and D are not legitimate acronyms (a word formed by initials of a term) referring to Medicare Participating Providers.

40. Which of the following is NOT true about the Outpatient Prospective Payment System?
    A. Known as the APC
    B. Was implemented in 2000
    C. Payment rates for each APC are published in the *Federal Register*
    D. Is applicable to non-Medicare and Medicare patients

Correct Answer: D.   **The OPPS is not used to report services to non-Medicare patients.**

Rationale: A, B, and C are all true statements about the OPPS.

Evaluation and Management

41. A second opinion is requested by a 90-year-old patient whose ophthalmologist recently diagnosed the patient with bilateral senile cataracts. Her regular ophthalmologist has recommended surgical removal of the cataracts and implantation of lens. The patient presents to the clinic stating that she is concerned about the necessity of the procedure at this time. During the detailed history, the patient states that she has had decreasing vision over the last year or two but has always had excellent vision. She cannot recall any eye trauma in the past. The physician conducted a detailed visual examination and confirmed the diagnosis of the patient's ophthalmologist. The medical decision making was of low complexity.
    A. 99263
    B. 92002
    C. 99243
    D. 99273

Correct Answer: D.   **99273 is a confirmatory consultation with a detailed history, detailed examination, and low complexity of medical decision making, which are the key components stated within the question.**

Rationale: A.   99263 is an inpatient follow-up consultation.
B.   92002 is a professional ophthalmologic service at an intermediate level for a new patient, not a consultation.
C.   99243 is an office consultation, not a confirmatory consultation.

42. The attending physician requests a confirmatory consultation from an interventional radiologist for a second opinion about a 63-year-old male with abnormal areas within the liver. The recommendation for a CT-guided biopsy is requested, which the attending has recommended be performed. During the comprehensive history, the patient reported right upper quadrant pain. His liver enzymes were elevated. Previous CT study revealed multiple low attenuation areas within the liver (infection versus tumor). The laboratory studies were creatine, 0.9; hemoglobin, 9.5; PT and PTT, 13.0/31.5 with an INR of 1.2. The comprehensive physical examination showed that the lungs were clear to auscultation and the heart had regular rate and rhythm. The mental status was oriented times three. Temperature, intermittent low-grade

fever, up to 101°F, usually occurred at night. The CT-guided biopsy was considered appropriate for this patient. The medical decision making was of high complexity.

A. 99245

B. 99255

C. 99275

D. 99274

Correct Answer: C. *99275 reports a confirmatory consultation, which is indicated by the fact that the attending has recommended that a liver biopsy be performed and is asking the interventional radiologist for an opinion to confirm the recommendation of the attending physician. The history was comprehensive, the physical examination was comprehensive, and the medical decision making was of high complexity.*

Rationale: A. 99245 describes an office or other outpatient consultation, not a confirmatory consultation, which can be conducted in any setting. The key components are at the correct level.

B. 99255 describes an initial inpatient consultation, not a confirmatory consultation. The key components are at the correct level.

D. 99274 is a confirmatory consultation, and the history and examination are at the comprehensive level; but the medical decision making is of moderate complexity, not a high complexity, as indicated in the question.

43. A cardiology consultation is requested for a 71-year-old inpatient for recent onset of dyspnea on exertion and chest pain. The comprehensive history reveals that the patient cannot walk three blocks without exhibiting retrosternal squeezing sensation with shortness of breath. She relates that she had the first episode 3 months ago, which she attributed to indigestion. Her medical history is negative for stroke, tuberculosis, cancer, or rheumatic fever but includes seborrheic keratosis and benign positional vertigo. She has no known allergies. A comprehensive physical examination reveals a pleasant, elderly female in no apparent distress. She has a blood pressure of 150/70 with a heart rate of 76. Weight is 131 pounds, and she is 5 foot 4 inches. Head and neck reveal JBP less than 5 cm. Normal carotid volume and upstroke without bruit. Chest examination shows clear to auscultation with no rales, crackles, crepitations, or wheezing. Cardiovascular examination reveals a normal PMI without RV lift. Normal S1 and S2 with an S3, without murmur, are noted. The medical decision making complexity is high based on the various diagnosis options.

A. 99275

B. 99245

C. 99255

D. 99274

Correct Answer: C. *99255 reports an initial inpatient consultation that included a comprehensive history and examination with high complexity of medical decision making.*

Rationale: A. 99275 is a confirmatory consultation, which was not indicated in the question. On a certification examination, you are not to make assumptions that are not stated; rather, you are to code the information presented in the case exactly as it appears.

B. 99245 describes an office or other outpatient consultation, not an inpatient consultation as was indicated in the case. The key components are at the correct level.

D. 99274 is a confirmatory consultation, which was not as indicated in the question.

44. A new patient presents to the emergency department with an ankle sprain received when he fell while roller blading. The patient is in apparent pain, and the ankle has begun to swell. He is unable to flex the ankle. The patient reports that he did strike his head on the sidewalk as a result of the fall. The physician completes an expanded problem-focused history and examination. The medical decision making complexity is low.
    A. 99232
    B. 99282
    C. 99202
    D. 99284

Correct Answer: B.   *99282 describes emergency department services with an expanded problem-focused history and examination with low complexity of medical decision making.*

Rationale: A.   *99232 is a subsequent hospital care service, and the patient in the question was treated in the emergency department.*

C.   *99202 describes a new patient service in an office or other outpatient services, but the service provided to the patient in the question was treated in the emergency department. The status of a new or established patient is not used within the emergency department services.*

D.   *99284 describes an emergency department service, but at a detailed level of examination and history and moderate medical decision making complexity; and the service described in the question indicates an expanded problem-focused history and examination with low complexity of medical decision making.*

45. An 89-year-old female patient is admitted to the skilled nursing facility after being seen in the office earlier today. The daughter brought the patient to the office. As a part of the detailed history, conducted with the patient's daughter, it is found that the patient was diagnosed with dementia last year. The patient was moved to this city from Anytown so that the daughter could care for her mother. The patient is noncontributory, and the physician relies on medical record documentation brought in by the daughter from her mother's previous physician. Of late, the patient has become more and more withdrawn and noncommunicative. She has wandered away from the daughter's home twice in the last week and on the last occasion was found walking on the street. After a comprehensive examination, it was decided that the patient would be admitted to the nursing facility today. The physician spent 45 minutes with the patient and in preparation of the medical documentation for admittance to the nursing facility. The level of medical decision making was of high complexity.
    A. 99313
    B. 99323
    C. 99302
    D. 99301

Correct Answer: C.   *99302 describes a detailed history, comprehensive examination, and moderate to high complexity of medical decision making.*

Rationale: A.   *99313 describes a subsequent nursing facility care and the patient was just admitted to the facility; so this would not be a subsequent service.*

B.   *99323 describes a service provided at a domiciliary or rest home, not at a skilled nursing facility. The key components are, however, at the correct level.*

D.   *99301 describes the right type of services but at the wrong levels: a detailed interval history, comprehensive examination, and a straightforward or low complexity of medical decision making.*

46. The physician provides a service to a new patient in a custodial care center. The patient is a paraplegic who has pneumonia of moderate severity. The physician performed an expanded problem-focused history and examination. The examination focused on the respiratory and cardiovascular systems, based on the patient's current complaint and past history of tachycardia. The medical decision making was of moderate complexity.
    A. 99332
    B. 99322
    C. 99342
    D. 99312

Correct Answer: B. **99322 indicates new patient service at a custodial care center with an expanded problem-focused history and examination with a moderate complexity of medical decision making.**

    Rationale: A.   *99332 is a service for an established patient at a custodial care center, although the level of the examination, history, and medical decision making complexity are at the correct level.*

          C.   *99342 describes a home service, not a custodial care center service, although the levels of services are at the correct level.*

          D.   *99312 describes a subsequent nursing facility care service not a custodial care center service, although the level of services is at the correct level.*

47. A 66-year-old male presents for a complete physical. There are no new complaints since my previous examination on 06/09 of last year. The patient spends 6 hours a week golfing and reports a brisk and active retirement. He does not smoke and has only an occasional glass of wine. He sleeps well but has been having nocturia times three. On physical examination, the patient is a well-developed, well-nourished male. The physician continues and provides a complete examination of the patient lasting 45 minutes.
    A. 99387
    B. 99403
    C. 99450
    D. 99397

Correct Answer: D. **99397 is correct because it describes a preventive medicine service to an established patient, and based on the age of the patient (66), the age 65 or over description in 99397 is the correct code.**

    Rationale: A.   *99387 is incorrect because it is for a preventive medicine service to a new patient, and the patient in the case is an established patient.*

          B.   *99403 describes a counseling service provided for risk reduction, not a physical examination service.*

          C.   *99450 is an examination for a basic life or disability evaluation, and the patient in the case had a physical.*

48. A new patient is seen in the office with complaints of a fever, chills, and difficulty breathing. The patient states that he has not been well for several weeks now and has progressively gotten weaker. He has not been able to work for the past week and before that was frequently absent from work over the course of 2 weeks. He is uncertain how long fever has been present but believes that it has been approximately 4 days. He does not have a thermometer at home and does not know what his temperature has been. He has been sleeping in a living room recliner because when he lies down, he has increased difficulty breathing. The detailed history and examination centered around the respiratory and cardiovascular systems. The upper respiratory findings included conjunctival injection, nasal discharge, and pharyngeal erythema.

A rapid test pack was used to diagnosis the viral infection. Chest x-ray showed patchy bilateral infiltrates. The physician diagnosed the patient with influenza A. The medical decision making complexity was low.

A. 99203
B. 99213
C. 99205
D. 99215

Correct Answer: A.   *99203 describes an office visit for a new patient service that included a detailed history and examination with a low complexity of medical decision making as stated in the question.*

Rationale: B.   *99213 is an office visit, but for an established patient, and the patient in the question was a new patient. The key components were not correct, as 99213 reports an expanded history and examination with low decision making. The case indicated that the history and examination were detailed with low medical decision making.*

C.   *99205 is an office visit for a new patient, but the key components are incorrect because the service was a detailed history and examination and low complexity of the medical decision making, and code 99205 describes a comprehensive history and examination and high complexity of medical decision making.*

D.   *99215 is an office visit for an established patient, and the patient in the case was a new patient. Also, this code is for a comprehensive history and examination with a high complexity of medical decision making rather than what the case stated, which was a detailed history and examination with low complexity of medical decision making.*

49. A new patient is admitted to the observation unit of the local hospital after a 10-foot fall from a ladder. The patient struck his head on the side of the garage as he fell into a hedge that somewhat broke his fall. He has significant bruising on the left side of his body and complains of a 5/10 pain under his left arm. A series of x-rays has been ordered in addition to an MRI. The physician completed a comprehensive history and physical examination. It was decided to admit the patient to observation based on some evidence that he may have hit the left side of his head during the fall. The medical decision making is moderately complex.

A. 99222
B. 99219
C. 99235
D. 99220

Correct Answer: B.   *99219 is correct because the service was an initial observation care service (not affected by new or established patient status) with a comprehensive history and examination and moderate medical decision making complexity.*

Rationale: A.   *99222 describes initial hospital inpatient care services (also not affected by new or established patient status), not an initial observation service. The levels of key components are correct.*

C.   *99235 describes an observation admission and discharge on the same day; however, the patient in the case was not discharged on the same day.*

D.   *99220 is an initial observation care service, but the key components are not at the correct level because the case indicated a comprehensive history and examination with moderate medical decision making complexity. 99220 is for a comprehensive history and examination with high complexity of medical decision making.*

50. An established patient is admitted to the hospital by his attending physician after a car accident in which the patient hit the steering wheel of the automobile with significant enough force to fold the wheel backwards. The patient complains of significant pain in the right shoulder. After a detailed history and physical examination, the physician believed the patient may have sustained a right rotator cuff injury. The medical decision was straightforward in complexity.
   A. 99283
   B. 99263
   C. 99221
   D. 99253

Correct Answer: C.   *99221 describes a initial hospital care service with a detailed history and physical examination and a straightforward medical decision making complexity.*

Rationale: A.   *99283 describes a service in the emergency department, and the patient in the case was admitted to the hospital. Even if the patient had been seen first in the emergency department and then admitted to the hospital by the same physician, the emergency department service would be bundled into the initial hospital admission service; but this patient had no mention of previous emergency department service. The key components were at the correct level.*

B.   *99263 describes a follow-up inpatient consultation service for an established patient rather than the initial hospital care service that the patient received.*

D.   *99253 is an initial inpatient service but it is a consultation and the service in the case was an admission service.*

SECTION 2

Questions 51-100

Anesthesia

51. If the anesthesia service was provided to a patient who had mild systemic disease, what would the physical status modifier be?
   A. P1
   B. P2
   C. P3
   D. P4

Correct Answer: B.   *P2 is a physical status modifier assigned based on the patient's condition at the time of surgery. P2 represents a patient with a mild systemic disease.*

Rationale: A.   *P1 is a normal healthy patient, not one with a mild systemic disease.*

C.   *P3 is a patient with a severe systemic disease, not one with a mild systemic disease.*

D.   *P4 is a patient with a severe systemic disease that is in constant threat of life, not one with a mild systemic disease.*

52. The qualifying circumstances code indicates a 72-year-old female:
   A. 99100
   B. 99116
   C. 99135
   D. 99140

Correct Answer: A. ***99100 describes anesthesia for patient of extreme age, under 1 or over 70 years of age. Qualifying circumstances codes identify situations that make administration of the anesthesia more difficult.***

Rationale: B. *99116 describes anesthesia complicated by utilization of total body hypothermia, not extreme age.*

C. *99135 is for anesthesia complicated by utilization of controlled hypotension, not extreme age.*

D. *99140 describes anesthesia complicated by emergency conditions, not extreme age.*

53. This type of sedation decreases the level of the patient's alertness but allows the patient to cooperate during the procedure:
    A. topical
    B. local
    C. regional
    D. conscious

Correct Answer: D. ***Conscious sedation decreases the level of the consciousness but is not general anesthesia.***

Rationale: A. *Topical is on the skin.*

B. *Local is insertion under the skin.*

C. *Regional is anesthesia of an area of the body.*

54. The national unit values for anesthesia services are listed in this publication:
    A. BVR by AS
    B. RVG by ASA
    C. ASA by RVG
    D. RVP by ASA

Correct Answer: B. ***Relative Value Guide by the American Society of Anesthesiology lists the national unit values for anesthesia services.***

Rationale: A. *There is no BVR or AS.*

C. *ASA is the American Society of Anesthesiology and RVG is the Relative Value Guide but the abbreviations are in the wrong order.*

D. *There is no RVP.*

55. When reporting anesthesia services performed for two procedures performed on the same patient during the same operative procedure, you would do the following to calculate the unit value of the services:
    A. Add the units of the two procedures together.
    B. Subtract the procedure with the lowest unit value from the procedure with the highest unit value.
    C. Report only the units for the lowest unit value procedure.
    D. Report only the units for the highest unit value procedure.

Correct Answer: D. ***When reporting anesthesia services performed, you would report only the units for the highest unit value procedure.***

Rationale: A, B, and C are not correct methods of calculating the unit value for a procedure.

56. Anesthesia provided for an anterior cervical diskectomy with decompression of a single interspace of the spinal cord and nerve roots and including osteophytectomy (63075).
    A. 00620
    B. 00630
    C. 00600
    D. 00640

Correct Answer: C.   ***00600 describes anesthesia for procedures on the cervical spine and cord.***
   Rationale: A.   *00620 is for anesthesia for procedures on the thoracic spine.*
          B.   *00630 is for anesthesia for procedures on the lumbar region.*
          D.   *00640 is for anesthesia for procedures involving manipulation of the cervical, thoracic, or lumbar spine.*

57. A 16-year-old female patient has a left thyroid mass, which is removed by total thyroidectomy. The anesthesia service would be reported with the following:
    A. 00320
    B. 00322
    C. 00326
    D. 00300

Correct Answer: A.   ***00320 is used to report anesthesia for all procedures on the thyroid on patients older than 1 year.***
   Rationale: B.   *00322 is for a needle biopsy of the thyroid.*
          C.   *00326 is a procedure on a patient younger than 1 year of age.*
          D.   *00300 is for anesthesia for all procedures on the integumentary system, not otherwise specified.*

58. General anesthesia for a limited ophthalmological examination and evaluation with the manipulation of the globe for range of motion (92019) using an ophthalmoscope:
    A. 00145
    B. 00140
    C. 00148
    D. 00147

Correct Answer: C.   ***00148 describes anesthesia for procedures on the eye using an ophthalmoscope.***
   Rationale: A.   *00145 is used to report vitreoretinal surgery, and no surgical procedure was indicated.*
          B.   *00140 is used to indicate anesthesia for procedures on the eye, not otherwise specified.*
          D.   *00147 is for an iridectomy, and no surgical procedure was indicated.*

59. The following indicates anesthesia for a procedure on the lower posterior abdominal wall for a patient with severe hypertension:
    A. 00820-P3
    B. 00820-P2
    C. 00800-P3
    D. 00800-P2

Correct Answer: A. ***00820 is correct for the anesthesia code, and P3 indicates a severe systemic disease.***

Rationale: B. *00820 is correct, but P2 is for a mild systemic disease.*

C. *00800 is for anesthesia for procedures on the lower anterior wall, but P3 is correct for a severe systemic disease.*

D. *00800 is, as in C, for anesthesia for procedures on the lower anterior wall, and P2 is for mild systemic disease.*

60. What combination of CPT code and modifier would you use to report anesthesia services for a patient who is 87 years of age and is not expected to survive without the surgical procedure being performed and for which anesthesia is being provided?
    A. 99116, P4
    B. 99100, P4
    C. 99100, P5
    D. 99140, P6

Correct Answer: C. ***99100 identifies patients under 1 year or over 70 years of age, and P5 identifies moribund patients who are not expected to survive without the procedure being performed.***

Rationale: A. *99116 is for anesthesia complicated by total body hypothermia, and P4 is for a patient with severe systemic disease that is in constant threat to life.*

B. *99100 is correct to indicate that a patient is over the age of 70 years, but P4 is for a patient with severe systemic disease that is in constant threat to life.*

D. *99140 is for anesthesia complicated by emergency conditions, and P6 is for brain-dead patients whose organs are being removed for donor purposes.*

Integumentary

61. A 24-year-old female is seen in the office for a single subcutaneous cyst that needs to be incised and drained:
    A. 10061
    B. 10080
    C. 10060
    D. 11400

Correct Answer: C. ***10060 is incision and drainage of subcutaneous cyst or abscess, single or simple.***

Rationale: A. *10061 is for complicated or multiple incision and drainage of subcutaneous cyst or abscess.*

B. *10080 is for simple incision and drainage of pilonidal cyst.*

D. *11400 is for excision of benign lesion.*

62. A 10-year-old boy presents for injuries caused by falling off his bike. All wounds were superficial. He has a 2-cm wound to his nose and a 1-cm wound to his cheek. He also has a 2.5-cm wound to his elbow. All injuries were simple repair by means of suture.
    A. 12011, 12001
    B. 12013, 12001
    C. 12013, 12002
    D. 12011, 12002

Correct Answer: B. *12013 describes a simple repair of superficial wounds to the face or nose (2.6 to 5.0 cm), and the superficial wounds to the patient were a 2-cm wound to the nose and a 1-cm wound to the cheek; so you add those two superficial wounds together (3 cm) before you choose the correct code (12013). 12001 describes the simple repair of superficial wounds to extremities (2.5 cm or smaller), and the patient's wound was a superficial wound to the elbow with a length of 2.5 cm. Note: Be certain always to add the lengths of repairs together for each group of anatomic sites of the same complexity.*

Rationale: A. *12011 is not correct because it is for simple repair of superficial wounds of the face or nose (2.5 cm or smaller), and the patient had a 2-cm repair of the nose and a 1-cm repair of the cheek (nose and face); these are added together (3 cm) before the correct code is chosen. Because 12011 is for wounds smaller than 2.5 cm, it is not the correct code. 12001 is the correct code because it describes simple repair of superficial wounds to extremities (2.5 cm or smaller), and the patient's wound was a superficial wound to the elbow with a length of 2.5 cm.*

C. *12013 is correct for the first code because it describes a simple repair of superficial wounds to the face or nose (2.6 to 5.0 cm), and the superficial wounds to the patient were a 2-cm wound to the nose and a 1-cm wound to the cheek; so you add those two superficial wounds together (3 cm) before you choose the correct code (12013). 12002 is not correct, however, because it describes a simple repair of superficial wound of extremities 2.6 cm to 7.5 cm, and the patient's elbow wound was 2.5 cm.*

D. *12011 is not correct because it is for simple repair of superficial wounds of the face or nose (2.5 cm or smaller), and the patient had a 2-cm repair of the nose and a 1-cm repair of the cheek (nose and face), which are added together (3 cm) before the correct code is chosen. Because 12011 is for wounds smaller than 2.5 cm, it is not the correct code. 12002 is not correct for the elbow repair because 12002 is a simple repair of superficial wounds of extremities 2.6 to 7.5 cm, and the patient's elbow wound was 2.5 cm.*

63. Dr. Smith performed a bilateral radical mastectomy, including the pectoral muscles and axillary lymph nodes, on a 63-year-old female with breast cancer:
    A. 19200, 174.9
    B. 19220-50, 174.9
    C. 19200-50, 174.9
    D. 19240-50, 174.9

Correct Answer: C. *19200-50 reports a radical mastectomy, including pectoral muscles and the axillary lymph nodes. Modifier -50 (bilateral) would be added to indicate that both breasts were removed. The diagnosis of breast cancer is correctly reported with 174.9, which is a unspecified malignant neoplasm of the female breast.*

Rationale: A. *19200 is correct for the mastectomy, but the case states that a bilateral procedure was performed; so modifier -50 must be added to indicate that both breasts were removed. The diagnosis code is correct.*

B. *19220-50 is a mastectomy code, but it includes the internal mammary lymph nodes, which was not stated as having been performed. The diagnosis code is correct.*

D. *19240-50 is a modified radical (axillary lymph nodes were done) mastectomy code, but it includes the axillary lymph nodes (with or without pectoralis minor muscle but excludes the pectoralis major muscle), which was not stated as having been performed. The diagnosis code is correct.*

64. What code(s) would you use to report chemosurgery, Mohs' micrographic technique, with six specimens of fresh tissue, first stage?
    A. 17304-51
    B. 17310-51
    C. 17304, 17307
    D. 17304, 17310

Correct Answer: D.   **17304 is for the first through the fifth specimens of a first stage (Mohs' micrographic technique); 17310, the add-on code, is used to report the sixth specimen.**

    Rationale: A.   *17304-51 reports the first stage of chemosurgery with up to five specimens. Modifier -51 is not used with the codes in the Chemosurgery, Mohs' micrographic technique section (17304-17310). Note the use of the circle with a line through it next to each of these codes to indicate a modifier -51 exempt code. Also, 17310 is required to report each additional specimen greater than five specimens.*

            B.   *17310-51 is the correct code but only for each additional specimen after the first specimen. 17310 is an add-on code that can be used only with another code and is also -51 exempt. Also, it is necessary to report the primary code for the chemosurgery (17306).*

            C.   *17304 is correct to report the first through the fifth specimens of the first stage, but 17307 is used to report an additional complete stage (up to five specimens).*

65. A 40-year-old male is in for layered closure of wounds due to a motor vehicle accident. The patient sustained injuries to the forehead, 1.5 cm, and a 1-cm wound to the eyebrow when his head hit the steering wheel. Code the service code only.
    A. 12011
    B. 12051
    C. 13131
    D. 12001

Correct Answer: B.   **12051 reports layer closure of wounds to face, ears, eyelids, nose, lips, 2.5 cm or smaller. Because the injury to the patient was a 1.5-cm wound to the forehead and a 1-cm wound to the eyebrow, you add the two wounds together (2.5 cm) and report the service with 12051.**

    Rationale: A.   *12011 is simple repair of superficial wounds of the face.*

            C.   *13131 is complex repair of the forehead (1.1 to 2.5 cm).*

            D.   *12001 is simple repair of superficial wounds of scalp, neck, trunk, or extremities, which is the wrong location for the injuries stated in the case (forehead and eyebrow).*

66. Which code would the surgeon use to report the shaving of an epidermal lesion of the arm when a lesion diameter is greater than 2.0 cm?
    A. 11402
    B. 11200
    C. 11303
    D. 11602

Correct Answer: **C.** **11303 correctly describes the shaving of a single epidermal or dermal lesion (larger than 2.0 cm) of the arms.**

Rationale: A. *11402 is for an excision of a benign lesion of the arm, but the case was for shaving of a lesion.*

B. *11200 is removal of skin tags, but the case was for shaving of a lesion.*

D. *11602 is excision of malignant lesion on the arm, but the case indicated shaving of a lesion.*

67. A 73-year-old male is admitted by Dr. Smith for an excision of a nail and nail matrix, complete, for permanent removal with amputation of a tuft of distal phalanx. A 2.0-cm single pinch skin graft was needed to cover the tip of the digit.
    A. 11752
    B. 11750
    C. 11750, 15050
    D. 11752, 15050

Correct Answer: **D.** **11752 is the partial or complete excision of nail and matrix for permanent removal and includes amputation of the tuft of distal phalanx. 15050 describes a skin graft, such as a pinch skin graft, up to a defect size 2 cm in diameter, which was the service performed.**

Rationale: A. *11752 is the correct code for the excision of nail and matrix with amputation, but the skin graft also needed to be coded to report the service completely.*

B. *11750 is excision of the complete nail and matrix but does not include the amputation of the tuft of the distal phalanx. The grafting service also needed to be reported.*

C. *11750 is excision of the complete nail and matrix but does not include the amputation of the tuft of the distal phalanx. 15050 describes a skin graft, such as a pinch skin graft, up to a defect size of 2 cm in diameter, which was the service performed.*

68. What code would you use for an initial large debridement of both arms resulting from burns, without general anesthesia?
    A. 16010
    B. 16025
    C. 16030-50
    D. 16030

Correct Answer: **D.** **16030 reports an initial debridement of a large area (e.g., more than one extremity) without anesthesia.**

Rationale: A. *16010 is for debridement of a small area under general anesthesia, and the patient had a large debridement.*

B. *16025. The code reports a debridement of a medium-sized area rather than the large area reported in the case.*

C. *16030 is the correct code for the initial debridement, but the use of modifier -50 is not necessary because the code states that the code that can be used to report more than one extremity, which makes the bilateral modifier, -50, unnecessary.*

69. Donna, a 41-year-old female, presents for biopsies of both breasts. Dr. Smith will be doing the biopsies using fine-needle aspiration with imaging guidance:
    A. 19102-50
    B. 10022-50
    C. 10021
    D. 19103-50

Correct Answer: B. *10022-50 is for bilateral fine-needle aspiration with the use of imaging guidance, which describes the service in the question.*

Rationale: A. *19102-50 is for a biopsy of breast, not a fine-needle aspiration.*

C. *10021 is for a fine-needle aspiration but without imaging guidance; also, because the service was a bilateral procedure, modifier -50 is necessary.*

D. *19103-50 describes a biopsy of both breasts by means of an automated vacuum-assisted or rotating biopsy device. The question did not indicate a vacuum or rotating biopsy device being used to perform the procedure and so is incorrect to report this service.*

70. Katie is seen in the clinic by Dr. Smith for several scars on her face caused by acne. Dr. Smith decides to do an epidermal chemical peel of the face.
    A. 15780
    B. 15781
    C. 15789
    D. 15788

Correct Answer: D. *15788 describes a facial (epidermal) chemical peel.*

Rationale: A. *15780 is for dermabrasion of the total face, which differs from a chemical peel in which an acid-based chemical is applied to the face, whereas dermabrasion is the sanding of the skin surface.*

B. *15781 is for dermabrasion on only a portion (segmental) of the face, which differs from a chemical peel in which an acid-based chemical is applied to the face, whereas dermabrasion is the sanding of the skin surface.*

C. *15789 is for a chemical peel of the dermal layer of the facial skin that involves a deeper layer (dermal, second layer) of the skin compared with an epidermal (first layer).*

Musculoskeletal System

71. Richard, a 34-year-old male, fell from a 4-foot scaffolding and hit his heel on the bottom rung of the support, fracturing his calcaneus in several locations. The orthopedic surgeon manipulated the bone pieces back into position and secured the fracture sites by means of percutaneous fixation.
    A. 28415
    B. 28405
    C. 28406
    D. 28456

Correct Answer: C. *28406 describes a percutaneous skeletal fixation of a calcaneal (heal bone) fracture that included manipulation.*

Rationale: A. *28415 describes an open treatment of a calcaneal fracture, but the case described a percutaneous treatment.*

B. *28405 describes a closed treatment of a calcaneal fracture, but the case described a percutaneous treatment.*

D. *28456 describes a percutaneous treatment, but of the tarsal bone, not of the calcaneal bone described in the case.*

72. Sammy, a 5-year-old male, tumbled down the stairs at daycare, striking and fracturing his coccygeal bone. The physician manually manipulated the bone into proper alignment and told Sammy's mother to have the child sit on a rubber ring to alleviate the pain.
    A. 27510
    B. 28445
    C. 27202
    D. 27200

Correct Answer: D.   ***27200 describes a closed treatment of a coccygeal fracture and includes manipulation.***
   Rationale: A.   27510 is used to report a closed treatment of a fracture of the femur, not of the coccygeal.
   B.   28445 reports an open treatment of a talus fracture, not a coccygeal fracture.
   C.   27202 is used to report an open treatment of the coccygeal, not a closed treatment.

73. Alice, a 42-year-old female, is a carpenter at the local college. While on a ladder repairing a window frame, the weld on the rung of the metal ladder loosened and she fell backwards a distance of 8 feet. She landed on her left hip, resulting in a dislocation. With the patient under general anesthesia, the Allis maneuver is used to repair an anterior dislocation of the right hip. The pelvis is stabilized and pressure applied to the thigh to reduce the hip and bring it into proper alignment.
    A. 27250
    B. 27252
    C. 27253
    D. 27254

Correct Answer: B.   ***27252 is a closed treatment of a traumatic hip dislocation with the use of general anesthesia. You know the treatment was closed by the statement "the Allis maneuver is used to repair an anterior dislocation to the right hip," which is used to maneuver the bone back into alignment from the outside (closed treatment).***
   Rationale: A.   27250 describes a closed treatment of a traumatic hip dislocation but without anesthesia, which was specified in the case (Under general anesthesia, . . .).
   C.   27253 is an open treatment of a traumatic hip dislocation, but the case was for a closed treatment.
   D.   27254 describes an open treatment of a traumatic hip dislocation, but the case was for a closed treatment.

74. A 13-year-old female sustained multiple tibial tuberosity fractures of the left knee while playing soccer at her local track meet. The physician extended the left leg and manipulated several fragments back into place. The knee was then aspirated. A long-leg knee brace was then placed on the knee.
    A. 27334
    B. 27550
    C. 27538
    D. 27330

Correct Answer: **C.**   *27538 describes a closed treatment of the knee with manipulation, which includes aspiration and a knee brace placed on the knee after surgery to immobilize the joint.*

   Rationale: *A.*   *27334 is an arthrotomy (open procedure) with removal of the synovial membrane of the knee, but the procedure in the case was indicated as being a closed procedure in which the physician manipulated the fragments back into place.*

   B.   *27550 describes a closed treatment of a dislocation, not of a fracture.*

   D.   *27330 is an open procedure in which a synovial biopsy is performed, but the case was a closed treatment of the knee with aspiration and application of a knee brace.*

75. Under general anesthesia, 5-year-old Michael's tarsal dislocation was reduced by means of manipulation. Two-view intraoperative x-rays demonstrated that the tarsus was in correct alignment, and a short leg cast was then applied. (Code only the reduction service.)
    A. 28545, 29405
    B. 28545, 29405, 73620
    C. 28540, 73620
    D. 28545

Correct Answer: **D.**   *28545 describes a closed treatment of a dislocated tarsal bone with the use of anesthesia. The cast is bundled into the repair service.*

   Rationale: *A.*   *28545 is correct for the closed treatment of the dislocated tarsal bone, but 29405, the short leg cast application, is not correct because the application of the cast is included in the treatment code. (See notes regarding Application of Casts and Strapping preceding code 29000 in the CPT manual.)*

   B.   *28545 is correct for the closed treatment of the dislocated tarsal bone, but 29405, the short leg cast application, is not correct because the application of the cast is included in the treatment code. (See notes regarding Application of Casts and Strapping preceding code 29000 in the CPT manual.) Also, the intraoperative x-ray was not to be coded, as indicated by the "Note: code only the reduction service."*

   C.   *28540 is a closed treatment of a dislocated tarsal bone, but without anesthesia, which was specified in the case (Under general anesthesia . . .), and you were not to code the intraoperative x-ray based on the ("Note code only the reduction service").*

76. Dr. Clark applied a cranial halo to Gordon to stabilize the cervical spine in preparation for x-rays and subsequent surgery. The scalp was sterilized and local anesthesia injected over the pin insertion sites. Posterior and anterior cranial pins are inserted and the halo device attached.
    A. 20664
    B. 20661, 90782
    C. 20661
    D. 20664, 90782

Correct Answer: **C.**   **20661 is used to report the application of a cranial halo, which was the service provided.**

Rationale: A.   *20664 describes the application of a cranial halo but for thin skull osteology (such as those with pediatric patients, hydrocephalus) and by means of general anesthesia; however, local anesthesia was used in the case.*

B.   *20661 is correct for the application of a cranial halo, but the injection, presumably for local anesthesia, is not necessary because the injection is included in the application service and is not reported separately.*

D.   *20664 describes the application of a cranial halo but for thin skull osteology (such as those with pediatric patients, hydrocephalus) and by means of general anesthesia; however, local anesthesia was used in the case. The injection, presumably for local anesthesia, is not necessary because the injection is included in the application service and is not reported separately.*

77. Samantha was playing in the back yard when her brother fired a pellet gun at her leg at close range. The pellet penetrated the skin and lodged in the muscle underlying the area. The physician removed the pellet without complication or incident.
   A. 20520
   B. 20525
   C. 10120
   D. 10121

Correct Answer: **A.**   **20520 reports a simple removal of a foreign body from the muscle.**

Rationale: B.   *20525 reports a removal of complicated or deep foreign body from the muscle. The statement that the physician removed the pellet without complication or incident is the indication that this is not a complicated or deep removal, as would be reported with 20525.*

C.   *10120 is used to report the simple removal of a foreign body from subcutaneous tissue, and the case indicated the removal was from the muscle.*

D.   *10121 reports a complicated removal of a foreign body from subcutaneous tissue, and the case indicated the removal was from the muscle.*

78. Kevin comes in with a deep hematoma on his shoulder that he has had for some time. After an exam was performed of the shoulder area, the physician decides that the hematoma needs to be incised and drained.
   A. 23030
   B. 10140
   C. 10060
   D. 10160

Correct Answer: **A.**   **23030 Incision and drainage, shoulder area; deep abscess or hematoma.**

Rationale: B.   *10140 is for an incision and drainage of hematoma of the skin, but the question stated "deep hematoma," which requires a code from the Musculoskeletal subsection.*

C.   *10060 is for an incision and drainage of simple subcutaneous abscess or cyst, which is skin-level I&D, and the question indicated a "deep hematoma," which requires a code from the Musculoskeletal subsection.*

D.   *10160 is for a puncture aspiration hematoma, but, again is of the skin when the question indicated a "deep hematoma," which requires a code from the Musculoskeletal subsection.*

79. Marsha is admitted to same-day surgery after having an abnormal shoulder x-ray in the clinic yesterday. The physician decides to do a diagnostic arthroscopy.
   A. 29806
   B. 29805
   C. 23066
   D. 23100

   Correct Answer: B. *29805 reports a diagnostic arthroscopy of the shoulder.*
   Rationale: A. *29806 is for a surgical arthroscopy, but this procedure was a diagnostic arthroscopy.*
   C. *23066 is a deep excisional biopsy of the shoulder area, and this procedure was only a diagnostic arthroscopy.*
   D. *23100 is for an arthrotomy of the glenohumeral joint that included biopsy, whereas the stated procedure was a diagnostic arthroscopy.*

80. Cole comes into the orthopedic department today with his mother after falling from the top bunk bed, where he and his brother were wrestling. Cole is having pain in his left lower leg and is unable to bear weight on it. Cole was taken to the x-ray department. After the physician talked with the radiologist regarding the diagnosis of sprained ankle, the physician decides to apply a walking short leg cast from just below his knee to his toes.
   A. 29405, 845.00, E884.4
   B. 29515, 845.00, E888.9
   C. 29355, 959.7, E884.4
   D. 29425, 845.00, E884.4

   Correct Answer: D. *29425 reports the application of short leg cast (below the knee to toes), walking or ambulatory type. 845.00 reports a sprained ankle, which is correct. E884.4 is the external cause code for falling from a bed.*
   Rationale: A. *29405 is only an application of short leg cast, which differs from a short leg walking cast in that a short leg cast does not have a special heel device that allows pressure to be applied to the cast when walking. 845.00 is the correct diagnosis. E884.4 is the correct external code for falling from a bed.*
   B. *29515 is for application of short leg splint (calf to foot), and the case specified a cast, not a splint. 845.00 reports a sprained ankle, which is the correct diagnosis. E888.9 is incorrect. It is the external code for an unspecified fall.*
   C. *29355 is application of long leg cast (thigh to toes), and the cast applied was a short leg walking cast. 959.7 is incorrect. This diagnosis is for a unspecified injury to the ankle.*

10,000 Respiratory System, Cardiovascular System, Mediastinum, and Diaphragm

81. PREOPERATIVE DIAGNOSIS: Deviated septum

   PROCEDURE PERFORMED:

   1. Septoplasty

   2. Resection of turbinates

   The patient was taken to the operating room and placed under general anesthesia. The fracture of the turbinates was first performed to do the septoplasty. Once this was done, the septoplasty was completed and the turbinates were placed back in their original position. The patient was taken to recovery in satisfactory condition. Code the procedure(s) and the diagnosis:

A. 30520, 30130, 470
B. 30520, 30130-51, 470
C. 30520, 30140-51, 478.1
D. 30520, 30140-51, 470

Correct Answer: D.   *30520 indicates septoplasty and 30140-51, submucous resection of turbinate with the -51 modifier showing multiple procedures. (See parenthetical note following 30140 in the CPT manual.) Both the septoplasty and the removal of the turbinate must be reported to describe completely the service provided. The diagnosis code 470 indicates a deviation of the septum.*

Rationale: A.   *30520 is the correct code for the septoplasty, and 30130 is for excision of turbinate. The operative report states that the turbinates were fractured (i.e., reduced), which is code 30140, not excised, code 30130. 470 is the correct diagnosis for a deviation of the septum.*

B.   *30520 is the correct code for the septoplasty, and 30130-51 is for excision of turbinate; the turbinates were fractured, not excised. The modifier -51 is correct (see comment under D rationale). 470 is the correct diagnosis.*

C.   *30520 is the correct code, and 30140-51 is the correct code with the incorrect modifier -51, as the parenthetical (in parenthesis) following 30140 in the CPT manual directs the coder to use modifier -52 for turbinate reduction. 478.1, nasal drainage, is the wrong diagnosis. As it states in the operative report, the diagnosis is deviated septum, 470; there was no mention of nasal drainage.*

82. The patient is seen in the clinic for chronic sinusitis. The physician decides to schedule an endoscopic sinus surgery for the next day. The patient arrives to same-day surgery, and the physician performs an endoscopic ethmoidectomy total with an endoscopic maxillary antrostomy with removal of maxillary tissue. Code the procedure(s) and diagnosis.

A. 31254, 31256-51, 473.9
B. 31255, 31267-51, 461.9
C. 31255, 31267-51, 473.9
D. 31200, 31225-51, 473.9

Correct Answer: C.   *31255, nasal/sinus endoscopy, surgical; with ethmoidectomy, total; 31267-51, nasal/sinus endoscopy, surgical, with maxillary antrostomy, with removal of tissue from maxillary sinus; the -51 modifier shows that a multiple procedure was performed. 473.9, chronic sinusitis, correctly describes the stated diagnosis.*

Rationale: A.   *31254 is for a nasal/sinus endoscopy, surgical, but with only a partial ethmoidectomy; the question stated a total ethmoidectomy. 31256-51 is for a surgical nasal/sinus endoscopy, with maxillary antrostomy without maxillary sinus tissue removal; 473.9, chronic sinusitis, is the correct diagnosis.*

B.   *31255, nasal/sinus endoscopy with total ethmoidectomy is the correct code. 31267-51, nasal/sinus endoscopy with maxillary antrostomy with -51 modifier is the correct code; 461.9 acute sinusitis is incorrect. The operative report states that the patient suffers from chronic sinusitis, 473.9.*

D.   *31200 is for ethmoidectomy, intranasal, anterior; 31225-51 is for maxillectomy without orbital exenteration, and 473.9 chronic sinusitis is the correct diagnosis.*

83. Faye, an 88-year-old female, is taken to same-day surgery for a possible small chicken bone stuck in her larynx. The physician does a direct laryngoscopy to check the larynx. On inspection, a small bone fragment is seen obstructing the larynx. The physician using an operating microscope removes the bone fragment. The patient is sent home in satisfactory condition.
A. 31526, 933.1, E915
B. 31531, 933.1, E912
C. 31530, 935.0, E912
D. 31511, 933.1, E912

Correct Answer: B. **31531, laryngoscopy, direct, operative, with foreign body removal with operating microscope; 933.1, foreign body, larynx, is the correct diagnosis. E912 is the external cause code for foreign body obstructing the air passage.**

Rationale: A. *31526 is for a laryngoscopy direct, with or without tracheoscopy diagnostic with operating microscope. 933.1 is the correct diagnosis. E915, the external cause code, states foreign body accidentally entering other orifice; this is not the case in this report.*

C. 31530 is for laryngoscopy, direct, operative, with foreign body removal without operating microscope. 935.0 is a foreign body entering the mouth, this is incorrect. E912 is the correct external cause code.

D. 31511 is for a laryngoscopy, indirect, with removal of foreign body. 933.1 is the correct diagnosis code, and E912 is the correct external cause code (e-code).

84. OPERATIVE REPORT

PREOPERATIVE DIAGNOSIS: Ventilator dependency, aspiration pneumonia

PROCEDURE PERFORMED: Tracheostomy

DESCRIPTION OF PROCEDURE: After consent was obtained, the patient was taken to the operating room and placed on the operating room table in the supine position. After an adequate level of general endotracheal anesthesia was obtained, the patient was positioned for tracheostomy. The patient's neck was prepped with Betadine and then draped in a sterile manner. A curvilinear incision was marked approximately a fingerbreadth above the sternal notch in any area just below the cricoid cartilage. This area was then infiltrated with 1% Xylocaine with 1:100,000 units of epinephrine. After several minutes, sharp dissection was carried down through the skin and subcutaneous tissue. The subcutaneous fat was removed down to the strap muscles. Strap muscles were divided in the midline and retracted laterally. The cricoid cartilage was then identified. The thyroid gland was divided in the midline with the Bovie, and then the two lobes were retracted laterally, exposing the anterior wall of the trachea. The space between the second and third tracheal rings was then identified. This was infiltrated with local solution. A cut was then made through the anterior wall. The endotracheal tube was then advanced superiorly. An inferior cut into the third tracheal ring was then done to make a flap. This was secured to the skin with 4-0 Vicryl suture. A no. 6 Shiley cuffed tracheotomy tube was then placed and secured to the skin with ties as well as the tracheostomy strap. The patient tolerated the procedure well and was taken to the critical care unit in stable condition. Report the procedure(s) and diagnosis.
A. 94656, 60220, 31600-51, 507.0
B. 31500, 31600-51
C. 31600, 507.0
D. 94656, 31502-51, 31600-51, 518.81, 507.0

Correct Answer: C. ***31600 reports a planned tracheostomy, and 507.0 is the correct diagnosis for aspiration pneumonia.***

Rationale: A. *94656 is for the first day of ventilation, although the patient is vent dependent; this is incorrect. 60220 is for a total thyroid lobectomy; this is incorrect. The thyroid was divided and retracted only. 31600 is the correct code for the tracheostomy. The -51 modifier would not be used because a multiple procedure was not done. 507.0 is the correct diagnosis for aspiration pneumonia.*

B. *31500 is for intubation. The patient, however, is already intubated because the patient is on a ventilator; this code is incorrect. 31600-51 is the correct code; however, this was the only procedure done in this case, and so a -51 modifier would not be added to the 31600.*

D. *94656 is incorrect because the patient is vent dependent, and this code is for first day of ventilation. 31502-51 is also incorrect. This code is for a tracheotomy tube change, and the procedure was for a tracheostomy. 31600-51 is the correct code; however, the -51 modifier would not be attached to codes 31502 or 31600 because multiple procedures were not done. 518.81 is the diagnosis for respiratory failure, which the patient is probably in; however, the diagnosis states aspiration pneumonia (507.0) only.*

85. Carl, a 58-year-old male, is taken to the operating room to remove his permanent pacemaker after successfully getting his heart back to normal sinus rhythm.
    A. 33236
    B. 33238
    C. 33243
    D. 33233

Correct Answer: D. ***33233 reports the removal of permanent pacemaker pulse generator.***

Rationale: A. *33236 is for removal of permanent epicardial pacemaker and electrodes.*

B. *33238 is for removal of permanent transvenous electrodes by thoracotomy.*

C. *33243 is for removal of a single- or dual-chamber pacing cardioverter-defibrillator electrode(s) by thoracotomy.*

86. This 70-year-old male is admitted for coronary ASHD. A prior cardiac catheterization showed numerous native vessels to be 70% to 100% blocked. The patient was taken to the operating room. After opening the chest and separating the rib cage, a coronary artery bypass was performed using five venous grafts and four coronary arterial grafts. Code the graft procedure(s) and the diagnosis:
    A. 33536, 33517-51, 414.9
    B. 33533, 33522, 414.05
    C. 33536, 33522, 414.01
    D. 33514, 414

Correct Answer: **C.**   *33536, coronary artery bypass, using arterial graft(s), four or more coronary arterial grafts; 33522, coronary artery bypass, using venous graft(s) and arterial graft(s), five venous grafts (list separately in addition to code for arterial graft); 414.01, coronary arteriosclerotic heart disease of the native vessels.*

Rationale: **A.**   *33536 is correct for the coronary artery bypass, but 33517-51 is for a single venous graft and is modifier exempt; 414.9 is an incorrect diagnosis, as the code reports ischemic heart disease.*

B.   *33533 is for a single arterial graft, 33522 is the correct code for the venous grafts, and 414.05 is incorrect, as it reports an unspecified type of bypass graft.*

D.   *33514 is for a coronary artery bypass, vein only, five coronary venous grafts; 414 is the correct three-digit code, but because a four-digit code is available, you must assign the four-digit code to code the greatest level of specificity.*

87. What code(s) would be used to report an arterial catheterization?
    A. 36600
    B. 36620, 36625
    C. 36620
    D. 3664

Correct Answer: **C.**   *36620 reports an arterial catheterization for sampling, monitoring, or transfusion; percutaneous.*

Rationale: **A.**   *36600, arterial puncture, withdrawal of blood for diagnosis.*

B.   *36620 is the correct code; 36625 is for arterial catheterization, cutdown, however, the procedure was percutaneous.*

D.   *36640 is for arterial catheterization for prolonged infusion therapy, cutdown.*

88. This patient is taken to the operating room for a ruptured spleen. Repair of the ruptured spleen with a partial splenectomy is done.
    A. 38101-58, 38115-51-58, 289.59
    B. 38115, 289.59
    C. 38120, 865.04
    D. 38129, 865.14

Correct Answer: **B.**   *38115 reports the repair of ruptured spleen with or without partial splenectomy. 289.59 is the correct code for a ruptured spleen.*

Rationale: **A.**   *38101-58 is for a staged splenectomy; partial. 38115-51-58 is the correct code; however, the -58 modifier would not be attached to 38101 or 38115 because the procedure does not indicate a staged procedure. Modifier -51 also would not be attached to code 38115, as this was not a multiple procedure. 289.59 is the correct code for a ruptured spleen.*

C.   *38120 is for a laparoscopic splenectomy and the report does not indicate laparoscopic approach. 865.04 is the code for a traumatic ruptured spleen, but traumatic is not stated in the report.*

D.   *38129 is the unlisted laparoscopic procedure of the spleen. 865.14 is the code for a traumatic ruptured spleen with open wound into cavity, which is not stated in the report.*

89. This 60-year-old female was seen previously for a laparoscopic biopsy of her cervical lymph nodes. The biopsy came back showing abnormal cells. The decision was made to do a lymphadenectomy.

    The patient was brought to the operating room and put under general anesthesia. After completing a radical neck dissection, the lymph nodes were excised. The patient was returned to recovery in satisfactory condition. Code the lymphadenectomy only.
    A. 38720, 38570-51
    B. 38720, 38500-51
    C. 38571
    D. 38724

Correct Answer: D.   ***38724 reports a cervical lymphadenectomy (modified radical neck dissection).***
    Rationale: A.   *38720 is for a cervical lymphadenectomy (complete), and 38570-51 is for the laparoscopic biopsy, which was not asked to be coded.*
    B.   *38720 is for a cervical lymphadenectomy (complete), and 38500-51 is for a biopsy of lymph nodes, which was done previously, not in this surgery.*
    C.   *38571 is for a laparoscopy, surgical, with bilateral total pelvic lymphadenectomy. Note: Remember to only code what is asked for.*

90. Connie is brought to the operating room for a diaphragmatic hernia. Transthoracic repair will be done to fix the hernia.
    A. 39520
    B. 39503
    C. 39530
    D. 39540

Correct Answer: A.   ***39520 reports the repair of a diaphragmatic hernia (esophageal hiatal) using a transthoracic approach.***
    Rationale: B.   *39503 is to repair a neonatal diaphragmatic hernia.*
    C.   *39530 is to repair a diaphragmatic hernia; combined, thoracoabdominal.*
    D.   *39540 is to repair a traumatic acute diaphragmatic hernia.*

40,000 Digestive System

91. OPERATIVE REPORT

    PROCEDURE: Excision of parotid tumor or gland or both

    Once the patient was successfully under general anesthetic, Dr. Green, assisted by Dr. Smith, opened the area in which the parotid gland is located. After carefully inspecting the gland, the decision was made to excise the total gland because of the size of the tumor (5.0 cm). With careful dissection and preservation of the facial nerve, the parotid gland was removed. The wound was cleaned and closed, and the patient was brought to recovery in satisfactory condition. Report only Dr. Smith's service.
    A. 42410-80, 11041, 142.0
    B. 42426-62, 210.2
    C. 42420-80, 239.0
    D. 11426, 239.0

Correct Answer: C.   *42420-80 is used to report the total excision of the parotid gland with dissection and preservation of the facial nerve. The cleaning and closure are included in the surgical package for 42420. Modifier -80 is attached to code 42420 to show that the physician served as an assistant surgeon. 239.0 indicates a neoplasm, parotid unspecified. This is the correct diagnosis code. The procedure does not specify the whether the tumor is malignant or benign.*

Rationale: A.   *42410-80 describes excision of only a portion (lateral lobe) of the parotid gland, not excision of the total gland as described in the report. 11041, which describes debridement, cannot be reported with the excision, as any debridement, and closure is bundled into 42410 and not reported separately. Modifier -80 indicates an assistant surgeon, 142.0 (malignant neoplasm, parotid) is incorrect. The report does not state whether the tumor is malignant.*

B.   *42426 is used to report the total removal of the parotid gland (which was done in this case), but the facial nerve is removed and in this case the facial nerve was preserved. Modifier -62 is incorrect. The case states that there was an assistant surgeon, meaning that he or she assisted with the surgery only. Modifier -62 is for two surgeons that complete the surgery together. 210.2 (benign neoplasm, parotid) is incorrect. The report does not state that the tumor is benign.*

D.   *11426 is the removal of a lesion of the skin, not the excision of an internally located tumor. 239.0 is the correct diagnosis.*

92. A 9-year-old boy is in for a tonsillectomy because of chronic tonsillitis and possible adenoidectomy. On inspection of the adenoids they were found not to be inflamed; then we did a tonsillectomy only. Code the tonsillectomy only:
A. 42820, 474.10
B. 42825, 474.00
C. 42830, 42825-51, 474.10
D. 42826, 42835-51, 474.02

Correct Answer: B.   *42825 is a tonsillectomy for a patient under 12 years of age. 474.00 (chronic tonsillitis) is the correct diagnosis code.*

Rationale: A.   *42820 is a tonsillectomy with an adenoidectomy, which was not indicated in the statement of the procedure. The code is for a patient under 12 years of age. 474.10 is the diagnosis for hypertrophy of tonsils and adenoids, but the patient had chronic tonsillitis.*

C.   *42830 is an adenoidectomy for a patient under 12 years of age, but the case indicated a tonsillectomy, not an adenoidectomy. 42525-51 is a tonsillectomy for a patient under age 12, using -51 modifier showing a multiple procedure, which was not done. 474.10 is the diagnosis for hypertrophy of tonsils and adenoids, but the patient had chronic tonsillitis.*

D.   *42826 is used to report a tonsillectomy, but for a patient over 12 years of age, and the patient in the case was under 12 years of age. 42835-51 is used to report a secondary adenoidectomy in a child under 12 years of age using a -51 modifier showing a multiple procedure, which was not done. 474.02 is the diagnosis for chronic tonsillitis and chronic adenoiditis, but the patient only had chronic tonsillitis.*

93. What code would you use to report a rigid proctosigmoidoscopy with guide-wire?
    A. 52260
    B. 45386
    C. 45339
    D. 45303

Correct Answer: D. *45303 is used to report a proctosigmoidoscopy with a guide-wire (dilation).*
    Rationale: A. *52260 is a cystourethroscopy with dilation of the bladder, but the case was for a proctosigmoidoscopy.*
    B. *45386 reports a colonoscopy, but the case was for a proctosigmoidoscopy.*
    C. *45339 is used to report ablation by means of a sigmoidoscopy.*

94. A 62-year-old female presents to Acute Surgical Care for a sigmoidoscopy. The physician inserts a flexible scope into the patient's rectum and determines the rectum is clear of any polyps. The scope is advanced to the sigmoid colon, and a total of three polyps are found. Using the snare technique, the polyps are removed. The remainder of the colon is free of polyps. The flexible scope is withdrawn.
    A. 45383, 211.3
    B. 44110, 153.9
    C. 45338, 211.3
    D. 44111, 153.3

Correct Answer: C. *45338 is a flexible sigmoidoscopy with snare removal of polyp(s). 211.3 is the correct code for polyps of the sigmoid colon. When looking up polyps, colon, in the ICD-9, it states to go to neoplasm, benign by site.*
    Rationale: A. *45383 is a colonoscopy with removal of polyp(s) that cannot be removed with a snare. Snare is the technique used to remove the polyps in this case. 211.3 is the correct diagnosis code.*
    B. *44110 describes removal of lesion(s) through an abdominal incision and then incision into the colon (colotomy), but the procedure described in the case is removal by means of a scope. 153.9 is the code for malignant neoplasm, colon. The report does not state the polyps were malignant.*
    D. *44111 is removal of a lesion(s) through an abdominal incision and then incision into the colon (colotomy), but the procedure described the case was removal by means of a scope. 153.3 is the code for malignant neoplasm, sigmoid colon. This code is also incorrect; the report says nothing about a malignancy.*

95. This patient is in for multiple external hemorrhoids. After inspection of the hemorrhoids, the physician decides to excise all the hemorrhoids.
    A. 46250, 455.3
    B. 46615, 455.0
    C. 46255, 455.3
    D. 46083, 455.5

Correct Answer: A. ***46250 describes the excision of external hemorrhoids. 455.3 is the correct code for external hemorrhoids.***

Rationale: B. *46615 is ablation of tumor, polyp, or other lesions by means of an endoscopy, and the case indicated the patient had external hemorrhoids, which would not require a scope. Also, a hemorrhoid is not a tumor, polyp, or lesion, but rather an engorged vein. 455.0 is the code for internal hemorrhoid, but the report states that the hemorrhoids are external.*

C. *46255 is the removal of internal and external hemorrhoids, but the case indicated only external hemorrhoids. 455.3 is the correct code for external hemorrhoids.*

D. *46083 is the incision of an external hemorrhoid, not an excision, as indicated in the case. 455.5 is a code for external hemorrhoids but with complications, and no complications are stated in the report.*

96. OPERATIVE REPORT

PREOPERATIVE DIAGNOSIS: Barrett's esophagus with severe dysplasia, possible carcinoma

POSTOPERATIVE DIAGNOSIS: Same

PROCEDURE PERFORMED: Exploratory laparotomy, biopsy of liver lesion, immobilization of stomach with pyloroplasty and placement of feeding tube

OPERATIVE NOTE: With the patient under general anesthesia, the abdomen was prepped and draped in a sterile manner. Midline incision was made from the xiphoid to below the pubis. Sharp dissection was carried down into the peritoneal cavity, and hemostasis was maintained with electrocautery. We began by exploring the abdominal cavity. The liver was carefully palpated. The area that had been identified on CT was at the very apex of the right lobe of the liver. We could feel this area, and it did not have a thickened feel to it but was more consistent with an area of hemangioma. There was a small secondary lesion on the undersurface of the right lobe. A biopsy was taken, and it did return a diagnosis of hemangioma. The rest of the liver appeared normal, and in my opinion we did not need to proceed with anything further. We thus began with mobilization of the stomach, taking down the greater curvature vessels, preserving the gastroepiploica. We carried our dissection all the way up into the hiatal hernia, preserving the blood supply to the spleen and not injuring it. We were then able to detach the left gastric artery such that the stomach was tethered on its other vasculature but appeared completely viable. All these vessels were taken down with clamps and ligatures of 2-0 silk. We then circumferentially went around the esophagus and carried our dissection all the back toward the pylorus. We then had the entire stomach freed up from the pylorus all the way up to the diaphragm. The stomach appeared viable with reasonable circulation. A Heineke-Mikulicz pyloroplasty then was performed to open the pylorus in one direction and close it in another using interrupted 3-0 silk sutures to complete the pyloroplasty. With this accomplished, we then picked up the jejunum, approximated 40 or 50 cm beyond the ligament of Treitz, and placed a red rubber feeding tube using a Witzel technique; this was a number 18-2. This was attached to the skin and brought out through a separate stab incision. The abdominal cavity was then checked for hemostasis, and everything appeared to be intact. We then closed the incision using running 0 loop nylon. We closed the skin with staples. A sterile dressing was applied. Code the biopsy of the liver lesion and pyloroplasty only.

A. 49000, 43830-51, 47000-51, 228.00, 150.9
B. 43800, 47001-51, 150.9
C. 43800, 47001
D. 43800, 47001-51

Correct Answer: C. **43800 is used to report a pyloroplasty, and 47001 is correct to report a liver biopsy.**

Rationale: A. *49000 is the code for an exploratory laparotomy, which was not asked to be coded. 43830-51 is the correct code for the pyloroplasty but does not require a -51 modifier. 47001-51 is the correct code for the liver biopsy, but it does not require a -51 modifier because this is an add-on code. 228.00 and 150.9 were not required to code for this case. Note that 150.9 is cancer of the esophagus, but the diagnosis states "possible carcinoma" and outpatient coders do not report possible diagnoses. Note: Remember to only code what you are directed to code when taking a certification examination.*

B. *43800 is the correct code for the pyloroplasty. 47001-51 is the correct code but does not require the -51 modifier because this code is an add-on code. 150.9 was not required to be coded for this report.*

D. *43800 is the correct code for the pyloroplasty. Although 47001-51 is the correct code, the -51 modifier is not required because it is an add-on code.*

97. OPERATIVE REPORT

PREOPERATIVE DIAGNOSIS: Upper gastrointestinal bleeding

POSTOPERATIVE DIAGNOSIS: Multiple serpiginous ulcers in the gastric antrum and body, not bleeding

FINDINGS: The video therapeutic double-channel endoscope was passed without difficulty into the oropharynx. The gastroesophageal junction was seen at 42 cm. Inspection of the esophagus revealed no erythema, ulceration, exudates, stricture, or other mucosal abnormalities. The stomach proper was entered. The endoscope was advanced to the second duodenum. Inspection of the second duodenum, first duodenum, duodenal bulb, and pylorus revealed no abnormalities. Retroflexion revealed no lesion along the cardia or lesser curvature. Inspection of the antrum, body, and fundus of the stomach revealed no abnormality except there were multiple serpiginous ulcerations in the gastric antrum and body. They were not bleeding. They had no recent stigmata of bleeding. Photographs and biopsies were obtained. The patient tolerated the procedure well.

A. 43258, 531.9
B. 43234, 531.30
C. 43239, 531.90
D. 43239, 532.9

Correct Answer: C. **43239 describes an upper gastrointestinal endoscopy to the furthest extent of the duodenum with multiple biopsies obtained. 531.90 is assigned for a gastric ulcer without mention of acute or chronic status and no mention of hemorrhage or perforation. The 5th digit "0" is assigned to indicate without mention of obstruction.**

Rationale: A.   *43258 identifies an endoscopy in which lesions are destroyed (ablation) by means of laser, electrocoagulation, or injection of a substance to dissolve the lesion, but the case indicated that only biopsies were performed. 531.9 is the correct four-digit code, but the 5th digit "0" must be added to indicate without mention of obstruction.*

        B.   *43234 describes a simple endoscopy in which the upper gastrointestinal tract is examined only. 531.30 is assigned to acute gastric ulcer, but the information in the case did not indicate "acute"; therefore, the unspecified as acute or chronic (531.90) is used.*

        D.   *43239 is correctly assigned to indicate the upper gastrointestinal endoscopy to the furthest extent of the duodenum with multiple biopsies obtained. 532.9 describes unspecified as acute or chronic duodenal ulcer, and the case indicated gastric ulcer.*

98. How would you code an excision of a ruptured appendix with generalized peritonitis?
    A. 44970
    B. 44950
    C. 44960
    D. 44960-22

Correct Answer: C.   **44960 describes an appendectomy for a ruptured appendix with generalized peritonitis.**

   Rationale: A.   *44970 describes an appendectomy by means of a laparoscopy.*

        B.   *44950 is used to report an appendectomy without mention of rupture or one that is incidental to another more major procedure.*

        D.   *44960 is the correct code to describe an appendectomy for a ruptured appendix with generalized peritonitis, but modifier -22, unusual procedural service, is not necessary because the case did not state that the service provided was greater than that usually provided.*

99. Kevin is admitted to same-day surgery today for a laparoscopic cholecystectomy.
    A. 47600
    B. 47562, 47550
    C. 47560
    D. 47562

Correct Answer: D.   **47562 describes removal of the gallbladder (cholecystectomy) by means of a laparoscope inserted through the abdominal wall.**

   Rationale: A.   *47600 is an open cholecystectomy, but the procedure indicated in the case was a laparoscopic cholecystectomy.*

        B.   *47562 is correct to describe removal of the gallbladder (cholecystectomy) by means of a laparoscope inserted through the abdominal wall, but the add-on code 47550, intraoperative biliary endoscopy, is a procedure in which the surgeon, during another biliary procedure, inserts an endoscope into the abdominal incision and inspects the biliary tract. This additional inspection was not indicated in the case description.*

        C.   *47560 describes a procedure in which the peritoneal cavity is inspected by laparoscopic means; however, the case indicated the removal of the gallbladder.*

100. INDICATION: Sean is a 2-year-old boy who was born with a cleft lip.

PROCEDURE: This 2-year-old male was taken to the operating room for plastic repair of a unilateral cleft lip.
A. 40701-52, 749.10
B. 40700, 749.10
C. 30460, 749.20
D. 40525, 749.20

Correct Answer: B.   **40700 is assigned to a unilateral plastic repair of a cleft lip. 749.10 is the code for a cleft lip.**

Rationale: A. *40701 describes a procedure that is completed in more than one stage. The use of the modifier -52, reduced service, would be appropriate, as a unilateral repair was performed in more than one stage. 749.10 is the correct code for a cleft lip.*

C. *30460 is a rhinoplasty, not repair of a cleft lip. 749.20 is the code for a cleft lip with a cleft palate, which is incorrect, as only the cleft lip was indicated.*

D. *40525 is full-thickness excision of the lip and reconstruction by means of a flap, but the case indicated plastic repair of a cleft lip. Also, there was no mention of repair by means of a flap. 749.20 is an incorrect diagnosis code. This code is for both a cleft lip and palate. Only the cleft lip had plastic repair.*

SECTION 3

Questions 101-150

50,000

101. OPERATIVE REPORT

DIAGNOSIS: Acute renal insufficiency

PROCEDURE: Renal biopsy

The patient was taken to the operating room for a percutaneous needle biopsy of the right and left kidneys.
A. 49000-50
B. 50555-50
C. 50542-LT, 50542-RT
D. 50200-50

Correct Answer: D.   **50200-50 describes percutaneous renal biopsy of both kidneys by means of a needle.**

Rationale: A. *49000 is an exploratory laparotomy with or without biopsy, but the procedure was stated to be by means of percutaneous biopsy. The bilateral modifier -50 could be used to indicate a right and left procedure, but the -LT and -RT HCPCS modifiers are more specific.*

B. *50555 describes an endoscopic biopsy performed using an established opening (nephrostomy or pyelostomy), but the case indicated a percutaneous biopsy. The bilateral modifier -50 could be used to indicate a right and left procedure, but the -LT and -RT HCPCS modifiers are more specific.*

C. *50542 is assigned when the procedure is a laparoscopic ablation of renal mass, not for a percutaneous renal biopsy. -LT and -RT HCPCS modifiers are correctly used to indicate left and right.*

102. What code(s) would you use to report a biopsy of the bladder?
     A. 52354
     B. 52204
     C. 52224
     D. 52250

Correct Answer: **B.**   **52204 is a biopsy of the bladder by means of a cystourethroscopy (scope inserted into the urethra and into the bladder).**

Rationale: *A.*   *52354 reports a cystourethroscopy with a biopsy of the kidney, not of the bladder as indicated in the case statement.*

C.   *52224 describes a fulguration (destruction of tissue) of the bladder with or without biopsy, and there was no mention of fulguration in the case.*

D.   *52250 describes the insertion of a radioactive substance into the bladder, with or without biopsy, and there was no mention of insertion in the case statement.*

103. OPERATIVE REPORT

DIAGNOSIS: Large bladder neck obstruction

PROCEDURE PERFORMED: Cystoscopy and transurethral resection of the prostate

The patient is a 78-year-old male with obstructive symptoms and subsequent urinary retention. The patient underwent the usual spinal anesthetic, was put in the dorsolithotomy position, prepped, and draped in the usual fashion. Cystoscopic visualization showed a marked high-riding bladder. Median lobe enlargement was such that it was difficult even to get the cystoscope over. Inside the bladder, marked trabeculation was noted. No stones were present.

The urethra was well lubricated and dilated. The resectoscopic sheath was passed with the aid of obturator with some difficulty because of the median lobe. TURP of the median lobe was performed, getting several big loops of tissue, which helped to improve visualization. Anterior resection of the roof was carried out from the bladder neck. Bladder-wall resection was taken from 10 to 8 o'clock. This eliminated the rest of the median lobe tissue as well. The patient tolerated the procedure well. Code the procedure(s) performed and the diagnosis.
     A. 52450, 52001-51, 596.0
     B. 52450, 52001-51, 753.6
     C. 52450, 52000-59, 596.0
     D. 52450, 52000, 753.6

Correct Answer: **C.**   **52450 reports the transurethral incision of the prostate. 52000-59 reports the cystourethroscopy, done independently of the main procedure with modifier -59. 596.0 is for obstruction bladder neck (acquired).**

Rationale: *A.*   *52450 is the correct code for the transurethral incision of the prostate. 52001-51 is the correct code for the cystourethroscopy because it states evacuation of clots that was not done. 596.0 is the correct diagnosis code.*

B.   *52450 reports the transurethral incision of the prostate, which is correct. 753.6 is the code for a congenital obstruction of the bladder neck, which this is a 78-year-old patient, and the report does not state that he has had this condition since birth.*

D.   *52450 reports the transurethral incision of the prostate, which is correct. 52000, although the right code, needs the -51 modifier to indicate a multiple procedure. 753.6 is the code for a congenital obstruction, which the report does not state.*

104. What code(s) would you use to code reconstruction of the penis for straightening of chordee?
   A. 54435
   B. 54328
   C. 54360
   D. 54300

Correct Answer: **D.**   ***54300 describes plastic repair of the penis for straightening of chordee, which is a downward bending of the penis.***

Rationale: A.   *54435 reports the repair of priapism, a condition in which the penis is abnormally erect, not a reconstruction of the penis for straightening of chordee (downward bending of the penis).*

   B.   *54328 is a repair for hypospadias (abnormal opening of the urethra on the underside of the penis) and chordee with use of flaps or grafts or both, not the plastic repair of the penis for straightening of chordee (downward bending of the penis).*

   C.   *54360 designates a plastic repair of an abnormal angulation of the penis, but not for straightening of chordee (downward bending of the penis).*

105. Clamp circumcision of a newborn:
   A. 54160
   B. 54150
   C. 54152
   D. 54161

Correct Answer: **B.**   ***54150 describes a newborn circumcision using a clamp or other device.***

Rationale: A.   *54160 is a circumcision for a newborn with other than a clamp or other device.*

   C.   *54152 is a circumcision using a clamp or other device, but not on a newborn, and the case stated the circumcision was for a newborn.*

   D.   *54161 is a circumcision not using a clamp or other device on other than a newborn patient, but the case stated that the procedure was conducted with a clamp.*

106. Jim is a 42-year-old male in for a bilateral vasectomy that will include three postoperative semen examinations:
   A. 52347 × 3
   B. 52648
   C. 55250
   D. 55250 × 3

Correct Answer: **C.**   ***55250 reports a bilateral vasectomy with postoperative semen examination(s).***

Rationale: A.   *52347 describes a cystourethroscopy with transurethral resection of the ejaculatory ducts; however, the case did not state that a scope was used for the procedure. Also, 52347 includes an inspection of the urethra, which was not indicated in the case.*

   B.   *52648 is a prostate procedure in which a laser is used to perform the procedure, and laser was not mentioned in the case.*

   D.   *55250 is the correct code to report a bilateral vasectomy, but the description indicates that postoperative semen examination(s) is included in the code and therefore not reported separately.*

107. Patient is seen for a Bartholin's gland abscess. The physician incised and drained the abscess.
   A. 56420
   B. 50600
   C. 53060
   D. 56405

Correct Answer: A.   **56420 describes the incision and drainage of the Bartholin's gland.**

Rationale: B.   *50600 is incision into the ureter (ureterotomy), not the incision and drainage of the Bartholin's gland.*

C.   *53060 is incision and drainage of the Skene's gland, not the Bartholin's gland.*

D.   *56405 is incision and drainage of the vulva or perineal abscess, not the Bartholin's gland.*

108. This 21-year-old female is seen at the clinic today for a colposcopy. The physician will take multiple biopsies of the cervix.
   A. 56821
   B. 57421
   C. 57455
   D. 57456

Correct Answer: C.   **57455 correctly reports a colposcopy of the cervix.**

Rationale: A.   *56821 describes a colposcopy of the vulva with biopsy(ies), not of the cervix.*

B.   *57421 is for biopsy(ies) of the vagina and there was no indication that the entire vagina was examined. The parenthetical note that follows 57421 indicates that you are to see codes 57452-57461 for colposcopic examination or biopsy(ies) of the cervix, and because the case you are coding indicates the cervix, you would reference these cervix codes.*

D.   *57456 is examination of the cervix with endocervical curettage (scraping), which was not indicated in the case.*

109. Sarah is a 37-year-old female diagnosed with an ectopic pregnancy. The patient was taken to the operating room for treatment of a tubal ectopic pregnancy, abdominal approach.
   A. 59130
   B. 59150
   C. 59120
   D. 59121

Correct Answer: D.   **59121 describes a surgical treatment of an ectopic pregnancy located in the fallopian tube (which this case was) or in the ovaries; the procedure can be performed either with an abdominal approach or a vaginal approach (which was used in the case).**

Rationale: A.   *59130 is surgical treatment of an abdominal ectopic pregnancy, not a tubal ectopic pregnancy.*

B.   *59150 is a laparoscopic approach for an ectopic pregnancy, not an abdominal approach.*

C.   *59120 reports a surgical treatment of an ectopic pregnancy located in the fallopian tube; however, it includes a salpingectomy (removal of uterine tube) or an oophorectomy (removal of ovary), which this case did not state.*

110. What code(s) do you use to report a cesarean delivery including the postpartum care?
  A. 58611, 59430
  B. 59400
  C. 59515
  D. 59622

Correct Answer: C.   **59515 is used to report a cesarean delivery with postpartum care.**
  Rationale: A.   *58611 is an add-on code used to report a tubal ligation done at the time of cesarean. 59430 reports only the postpartum care after a vaginal delivery.*
  B.   *59400 is routine obstetric care including antepartum care, a vaginal delivery, and postpartum care.*
  D.   *59622 is a cesarean delivery following an attempted vaginal delivery after a previous cesarean delivery and including postpartum care.*

60,000

111. OPERATIVE REPORT

  DIAGNOSIS: Malignant tumor, thyroid

  PROCEDURE: Thyroidectomy, total

  The patient was prepped and draped. The neck area was opened. With careful radical dissection of the neck completed, one could visualize the size of the tumor. The decision was made to do a total thyroidectomy. Note: The pathology report later indicated that the tumor was malignant.
  A. 60240, 193
  B. 60271, 193
  C. 60220, 164.0
  D. 60254, 193

Correct Answer: D.   **60254 is used to report a total thyroidectomy that included a radical neck dissection and one that is performed due to malignancy. 193 is the code for malignant neoplasm of the thyroid gland.**
  Rationale: A.   *60240 is used to report a total thyroidectomy but without radical neck dissection, which was specified in this case ("With careful radical dissection of the neck . . ."). 193 is the correct diagnosis code.*
  B.   *60271 reports a thyroidectomy but not one performed for reason of a tumor, and in this case there was a tumor; so the more specific code is 60254. 193 is the correct diagnosis code.*
  C.   *60220 reports the removal of one lobe of the thyroid and did not include radical neck dissection (which the case specified), nor does this code (60220) include removal of the thyroid due to malignancy (which was specified in the case), nor does this code (60220) include the removal of all of the thyroid (total thyroidectomy). 164.0 is the code for malignant neoplasm of the thymus gland, which is incorrect. The report stated thyroid.*

112. What code(s) would you use to report burr hole(s) to drain an abscess of the brain?
  A. 61253
  B. 61150
  C. 61156
  D. 61151

Correct Answer: B.   ***61150 is used to report the initial drainage of a brain abscess by means of burr holes drilled into the skull to access the brain.***

> *Rationale:* *A.*   *61253 describes infratentorial exploration by means of burr holes in the skull.*
>
> *C.*   *61156 reports aspiration of a hematoma by means of burr holes.*
>
> *D.*   *61151 is used to report a subsequent drainage of an abscess of the brain.*

113. This patient was brought to the operating room to repair an aneurysm of the intracranial artery by balloon catheter:
    A. 61698
    B. 61697
    C. 61710
    D. 61700

Correct Answer: C.   ***61710 describes surgery for an intracranial aneurysm by means of a balloon catheter.***

> *Rationale:* *A.*   *61698 is used to report repair of a basilar artery by means of an open surgical procedure, which involves opening the skull and exposing the interior to the surgeon's view, but the case indicated a balloon catheter as the method of repair.*
>
> *B.*   *61697 is surgery for a complex intracranial aneurysm during an open surgical procedure, which involves opening the skull and exposing the interior to the surgeon's view, but the case indicated a balloon catheter as the method of repair.*
>
> *D.*   *61700 is an open procedure for the simple removal of an intracranial aneurysm, but the case indicated a balloon catheter as the method of repair.*

114. OPERATIVE REPORT

PREOPERATIVE DIAGNOSIS: Obstructed ventriculoperitoneal shunt

PROCEDURE PERFORMED: Revision of shunt. Replacement of ventricular valve and peritoneal end. Entire shunt replacement.

PROCEDURE: Under general anesthesia, the patient's head, neck, and abdomen were prepped and draped in the usual manner. An incision was made over the previous site where the shunt had been inserted in the posterior right occipital area. This shunt was found to be nonfunctioning and was removed. The problem was that we could not get the ventricular catheter out without probably producing bleeding, so it was left inside. The peritoneal end of the shunt was then pulled out through the same incision. Having done this, I placed a new ventricular catheter into the ventricle. I then attached this to a medium pressure bulb valve and secured this with 3-0 silk to the subcutaneous tissue. We then went to the abdomen and made an incision below the previous site, and we were able to trocar the peritoneal end of the shunt by making a stab wound in the neck and then connecting it up to the shunt. This was then connected to the shunt. Pumping on the shunt, we got fluid coming out the other end. I then inserted this end of the shunt into the abdomen by dividing the rectus fascia, splitting the muscle, and dividing the peritoneum and placing the shunt into the abdomen. One 2-0 chromic suture was used around the peritoneum. The wound was then closed with 2-0 Vicryl, 2-0 plain in the subcutaneous tissue, and surgical staples on the skin. The stab wound on the neck was closed with surgical staples. The head wound was closed with 2-0 Vicryl on the galea and surgical staples on the skin. A dressing was applied. The patient was discharged to the recovery room.

A. 63740, 996.2
B. 62256, 996.59
C. 62160, 996.2
D. 62230, 996.2

Correct Answer: D. *62230 reports the replacement of cerebrospinal fluid (CSF) shunt, obstructed valve, or distal catheter in shunt system. 996.2 is mechanical complication of a nervous system device, implant (ventricular shunt).*

Rationale: A. *63740 is used to report the creation of a shunt, not the removal and replacement of a CSF shunt. 996.2 is the correct diagnosis.*

B. *62256 is the removal of a CFS system, but without replacement, which was specified in the case. 996.59 is the code for a mechanical complication of a peritoneal dialysis catheter, which is incorrect. The report states obstructed shunt, which is a complication of a nervous system device or implant.*

C. *62160 reports a neuroendoscopic procedure for placement or replacement of a ventricular catheter that is attached to a shunt system or for external drainage and is an add-on code that cannot be reported alone. 996.2 is the correct diagnosis code.*

115. OPERATIVE REPORT

DIAGNOSIS: Herniated disk

PROCEDURE: Hemilaminectomy L4-5 and L5-S1

The patient was taken to the operating room prepped and draped in the usual fashion. Once the lower back area was opened, after decompression of the nerve roots, the interspace at L4-5 disk was excised. Next the interspace at L5-S1 disk was excised. The patient tolerated the procedure well.

A. 63045, 63048, 722.2
B. 63040, 63043, 839.00
C. 63030, 63035, 722.10
D. 63040, 63043, 722.10

Correct Answer: C. *63030 reports one lumbar interspace (L4-5) repair, 63035 reports each additional lumbar interspace (L5-S1) repair, and 722.10 is used to report displacement of a lumbar intervertebral disk.*

Rationale: A. *63045 reports one cervical interspace repair, and 63048 reports each additional cervical interspace repair, but the case indicated repair of lumbar interspaces. 722.2 is the displacement of an intervertebral disk with an unspecified site, but the site is known in the case as L5-S1 and L4-5.*

B. *63040 reports repair of a cervical interspace, and 63043 reports each additional cervical interspace. 839.00 is cervical dislocation of the spine, not displacement of a lumbar intervertebral disk.*

D. *63040 reports repair of a cervical interspace, and 63043 reports each additional cervical interspace, but the case indicated lumbar interspace repair, not cervical. The diagnosis code 722.10 is correctly used to report displacement of a lumbar intervertebral disk, the condition in this case.*

116. Delores, a 67-year-old female, is seen today for destruction of a lesion of her cornea. The lesion is removed by thermocauterization.
    A. 65400
    B. 65450
    C. 65435
    D. 65410

Correct Answer: **B.**   ***65450 reports destruction of a corneal lesion by means of thermocautery, which was the method used in this case.***

Rationale: A.   *65400 reports the excision of a corneal lesion by means of sharp dissection (blade, forceps, scissors), not thermocautery.*

    C.   *65435 is removal of the corneal epithelium by scraping or cutting.*

    D.   *65410 is biopsy of the cornea, not destruction of a lesion.*

117. What code(s) would you use to code the removal of a foreign body embedded in the eyelid?
    A. 67830
    B. 67413
    C. 67801
    D. 67938

Correct Answer: **D.**   ***67938 reports removal of a foreign body embedded in the eyelid.***

Rationale: A.   *67830 reports correction of ingrown eyelashes by incision of the lid margin.*

    B.   *67413 is removal of a foreign body from the eyeball (orbitotomy), not the eyelid, as indicated in the case*

    C.   *67801 reports the excision of multiple chalazion, which is a small mass on the eyelid that remains inflamed; however, the case indicated that a foreign body was removed from the eyelid, not a mass.*

118. Kristie is a 14-year-old female with a diagnosis of chronic otitis media. The patient was taken to same-day surgery and placed under general anesthesia. Dr. White performed a bilateral tympanostomy with the insertion of ventilating tubes. The patient tolerated the procedure well.
    A. 69421-50, 69433-51, 382.1
    B. 69420-50, 382.4
    C. 69436-50, 382.9
    D. 69436-50, 382.02

Correct Answer: C. *69436-50 is assigned when reporting a tympanostomy performed with general anesthesia. Modifier -50 indicates a bilateral procedure. 382.9 is assigned to indicate unspecified chronic otitis media.*

Rationale: A. *69421-50 is used to report a procedure, using general anesthesia, in which an incision is made in the eardrum and fluid suctioned out, but the procedure in the case was insertion of ventilation tubes with no mention of fluid aspiration. 69433-51 reports insertion of ventilating tubes using local or topical anesthesia, but general anesthesia was indicated in the case; further, -51 is multiple procedures, and this was a bilateral procedure (-50). 382.1 reports chronic tubotympanic suppurative otitis media, which is a condition that includes discharge of pus and perforation of eardrum, and this is not the condition specified in the case (chronic otitis media).*

B. *69420 is a procedure in which an incision is made in the eardrum and fluid is suctioned out, but in the procedure identified in the case, ventilation tubes were inserted and there was no mention of fluid aspiration. 382.4 is unspecified suppurative (discharge of pus) otitis media, but suppurative was not indicated; rather, chronic otitis media was indicated.*

D. *69436-50 is correct; however, the diagnosis code is incorrect because 382.02 is acute suppurative otitis media in disease classified elsewhere and would be reported only with the underlying disease, such as influenza or scarlet fever, being reported first.*

119. Kristie, a 15-year-old female, is seen today for removal of bilateral ventilating tubes that Dr. White inserted 1 year ago.
    A. 69205-50
    B. 69424-79
    C. 69424-50
    D. 69424-50-78

Correct Answer: C. *69424-50 correctly describes the bilateral removal of ventilation tubes. According to third-party payers, you would not report the removal of the ventilating tubes for the same physician who put them in, but on the certification examination, you do not consider what the third-party payers would do—you do not consider reimbursement for any of the coding questions.*

Rationale: A. *69205-50 is for a bilateral foreign body removal; it states that the physician was removing ventilating tubes.*

B. *69424-79 is the correct code, but the -79 modifier is attached to the code when a same physician performs an unrelated procedure during the postoperative period.*

D. *69424-50-78 has the correct code; it has the correct -50 modifier, stating that the procedure was bilateral, but the -78 modifier is incorrect. The -78 modifier is reported when a patient returns to the operating room for a related procedure during the postoperative period.*

120. What code would you use for a revision mastoidectomy resulting in a radical mastoidectomy?
    A. 69502
    B. 69511
    C. 69602
    D. 69603

Correct Answer: D. *69603 reports a revision mastoidectomy (repair of previous procedure) that resulted in a radical mastoidectomy (removal of mastoid and surrounding tissue).*

Rationale: *A.* *69502 is a complete mastoidectomy, which is an excision procedure, not a repair procedure as described in the case statement (revision mastoidectomy).*

B. *69511 is a radical mastoidectomy, which is an excision procedure, not a repair procedure as described in the case statement (revision mastoidectomy).*

C. *69602 is a repair of previous procedure (revision mastoidectomy) resulting in a modified radical mastoidectomy, not as stated in the case "resulting in a radical mastoidectomy."*

70,000 Radiology

121. A 62-year-old male comes into the clinic complaining of shortness of breath. The physician orders a chest x-ray, frontal and lateral.
    A. 71015, 786.09
    B. 71020, 786.05
    C. 71035, 786.9
    D. 71020 × 2, 786.05

Correct Answer: B. *71020 reports a two-view (frontal and lateral) chest x-ray; 786.05 reports shortness of breath.*

Rationale: *A.* *71015 reports a stereo (two-view) frontal x-ray, and the case indicated a two-view x-ray, but one view frontal and one lateral (side). 786.09 is assigned to dyspnea that is not otherwise specified, which is not as specific a code as 786.05, which specifically indicates shortness of breath.*

C. *71035 reports a chest x-ray with special views, such as lateral decubitus, or Bucky studies. 786.9 reports other symptoms involving the respiratory system and chest, such as breath-holding spells, and is not related to shortness of breath, which is indicated in the case.*

D. *71020 is the correct service code for a two-view (frontal and lateral) chest x-ray, but the "2" units is not necessary because the code already specifies two views. 786.05 is the correct diagnosis code for shortness of breath.*

122. A patient is in for an MRI (magnetic resonance imaging) of the pelvis with contrast material(s):
    A. 72125
    B. 72198
    C. 72196
    D. 72159

Correct Answer: C. *72196 correctly reports an MRI of the pelvis with contrast.*

Rationale: *A.* *72125 is a CT (computed tomography) of the cervical spine, not an MRI of the pelvis, with contrast.*

B. *72198 is an MRI of a pelvic artery (angiography) either with or without contrast, not an MRI of the pelvis with contrast.*

D. *72159 is an MRI of an artery (angiography) of the spinal canal and contents, not an MRI of the pelvis with contrast.*

123. What code(s) would you use for an endoscopic catheterization of the biliary ductal system for the professional radiology component only?
    A. 43271, 74328
    B. 74328-26
    C. 74300-26
    D. 74330-26

Correct Answer: B. *74328-26 is an endoscopic catheterization of the biliary ductal system, and modifier -26 is added to indicate the professional component only.*

Rationale: A. *43271 is the surgeon's portion of the service, and the case stated that you were to report only the professional radiology component of the service, not the surgical procedural service. 74328 is the correct code for an endoscopic catheterization of the biliary ductal system but without modifier -26; code 74328 reports both the technical (technician and equipment) portion of the service, and you were to report only the professional (physician) component of the service.*

C. *74300 is an intraoperative radiology service, but the case did not indicate a radiology service during an operative session. Modifier -26 is correct to indicate the professional component of the service.*

D. *74330 is a combination of biliary and pancreatic ductal catheterization, but the case did not indicate pancreatic ductal catheterization. Modifier -26 is correct to indicate the professional component of the service.*

124. Jennifer is a 29-year-old pregnant female in for a follow-up ultrasound with image documentation of the uterus.
    A. 74740
    B. 76816
    C. 74710
    D. 76856

Correct Answer: B. *76816 is an ultrasound of a pregnant uterus with image documentation.*

Rationale: A. *74740 is an x-ray of the uterus and fallopian tubes, but the case indicated ultrasound, not an x-ray.*

C. *74710 is an x-ray of the pelvis, without or without placental location, not an ultrasound.*

D. *76856 is an ultrasound of a nonobstetric pelvis, and the case indicated a pregnant uterus.*

125. What codes would you use for complex brachytherapy isodose calculation for a patient with prostate cancer?
    A. 77776, 184
    B. 77300, 185
    C. 77327-22, 186
    D. 77328, 185

Correct Answer: D. *77328 is used to report a complex brachytherapy isodose plan; 185 indicates a neoplasm of the prostate.*

Rationale: A. *77776 reports the clinical brachytherapy (treatment), not the planning of the therapy as indicated in this case. 184 indicates a malignant neoplasm of the female genital, not the prostate, and requires a 4th digit.*

B. *77300 reports basic radiation dosimetry calculation, not clinical brachytherapy isodose planning. Dosimetry calculations measure the axis depth-dose calculations and nonionizing radiation surface as required during the course of treatment. 185 is the correct diagnosis code.*

C. *77327 is an intermediate brachytherapy plan, but the case indicated a complex calculation. Modifier -22 is used to indicate an unusual service; for example, if there was not a complex calculation code (77328), but a complex service was provided, the addition of modifier -22 would indicate a service over that specified in the code description. 186 is a malignant neoplasm of the testes, not the prostate as indicated in the case, and requires a 4th digit.*

126. Therapeutic radiology treatment planning is the "prescription" for a patient who will start radiation therapy for a cancerous neoplasm of the adrenal gland. What code would you use for a complex treatment planning?
     A. 60540
     B. 77315
     C. 77263
     D. 77401

Correct Answer: C.   *77263 describes a complex clinical treatment plan.*
     Rationale: A.   60540 is the surgical removal of the adrenal gland, not the development of a treatment plan.
     B.   77315 is a complex teletherapy isodose plan, not a complex clinical treatment plan.
     D.   77401 is radiation treatment delivery, not a complex clinical treatment plan.

127. Because of the number of headaches this 50-year-old female had been experiencing, her physician ordered a CT of her head, without contrast materials.
     A. 70450
     B. 70460
     C. 70470
     D. 70496

Correct Answer: A.   *70450 is a CT or computerized axial tomography of the head without contrast.*
     Rationale: B.   70460 is a CT with contrast, and the case indicated without contrast.
     C.   70470 is a CT without contrast but followed by contrast material and further sections, but the case did not indicate that the CT was followed by contrast material and further sections.
     D.   70496 reports a CT of an artery of the head without contrast material, followed by contrast material and further sections, but the case did not indicate the CT was followed by contrast material and further sections.

128. A patient presents to the clinic for a barium enema that was ordered by his physician. Once the patient drinks the barium, the patient will be taken to radiology for a colon x-ray, including KUB.
     A. 74000
     B. 74241
     C. 74270
     D. 74247

Correct Answer: C.   *74270 reports an x-ray of the colon after barium enema and including KUB (kidney, ureters, and bladder).*
     Rationale: A.   74000 is an x-ray of the abdomen, not specifically the colon as indicated in the case.
     B.   74241 is an x-ray of the upper gastrointestinal tract with KUB, but without mention of barium enema and not specifically the colon.
     D.   74247 reports an x-ray of the upper gastrointestinal tract and not specifically the colon.

129. Margie is a 62-year-old female in to see her primary physician with complaints of chest pain and shortness of breath. She has been experiencing these symptoms on and

off for the last 2 months. Her primary physician refers Margie to a cardiologist to consult her about her symptoms.

Dr. Tom, a cardiologist, consults Margie for chest pain and shortness of breath. He performs a comprehensive history and exam; the medical decision making is of moderate complexity. Dr. Tom calls the hospital to set up a tomographic chemical stress test (myocardial perfusion imaging single study at rest). When the test is completed, he will interpret the results. Code the consult, the supervision and interpretation of the stress test, the diagnosis(s), and the radiologist's part of the stress test.

A. 99244-57, 93016, 93018, 78464-26, 786.50, 786
B. 99243, 78460, 786.50, 786.05
C. 99244, 78461-76, 78480-26, 786, 786.05
D. 99244-25, 93016, 93018, 78464-26, 786.50, 786.05

Correct Answer: D.   *99244 reports an office or other outpatient consult with a comprehensive history and examination with moderate medical decision making complexity, and the service is reported with modifier -25 because the patient is having the procedure on the same day as the examination. 93016 and 93018 are the codes for the physician supervising and preparing a report for the stress test. 78464-26 is the radiologist's part of the tomography stress test. 786.50 is the code for chest pain and 786.05 for shortness of breath, and these are the correct diagnosis codes.*

Rationale: A.   *99244-57 is the correct consult code, but the -57 modifier is incorrect. The physician did not make a decision to perform surgery. 93016 and 93018 are the correct codes for the cardiologist supervising and preparing the report for the stress test. 78464-26 is the correct code for the tomography myocardial perfusion imaging, single study with a -26 modifier, in which the radiologist did the interpretation only. 786.50 is the correct diagnosis code for chest pain, but 786 needs all five-digits to be correct. Always code to the furthest specificity, which means you cannot use a three-digit code if a four-digit code is available, and you cannot use a four-digit code if a five-digit one is available.*

B.   *99243 is a consult with detailed history and examination. The medical decision making complexity is low. The physician did a comprehensive history and examination, and the decision making complexity was moderate. 78460 is an incorrect code for a planar stress test, but the physician performed the interpretation, indicating that a -26 modifier must be attached to 78460. 786.50 and 786.05 are the correct diagnosis codes.*

C.   *99244 is the correct code for the consult. 78461-26 is a myocardial perfusion imaging with multiple studies and at rest with interpretation only. 78478-26 is an add-on code, which is listed separately from the primary code 78464-26. 78478-26 indicates that the patient comes back the next day to have additional imaging. 786.05 is the correct diagnosis code for the shortness of breath, but 786 is not correct for the chest pains because a five-digit code is available. Always code to the furthest specificity, which means you cannot use a three-digit code if a four-digit one is available, and you cannot use a four-digit code if a five-digit one is available.*

130. Tina is a patient who suffers from lower back pain. Her physician has ordered an x-ray of her lumbar spine, four views.
A. 72110, 724.2
B. 72074, 724.5
C. 72110, 307.89
D. 72080, 721.42

Correct Answer: A.   *72110 is used to report an x-ray of the lumbosacral spine, four views. 724.2 indicates that the chief complaint is lower back pain because no diagnosis has yet been made and is reported with 724.2 for lumbago, including lower back pain.*

   Rationale: B.   *72074 is the code of the thoracic spine, not of the lumbar spine as indicated in the case statement. 724.5 is an unspecified backache.*

            C.   *72110 is used to report an x-ray of the lumbosacral spine, four views, and is correct; but 307.89 is psychogenic back pain, not the correct diagnosis code.*

            D.   *72080 is a two-view thoracolumbar x-ray of the spine, not the service indicated in the case (four views). 721.42 is spondylosis with myelopathy of the lumbar region, which is not a stated diagnosis in this case.*

80,000 Pathology and Laboratory

131. A patient presents to the laboratory at the clinic for the following tests: thyroid stimulating hormone, comprehensive metabolic panel, and an automated hemogram with manual differential WBC count (CBC). How would you code this lab?
A. 84443, 80053, 85027, 85007
B. 80050
C. 84443
D. 84445, 80051, 85025

Correct Answer: B.   *80050 is a panel code that correctly reports each of the tests performed by the laboratory.*

   Rationale: A.   *84443 (thyroid stimulating hormone), 80053 (comprehensive metabolic panel), 85027 (automated hemogram), and 85007 (manual differential) are the correct codes, but all these codes are listed together as a panel in code 80050, and if a panel code is available, it must be used.*

            C.   *84443 is a thyroid stimulating hormone.*

            D.   *84445 is thyroid stimulating immune globulins, 80051 is an electrolyte panel, and 85025 is a hemogram and platelet count, automated and complete CBC.*

132. An 80-year-old female patient presented to the laboratory for a lipid panel that includes measurement of total serum cholesterol, lipoprotein (direct measurement, HDL), and triglycerides.
A. 82465, 83718, 84478
B. 82465-52, 83718, 84478
C. 80061-52
D. 80061

Correct Answer: D.   *80061 reports a total serum cholesterol, direct lipoprotein, and triglycerides in one panel code.*

   Rationale: A.   *82465, total serum cholesterol; 83718, lipoprotein (direct measurement, HDL); and 84478, triglycerides, are all correct codes, but each can be correctly reported with the use of a panel code (80061) and as such must be used if available.*

            B.   *82465, total serum cholesterol with modifier -52 to indicate a reduced service; 83718, lipoprotein (direct measurement, HDL); and 84478, triglycerides, are all correct codes, but each can be correctly reported with the use of a panel code (80061) and as such must be used if available.*

            C.   *80061 is the correct code, but modifier -52 for a reduced service has no purpose in this case.*

133. Philip has end-stage renal failure and comes to the clinic lab today for his monthly urinalysis (qualitative, microscopic only).
    A. 81015, 586
    B. 81001, 584.9
    C. 81015, 585
    D. 81003, 585

Correct Answer: C. **81015 reports a qualitative microscopic urinalysis, and 585 is assigned to chronic renal failure because end-stage renal failure is a chronic condition.**

   Rationale: A. *81015 is correct for the urinalysis, but 586 reports unspecified renal failure and because end-stage renal failure is a chronic condition, code 585 would be the correct diagnosis code.*

   B. *81001 is an automated urinalysis, but the case indicated a microscopic urinalysis, which is a nonautomated method of inspecting the urine sample. An automated method would include the sample being placed into a machine that would analyze the specimen and generate a report of the analysis. 584.9 is acute renal failure, and end-stage renal failure is a chronic condition.*

   D. *81003: A chemical strip is placed into the urine and the chemical reaction is processed by a machine with a readout of the results, no microscopy performed. 585 is the correct diagnosis code.*

134. This 33-year-old male has been suffering from chronic fatigue. His physician has ordered a TSH test.
    A. 80418, 780.71
    B. 80438, 780.79
    C. 80440, 780.71
    D. 84443, 780.79

Correct Answer: D. **84443 correctly reports a TSH (thyroid stimulating hormone) measurement, and 780.79 is other malaise and fatigue.**

   Rationale: A. *80418 is used to report a pituitary evaluation, not a thyroid stimulating hormone test. 780.71 is chronic fatigue syndrome, and the case did not state that this was a syndrome.*

   B. *80438 is a thyrotropin releasing hormone (TRH) stimulating hormone. 780.79 is correct for the diagnosis of chronic fatigue.*

   C. *80440 is a thyrotropin releasing hormone for hyperprolactinemia, which is not stated in the case. 780.71 is chronic fatigue syndrome, and the case did not state this was a syndrome.*

135. Surgical pathology, gross examination, or microscopic examination is most often required when a sample of an organ, tissue, or body fluid is taken from the body. What code(s) would you use to report biopsy of the colon, hematoma, pancreas, and a tumor of the testis?
    A. 88304, 88304, 88309, 88309
    B. 88305, 88303, 88307, 88309
    C. 88305, 88304, 88307, 88309
    D. 88307, 88304, 88309, 88309

Correct Answer: C.   *88305, colon; 88304, hematoma; 88307, pancreas; and 88309, tumor of testis. Note: Read the description carefully. When coding the biopsy of a tumor of the testis 88309, there is also a code for biopsy of the testis, 88307.*

Rationale: A.   *88304 is incorrect because this code reports colostomy stoma, not colon biopsy; 88304 is correct for hematoma; 88309 is incorrect because this code reports resection of pancreas, not biopsy; 88309 is correct for tumor of testis.*

B.   *88305 is correct for the biopsy of the colon; 88303 is not a valid CPT code; hematoma, is correctly reported with 88304; 88307 is correct for pancreas; 88309 is correct for tumor of testis.*

D.   *88307 is for a resection of the colon, not a biopsy; 88304 is correct for hematoma biopsy; 88309 is the total resection of the pancreas, not a biopsy; 88309 is correct for biopsy of a tumor of the testis.*

136. A patient presents to the clinic laboratory for a prothrombin time measurement because of long-term use of Coumadin.
   A. 85210, V58.62
   B. 85610, V58.61
   C. 85230, V58
   D. 85210, V58.61

Correct Answer: B.   *85610 is located in the index of the CPT under "Prothrombin Time." When referenced in the main portion of the CPT, the code is correct to report the prothrombin time. The test is ordered as a prothrombin, prothrombin time, or PT and is usually used to monitor anticoagulant drugs, which are prescribed to patients with myocardial infarction. V58.61 correctly reports the long-term (current) use of anticoagulants.*

Rationale: A.   *85210 is a clotting factor prothrombin and would be ordered as a prothrombin factor assay, clotting factor, or factor II test. V58.62 is long-term and current use of antibiotics, not long-term and current use of the anticoagulant Coumadin.*

C.   *85230 is a factor VII assay or a clotting factor VII assay and is not a prothrombin time. V58 must be reported with fourth or fifth digits if available; V58 does have both fourth and fifth digits available.*

D.   *85210 is a clotting factor prothrombin and would be ordered as a prothrombin factor assay, clotting factor, or factor II test. V58.61 correctly reports the long-term (current) use of anticoagulants.*

137. The patient presented to the laboratory at the clinic for the following blood tests ordered by her physician: albumin (serum), bilirubin (total), and BUN (quantitative):
   A. 82044, 82248, 84520
   B. 82040, 82252, 84525
   C. 82040, 82247, 84520
   D. 82044, 82247, 84540

Correct Answer: C. ***82040 reports the serum albumin, 82247 reports the total bilirubin, and 84520 reports the BUN (blood urea nitrogen).***

Rationale: A. *82044 reports an albumin using urine as the sample rather than blood as indicated in the case. 82248 is used to report a direct bilirubin rather than the total bilirubin indicated. 84520 is correct for the BUN.*

B. *82040 is correct for the albumin, 82252 reports a qualitative fecal bilirubin, not the total bilirubin indicated in the case, and 84525 reports a semiquantitative BUN, not the quantitative BUN specified.*

D. *82044 reports a semiquantitative microalbumin by means of urine, 82247 is correct for the total bilirubin, and 84540 is a urea nitrogen by means of urine.*

138. A 70-year-old male who suffers from atrial fibrillation has been on long-term use of digoxin. He comes into the lab today to have a quantitative drug assay performed for digoxin:
    A. 80100
    B. 80102
    C. 80299
    D. 80162

Correct Answer: D. ***80162 is the correct code for digoxin and can be located in the index of the CPT manual under the main term Digoxin.***

Rationale: A. *80100 is a qualitative drug-screening code to identify only the presence of a drug, not a quantitative (amount of drug present) test as indicated in the case.*

B. *80102 is a drug-screening code to identify only the presence of the drug, not a quantitative (amount of drug present) test as indicated in the case.*

C. *80299 is used to report the amount of a drug, but a drug for which there is no more specific code, and because 80160 specifies digoxin that code is correct.*

139. This 68-year-old female suffers from chronic liver disease and needs a hepatic function panel performed every 6 months. Tests include total bilirubin (82247), direct bilirubin (82248), total protein (84155), alanine aminotransferases [ALT and SGPT] (84460), aspartate aminotransferases [AST and SGOT] (84450), and what other lab tests?
    A. 80061, 83718
    B. 82040, 82247
    C. 84295, 84450
    D. 82040, 84075

Correct Answer: D. ***Hepatic function panel code is 80076 and also includes albumin, 82040, as well as 84075 for alkaline phosphatase.***

Rationale: A. *80061 is a lipid panel and is not included in a hepatic function panel; 83718 is a lipoprotein and is not included in a hepatic function panel, 80076.*

B. *82040 is for albumin and is also included in a hepatic function panel. 82247 is bilirubin and was stated in the question as having been included in the hepatic function.*

C. *84295 is for sodium and is not in the hepatic function panel; 84450 is transferase, aspartate amino, and is already included in the question as being a part of the hepatic function.*

140. Edgar is status post kidney transplant and comes into the clinic lab for a follow-up creatinine clearance:
  A. 82540, V42.0
  B. 82575, V42.0
  C. 82565, 586
  D. 82570, 585

Correct Answer: B.   **82575 is a creatinine clearance, which was the test ordered, and measures the serum creatinine in urine, which indicates the kidney filtration function. V42.0 reports the kidney transplantation as a condition influencing health status.**

Rationale: A.   *82540 reports creatine not creatinine clearance. V42.0 correctly reports the kidney transplantation as a condition influencing health status.*

       C.   *82565 reports a blood creatinine. 586 reports unspecified renal failure; the patient is no longer in renal failure due to his kidney transplant. The creatinine clearance is ordered to check the transplanted kidney in this instance.*

       D.   *82570 reports creatinine from other source and is not a clearance. 585 reports chronic renal failure, and the patient no longer has renal failure due to kidney transplant. The reason a physician orders this lab is to make sure the patient is not having any type of renal insufficiency or failure.*

90,000 Medicine

141. An elderly male comes in for his flu (split virus, IM) and pneumonia (23-valent, IM) vaccines. Code only the immunization administration and diagnoses for the vaccines:
  A. 90471, 90658, 90472, 90732, V04.8, V03.82
  B. 90471 × 2, 90658, 90732, V04.8
  C. 90471, 90472, V04.8, V03.82
  D. 90658, 90732, V05.8, V04.8

Correct Answer: C.   **90471 reports the first administration. 90472 reports the second administration and for the diagnoses V04.8, influenza vaccination; V03.82, pneumococcal vaccination.**

Rationale: A.   *90471 and 90472 report the first and second administration and are correct. 90658 reports the vaccine, whole-vaccine IM, but the directions indicated to code only the administration and diagnoses and did not direct the report of the vaccine substance. 90732 is the pneumococcal vaccine (23-valent), but again the directions did not indicate to code the vaccine substance, but rather the administration and diagnoses only.*

       B.   *90471 is not used with units (-2) but rather is used only to report the first administration. 90658 reports the vaccine, split-vaccine IM, but the directions indicated to code only the administration and diagnoses and did not direct the report of the vaccine substance. 90732 is the pneumococcal vaccine (23-valent), but again the directions did not indicate to code the vaccine substance, but rather the administration and diagnoses only. V04.8 reports only the influenza vaccination code. This answer is missing the V03.82 used to report the pneumococcal vaccination.*

       D.   *90658 reports the vaccine, split-vaccine IM, but the directions indicated to code only the administration and diagnoses and did not direct the report of the vaccine substance. 90732 is the pneumococcal vaccine (23-valent), but again the directions did not indicate to code the vaccine substance, but rather the administration and diagnoses only. V05.8 is used to report vaccination for and other specified disease and is not correct when a more specific code (V03.82) is available to report the pneumococcal vaccination. V04.8 correctly reports the influenza vaccination code.*

142. Code the substance of DTP given intramuscularly:
    A. 90700, 90471
    B. 90702
    C. 90701, 90471
    D. 90701

Correct Answer: D.   *90701 correctly reports only the substance given—DTP (diphtheria, tetanus, and pertussis)—not the administration.*
    Rationale: A.   *90700 is DTaP or diphtheria, tetanus toxoids, and acellular pertussis vaccine. 90471 is an administration code, but the question did not specify that you were to code the administration, and so this code is not required.*
    B.   *90702 is used to report diphtheria and tetanus toxoids (DT).*
    C.   *90701 is correct for the DTP. 90471 is an administration code, but the question did not specify that you were to code the administration, and so this code is not correct.*

143. Katie is a 9-year-old female who comes into the clinic to have her first ophthalmological exam. The exam was intermediate.
    A. 99203
    B. 92002
    C. 92002, 99203
    D. 92004

Correct Answer: B.   *92002 is correct to report an intermediate ophthalmological examination for a new patient.*
    Rationale: A.   *99203 is an E/M code for a new patient for an office or other outpatient service, but it is not used to report an ophthalmological examination.*
    C.   *92002 is correct for a new patient for an intermediate ophthalmological examination, but the E/M code to report an office or other outpatient service is not necessary.*
    D.   *92004 is an ophthalmological examination but at a comprehensive level, and the case indicated an intermediate level of service.*

144. Katie is back for a 2-year follow-up comprehensive ophthalmological exam. The physician gives her contact lenses. She is to follow-up in 1 week to see how her contacts are working. Code the exam and the supply of contact lenses.
    A. 92014, 92391
    B. 92391
    C. 92014, 92396
    D. 92014, 92393

Correct Answer: A.   *92014 reports a comprehensive ophthalmological service for an established patient. 92391 reports the supply of the contact lenses.*
    Rationale: B.   *92391 is correct for the supply of the contact lenses, but you also need a code for the examination (92014).*
    C.   *92014 is the correct code for the examination, but 92396 is dispensing of contact lenses for a patient who has had an eyeball removed.*
    D.   *92014 is correct to report the comprehensive examination, but 92393 is supply of an artificial eye.*

145. This 70-year-old male is taken to the emergency room with severe chest pain. The physician provided an expanded problem-focused history and examination. While the physician is examining the patient, his pressures drop and he goes into cardiac arrest. Cardiopulmonary resuscitation is given to the patient, and his pressure returns to normal; he is transferred to the intensive care unit in critical condition. Code the cardiopulmonary resuscitation and the diagnosis. The medical decision making was of low complexity.
    A. 99282, 92950, 427.5
    B. 99238, 92970, 427.5
    C. 92950, 427.5
    D. 92960, 427.5

Correct Answer: C.   *92950, correctly reports only the cardiopulmonary resuscitation. 427.5 is the code for cardiac arrest.*
   Rationale: A.   *99282 is incorrect because the question directed you to code only the cardiopulmonary resuscitation. 92950 is correct, however, for the cardiopulmonary resuscitation. 427.5 is coded correctly.*
            B.   *99283 is incorrect because the question directed you to code only the cardiopulmonary resuscitation. 92970 is used to report cardioassist method of circulatory assist, internal, and was not specified in the case. 427.5 is the correct diagnosis for cardiac arrest.*
            D.   *92960 is cardioversion that is performed on an elective basis, and the case indicated CPR, not cardioversion. 427.5 is the correct diagnosis code.*

146. The patient is taken to the operating room for insertion of a Swan-Ganz catheter. The physician inserts the catheter for monitoring cardiac output measurements and blood gases.
    A. 36013, 93503
    B. 36013
    C. 93508
    D. 93503

Correct Answer: D.   *93503 is correct for insertion of a Swan-Ganz catheter. A Swan-Ganz is a catheter that is inserted into the right side of the heart to monitor blood pressure, take blood samples, and perform other tests. The code is initially located in the CPT index under the main term catheter.*
   Rationale: A.   *36013 is a catheterization of the right side of the heart, but in this case the insertion was for a Swan-Ganz, which can be reported with 93503 alone.*
            B.   *36013 is a catheterization of the right side of the heart, but in this case the insertion was for a Swan-Ganz, which is reported with 93503.*
            C.   *93508 is used to report insertion of a catheter into a coronary artery for angiography without left-sided heart catheterization and is not the service identified in the case.*

147. Dr. Green orders a sleep study for Dan, a 51-year-old male who has been diagnosed with obstructive sleep apnea. The sleep study will be done with C-PAP (continuous positive airway pressure).
    A. 95806, 786.03
    B. 95807, 780.53
    C. 95811, 780.57
    D. 95806, 780.57

Correct Answer: **C.** *95811 reports a polysomnography with a continuous positive airway pressure. 780.57 reports the sleep disturbance of "Other and unspecified sleep apnea."*

Rationale: **A.** *95806 reports a sleep study that is done at the same time as a ventilation, respiratory effort, ECG, heart rate, or oxygen saturation, unattended by a technician, which was not indicated in the case. 786.03 reports apnea but excludes sleep apnea (see the Excludes note that follows 786.03).*

B. *95807 reports a sleep study done at the same time as a ventilation, respiratory effort, ECG, heart rate, or oxygen saturation, attended by a technician, which was not indicated in the case. 780.53 reports hypersomnia with sleep apnea, which is an excess need for sleep in addition to sleep apnea, which was not indicated in the case.*

D. *95806 reports a sleep study that is done at the same time as a ventilation, respiratory effort, ECG, heart rate, or oxygen saturation, unattended by a technician, which was not indicated in the case. 780.57 reports the sleep disturbance of "Other and unspecified sleep apnea."*

148. Ann is a 58-year-old female with end-stage renal failure. She receives dialysis Tuesdays, Thursdays, and Saturdays each week. Code a full month of dialysis for the month of December.
     A. 90918, 593.9
     B. 90921, 585
     C. 90921-52, 585
     D. 90935, 586

Correct Answer: **B.** *90921 correctly reports a full month of end-stage renal disease (ESRD) for a patient 20 years of age or older, and 585 correctly reports chronic renal failure/end-stage renal failure.*

Rationale: **A.** *90918 correctly reports a full month of end-stage renal disease but for a patient under 2 years of age. 593.9 reports unspecified disorder of kidney and ureter, which is incorrect. The case states the patient has end-stage renal failure.*

C. *90921-52 correctly reports the full month of dialysis; however, the -52 modifier is attached, telling you to reduce the services, which is incorrect. 585 correctly reports end-stage renal failure.*

D. *90935 reports hemodialysis procedure with a single physician evaluation, most commonly used in the inpatient setting. 586 is reported incorrectly. This code is for unspecified chronic renal failure. The case specifies end-stage renal failure.*

149. OPERATIVE REPORT

PROCEDURE PERFORMED: Primary stenting of 70% proximal posterior descending artery stenosis

INDICATIONS: Atherosclerotic heart disease

DESCRIPTION OF PROCEDURE: Please see the computer report. Please note that a 2.5 × 13-mm pixel stent was deployed.

COMPLICATIONS: None

RESULTS: Successful primary stenting of 70% proximal posterior descending artery stenosis with no residual stenosis at the end of the procedure.
A. 92980-RC, 92981, 414.01
B. 92982-RC, 414.9
C. 92980-RC, 413.9
D. 92980-RC, 414.01

Correct Answer: D.   ***92980 correctly reports insertion of a coronary stent. To find the stent procedure in your CPT correctly, go to "Insertion" in the index and look for stent, coronary. It is also known as a transcatheter placement of an intracoronary stent. 414.01 correctly identifies atherosclerotic heart disease.***

Rationale: A.   *92980 correctly reports the stenting; however, 92981 is listed in addition to code for primary procedure. This code is to list each additional vessel, but the case states that only one vessel was stented. 414.01 is the code atherosclerotic heart disease, which is correct.*

B.   *92982 is to report a percutaneous transluminal coronary balloon angioplasty: single vessel. Only a stent was performed, and no mention was made of balloon angioplasty. 414.9 is the incorrect code because it reports unspecified ischemic heart disease.*

C.   *92980 correctly reports the insertion of a coronary stent. 413.9 is an incorrect diagnosis code.*

150. Dr. Barrette is a neurosurgeon who has taken Betty, a 42-year-old female, with a diagnosis of carotid stenosis, to the operating room to perform a thromboendarterectomy, unilateral. During the surgery, the patient is monitored by electroencephalogram (EEG). Code the monitoring only:
A. 35301, 95955, 433.10
B. 35301-50, 433.30
C. 95955, 433.10
D. 95955

Correct Answer: D.   ***95955 reports an EEG (electroencephalogram). No other codes should have been listed.***

Rationale: A.   *35301 reports the thromboendarterectomy; however, you were asked to code only the monitoring. 95955 correctly reports the EEG. Although 433.10 is the correct diagnosis, you were only asked to code the monitoring.*

B.   *35301-50 reports a bilateral thromboendarterectomy. The case states unilateral; however, you were to code only the monitoring, 95955. 433.30 is the diagnosis code for bilateral stenosis, which is incorrectly coded for this case and was not required to be coded.*

C.   *95955 correctly reports the monitoring. Although 433.10 is the correct diagnosis, you were asked to code only the monitoring.*

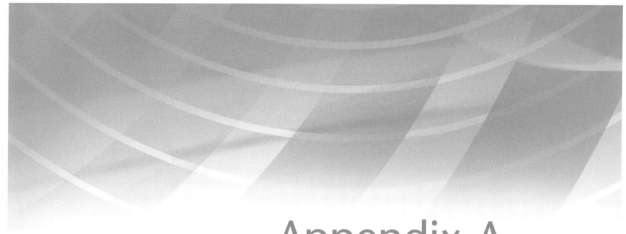

Appendix A

*ICD-9-CM Official Guidelines
for Coding and Reporting*

Effective October 1, 2002

The Centers for Medicare and Medicaid Services (CMS) formerly the Health Care Financing Administration (HCFA) and the National Center for Health Statistics (NCHS), two departments within the Department of Health and Human Services (DHHS) present the following guidelines for coding and reporting using the International Classification of Diseases, 9th Revision, Clinical Modification (ICD-9-CM). These guidelines should be used as a companion document to the official version of the ICD-9-CM as published on CD-ROM.

These guidelines for coding and reporting have been developed and approved by the Cooperating Parties for ICD-9-CM: the American Hospital Association, the American Health Information Management Association, CMS, and the NCHS. These guidelines, published by the Department of Health and Human Services have also appeared in the Coding Clinic for ICD-9-CM, published by the American Hospital Association.

These guidelines have been developed to assist the user in coding and reporting in situations where the ICD-9-CM does not provide direction. Coding and sequencing instructions in volumes I, II, and III of ICD-9-CM take precedence over any guidelines. The conventions, general guidelines and chapter-specific guidelines apply to the proper use of ICD-9-CM, regardless of the health care setting. A joint effort between the attending physician and coder is essential to achieve complete and accurate documentation, code assignment, and reporting of diagnoses and procedures. These guidelines have been developed and approved by the Cooperating Parties to assist both the physician and the coder in identifying those diagnoses that are to be reported. The importance of consistent, complete documentation in the medical record cannot be overemphasized. Without such documentation the application of all coding guidelines is a difficult, if not impossible, task.

These guidelines are not exhaustive. The cooperating parties are continuing to conduct reviews of these guidelines and develop new guidelines as needed. Users of the ICD-9-CM should be aware that only guidelines approved by the cooperating parties are official. Revision of these guidelines and new guidelines will be published by the U.S. Department of Health and Human Services when they are approved by the cooperating parties. The term "admitted" is used generally to mean a health care encounter in any setting.

The guidelines have been reorganized into several new sections including an enhanced introduction that provides more detail about the structure and conventions of the classification usually found in the classification itself. The other new section, General Guidelines, brings together overarching guidelines that were previously found throughout the various sections of the guidelines. The new format of the guidelines also includes a resequencing of the disease-specific guidelines. They are sequenced in the same order as they appear in the tabular list chapters (Infectious and Parasitic diseases, Neoplasms, etc.)

These changes will make it easier for coders, experienced and beginners, to more easily find the specific portion of the coding guideline information they seek.

Table of Contents

C. Chapter-specific Guidelines

   C1. Infectious and Parasitic diseases

      A. Human Immunodeficiency Virus (HIV) Infections

         Asymptomatic HIV Infection

         Confirmed Cases of HIV Infection/Illness

         HIV Infection in Pregnancy, Childbirth and the Puerperium

         Inconclusive Lab Test for HIV

         Previously Diagnosed HIV-related Illness

         Selection and Sequencing of HIV Code

         Testing for HIV

      B. Septicemia and Shock

   C2. Neoplasms

   C3. Endocrine, Nutritional, and Metabolic Diseases and Immunity Disorders

      Reserved for future guidelines expansion

   C4. Diseases of Blood and Blood Forming Organs

      Reserved for future guideline expansion

   C5. Mental Disorders

      Reserved for future guideline expansion

   C6. Diseases of Nervous System and Sense Organs

      Reserved for future guideline expansion

   C7. Diseases of Circulatory System

      A. Hypertension

         Controlled Hypertension

         Elevated Blood Pressure

         Essential Hypertension

         Hypertension with Heart Disease

         Hypertensive Cerebrovascular Disease

         Hypertensive Heart and Renal Disease

         Hypertensive Renal Disease with Chronic Renal Failure

         Hypertensive Retinopathy

         Secondary Hypertension

         Transient Hypertension

         Uncontrolled Hypertension

      B. Late Effect of Cerebrovascular Accident

   C8. Diseases of Respiratory System

      Reserved for future guideline expansion

SECTION I CONVENTIONS, GENERAL CODING GUIDELINES AND CHAPTER-SPECIFIC GUIDELINES

The conventions, general guidelines and chapter-specific guidelines are applicable to all health care settings unless otherwise indicated.

A. Conventions for the ICD-9-CM

The conventions for the ICD-9-CM are the general rules for use of the classification independent of the guidelines. These conventions are incorporated within the index and tabular of the ICD-9-CM as instructional notes. The conventions are as follows:

1. Format: The ICD-9-CM uses an indented format for ease in reference

2. Abbreviations

   a. Index Abbreviations

      NEC "Not elsewhere classifiable"

      This abbreviation in the index represents "other specified" When a specific code is not available for a condition the index directs the coder to the "other specified" code in the tabular.

   b. Tabular Abbreviations

      NEC "Not elsewhere classifiable"

      This abbreviation in the tabular represents "other specified" When a specific code is not available for a condition the tabular includes an NEC entry under a code to identify the code as the "other specified" code. (see "Other" codes)

      NOS "Not otherwise specified" This abbreviation is the equivalent of unspecified. (see "Unspecified" codes)

3. Punctuation

   [ ] Brackets are used in the tabular list to enclose synonyms, alternative wording or explanatory phrases. Brackets are used in the index to identify manifestation codes. (see etiology/manifestations)

   ( ) Parentheses are used in both the index and tabular to enclose supplementary words which may be present or absent in the statement of a disease or procedure without affecting the code number to which it is assigned. The terms within the parentheses are referred to as nonessential modifiers.

: Colons are used in the Tabular list after an incomplete term which needs one or more of the modifiers following the colon to make it assignable to a given category.

4. Includes and Excludes Notes and Inclusion terms

Includes: This note appears immediately under a three-digit code title to further define, or give examples of, the content of the category.

Excludes: An excludes note under a code indicate that the terms excluded from the code are to be coded elsewhere. In some cases the codes for the excluded terms should not be used in conjunction with the code from which it is excluded. An example of this is a congenital condition excluded from an acquired form of the same condition. The congenital and acquired codes should not be used together. In other cases, the excluded terms may be used together with an excluded code. An example of this is when fractures of different bones are coded to different codes. Both codes may be used together if both types of fractures are present.

Inclusion terms: List of terms are included under certain four and five digit codes. These terms are the conditions for which that code number is to be used. The terms may be synonyms of the code title, or, in the case of "other specified" codes, the terms are a list of the various conditions assigned to that code. The inclusion terms are not necessarily exhaustive. Additional terms found only in the index may also be assigned to a code.

5. Other and Unspecified codes

a. "Other" codes

Codes titled "other" or "other specified" (usually a code with a 4th digit 8 or fifth-digit 9 for diagnosis codes) are for use when the information in the medical record provides detail for which a specific code does not exist. Index entries with NEC in the line designate "other" codes in the tabular. These index entries represent specific disease entities for which no specific code exists so the term is included within an "other" code.

b. "Unspecified" codes

Codes (usually a code with a 4th digit 9 or 5th digit 0 for diagnosis codes) titled "unspecified" are for use when the information in the medical record is insufficient to assign a more specific code.

6. Etiology/manifestation convention ("code first", "use additional code" and "in diseases classified elsewhere" notes)

Certain conditions have both an underlying etiology and multiple body system manifestations due to the underlying etiology. For such conditions the ICD-9-CM has a coding convention that requires the underlying condition be sequenced first followed by the manifestation. Wherever such a combination exists there is a "use additional code" note at the etiology code, and a "code first" note at the manifestation code. These instructional notes indicate the proper sequencing order of the codes, etiology followed by manifestation.

In most cases the manifestation codes will have in the code title, "in diseases classified elsewhere." Codes with this title are a component of the etiology/manifestation convention. The code title indicates that it is a manifestation code. "In diseases classified elsewhere" codes are never permitted to be used as first listed or principal diagnosis codes. They must be used in conjunction with an underlying condition code and they must be listed following the underlying condition.

There are manifestation codes that do not have "in diseases classified elsewhere" in the title. For such codes a "use additional code" note will still be present and the rules for sequencing apply.

In addition to the notes in the tabular, these conditions also have a specific index entry structure. In the index both conditions are listed together with the etiology code first followed by the manifestation codes in brackets. The code in brackets is always to be sequenced second.

The most commonly used etiology/manifestation combina-tions are the codes for Diabetes mellitus, category 250. For each code under category 250 there is a use additional code note for the manifestation that is specific for that particular diabetic manifestation. Should a patient have more than one manifesta-tion of diabetes more than one code from category 250 may be used with as many manifestation codes as are needed to fully describe the patient's complete diabetic condition. The 250 diabetes codes should be sequenced first, followed by the manifestation codes.

"Code first" and "Use additional code" notes are also used as sequencing rules in the classification for certain codes that are not part of an etiology/manifestation combination. See—Other multiple coding for a single condition in the General Guidelines section.

B. General Coding Guidelines

1. Use of Both Alphabetic Index and Tabular List

   Use both the Alphabetic Index and the Tabular List when locating and assigning a code. Reliance on only the Alphabetic Index or the Tabular List leads to errors in code assignments and less specificity in code selection.

2. Locate each term in the Alphabetic Index and verify the code selected in the Tabular List. Read and be guided by instructional notations that appear in both the Alphabetic Index and the Tabular List.

3. Level of Detail in Coding

   Diagnosis and procedure codes are to be used at their highest number of digits available.

   ICD-9-CM diagnosis codes are composed of codes with 3, 4, or 5 digits. Codes with three digits are included in ICD-9-CM as the heading of a category of codes that may be further subdivided by the use of fourth and/or fifth digits, which provide greater detail.

   A three-digit code is to be used only if it is not further subdivided. Where fourth-digit subcategories and/or fifth-digit subclassifications are provided, they must be assigned. A code is invalid if it has not been coded to the full number of digits required for that code. For example, Acute myocardial infarction, code 410, has fourth digits that describe the location of the infarction (e.g., 410.2, Of inferolateral wall), and fifth digits that identify the episode of care. It would be incorrect to report a code in category 410 without a fourth and fifth digit.

   ICD-9-CM Volume 3 procedure codes are composed of codes with either 3 or 4 digits. Codes with two digits are included in ICD-9-CM as the heading of a category of codes that may be further subdivided by the use of third and/or fourth digits, which provide greater detail.

4. The appropriate code or codes from 001.0 through V83.89 must be used to identify diagnoses, symptoms, conditions, problems, complaints or other reason(s) for the encounter/visit.

5. The selection of codes 001.0 through 999.9 will frequently be used to describe the reason for the admission/encounter. These codes are from the section of ICD-9-CM for the classification of diseases and injuries (e.g., infectious and parasitic diseases; neoplasms; symptoms, signs, and ill- defined conditions, etc.).

6. Codes that describe symptoms and signs, as opposed to diagnoses, are acceptable for reporting purposes when a related definitive diagnosis has not been established (confirmed) by the physician. Chapter 16 of ICD-9-CM, Symptoms, Signs, and Ill-defined conditions (codes 780.0-799.9) contain many, but not all codes for symptoms.

7. Conditions that are an integral part of a disease process

   Signs and symptoms that are integral to the disease process should not be assigned as additional codes.

8. Conditions that are not an integral part of a disease process

   Additional signs and symptoms that may not be associated routinely with a disease process should be coded when present.

9. Multiple coding for a single condition

   In addition to the etiology/manifestation convention that requires two codes to fully describe a single condition that affects multiple body systems, there are other single conditions that also require more than one code. "Use additional code" notes are found in the tabular at codes that are not part of an etiology/manifestation pair where a secondary code is useful to fully describe a condition. The sequencing rule is the same, "use additional code" indicates that a secondary code should be added.

   For example, for infections that are not included in chapter 1, a secondary code from category 041, Bacterial infection in condi-tions classified elsewhere and of unspecified site, may be required to identify the bacterial organism causing the infection. A "use additional code" note will normally be found at the infection code indicates a need for the organism code to be added as a secondary code.

   "Code first" notes are also under certain codes that are not specifically manifestation codes but may be due to an underlying cause. When a "code first" note is present and an underlying condition is present the underlying condition should be sequenced first.

   "Code, if applicable, any causal condition first", notes indicate that this code may be assigned as a principal diagnosis when the causal condition is unknown or not applicable. If a causal condition is known, then the code for that condition should be sequenced as the principal or first-listed diagnosis.

   Multiple codes may be needed for late effects, complication codes and obstetric codes to more fully describe a condition. See the specific guidelines for these conditions for further instruction.

10. Acute and Chronic Conditions

   If the same condition is described as both acute (subacute) and chronic, and separate subentries exist in the Alphabetic Index at the same indentation level, code both and sequence the acute (subacute) code first.

11. Combination Code

A combination code is a single code used to classify:
two diagnoses, or
A diagnosis with an associated secondary process (manifestation) A diagnosis with an associated complication.

Combination codes are identified by referring to subterm entries in the Alphabetic Index and by reading the inclusion and exclusion notes in the Tabular List.

Assign only the combination code when that code fully identi-fies the diagnostic conditions involved or when the Alphabetic Index so directs. Multiple coding should not be used when the classification provides a combination code that clearly identifies all of the elements documented in the diagnosis. When the combination code lacks necessary specificity in describing the manifestation or complication, an additional code may be used as a secondary code.

12. Late Effects

A late effect is the residual effect (condition produced) after the acute phase of an illness or injury has terminated. There is no time limit on when a late effect code can be used. The residual may be apparent early, such as in cerebrovascular accident cases, or it may occur months or years later, such as that due to a previous injury. Coding of late effects generally requires two codes sequenced in the following order: The condition or nature of the late effect is sequenced first. The late effect code is sequenced second.

An exception to the above guidelines are those instances where the code for late effect is followed by a manifestation code identified in the Tabular List and title, or the late effect code has been expanded (at the fourth and fifth-digit levels) to include the manifestation(s). The code for the acute phase of an illness or injury that led to the late effect is never used with a code for the late effect.

13. Impending or Threatened Condition

Code any condition described at the time of discharge as "impending" or "threatened" as follows:

If it did occur, code as confirmed diagnosis.

If it did not occur, reference the Alphabetic Index to determine if the condition has a subentry term for "impending" or "threatened" and also reference main term entries for "Impending" and for "Threatened."

If the subterms are listed, assign the given code. If the subterms are not listed, code the existing underlying condition(s) and not the condition described as impending or threatened.

C. Chapter-Specific Coding Guidelines

In addition to general coding guidelines, there are guidelines for specific diagnoses and/or conditions in the classification. Unless otherwise indicated, these guidelines apply to all health care settings.

C1. Infectious and Parasitic Diseases

A. Human Immunodeficiency Virus (HIV) Infections

1. Code only confirmed cases of HIV infection/illness. This is an exception to the hospital inpatient guideline Section II, H.

In this context, "confirmation" does not require documentation of positive serology or culture for HIV; the physician's diagnostic statement that the patient is HIV positive, or has an HIV-related illness is sufficient.

2. Selection and sequencing

   a. If a patient is admitted for an HIV-related condition, the principal diagnosis should be 042, followed by additional diagnosis codes for all reported HIV-related conditions.

   b. If a patient with HIV disease is admitted for an unrelated condition (such as a traumatic injury), the code for the unrelated condition (e.g., the nature of injury code) should be the principal diagnosis. Other diagnoses would be 042 followed by additional diagnosis codes for all reported HIV-related conditions.

   c. Whether the patient is newly diagnosed or has had previous admissions/encounters for HIV conditions is irrelevant to the sequencing decision.

   d. V08 Asymptomatic human immunodeficiency virus [HIV] infection, is to be applied when the patient without any documentation of symptoms is listed as being "HIV positive," "known HIV," "HIV test positive," or similar terminology. Do not use this code if the term "AIDS" is used or if the patient is treated for any HIV-related illness or is described as having any condition(s) resulting from his/her HIV positive status; use 042 in these cases.

   e. Patients with inconclusive HIV serology, but no definitive diagnosis or manifestations of the illness, may be assigned code 795.71, Inconclusive serologic test for Human Immunodeficiency Virus [HIV].

   f. Previously diagnosed HIV-related illness

      Patients with any known prior diagnosis of an HIV-related illness should be coded to 042. Once a patient had developed an HIV-related illness, the patient should always be assigned code 042 on every subsequent admission/encounter. Patients previously diagnosed with any HIV illness (042) should never be assigned to 795.71 or V08.

   g. HIV Infection in Pregnancy, Childbirth and the Puerperium

      During pregnancy, childbirth or the puerperium, a patient admitted (or presenting for a health care encounter) because of an HIV-related illness should receive a principal diagnosis of 647.6X, Other specified infectious and parasitic diseases in the mother classifiable elsewhere, but complicating the pregnancy, childbirth or the puerperium, followed by 042 and the code(s) for the HIV-related illness(es). Codes from Chapter 15 always take sequencing priority.

      Patients with asymptomatic HIV infection status admitted (or presenting for a health care encounter) during pregnancy, childbirth, or the puerperium should receive codes of 647.6X and V08.

   h. Encounters for Testing for HIV

      If a patient is being seen to determine his/her HIV status, use code V73.89, Screening for other specified viral disease. Use code V69.8,

Other problems related to lifestyle, as a secondary code if an asymptomatic patient is in a known high risk group for HIV. Should a patient with signs or symptoms or illness, or a confirmed HIV related diagnosis be tested for HIV, code the signs and symptoms or the diagnosis. An additional counseling code V65.44 may be used if counseling is provided during the encounter for the test.

When a patient returns to be informed of his/her HIV test results use code V65.44, HIV counseling, if the results of the test are negative.

If the results are positive but the patient is asymptomatic use code V08, Asymptomatic HIV infection. If the results are positive and the patient is symptomatic use code 042, HIV infection, with codes for the HIV related symptoms or diagnosis. The HIV counseling code may also be used if counseling is provided for patients with positive test results.

B. Septicemia and Septic Shock

1. When the diagnosis of septicemia with shock or the diagnosis of general sepsis with septic shock is documented, code and list the septicemia first and report the septic shock code as a secondary condition. The septicemia code assignment should identify the type of bacteria if it is known.

2. Sepsis and septic shock associated with abortion, ectopic pregnancy, and molar pregnancy are classified to category codes in Chapter 11 (630-639).

3. Negative or inconclusive blood cultures do not preclude a diagnosis of septicemia in patients with clinical evidence of the condition.

C2. Neoplasms

Chapter 2 of the ICD-9-CM contains the code for most benign and all malignant neoplasms. Certain benign neoplasms, such as prostatic adenomas, may be found in the specific body system chapters. To properly code a neoplasm it is necessary to determine from the record if the neoplasm is benign, in-situ, malignant, or of uncertain histologic behavior. If malignant, any secondary (metastatic) sites should also be determined.

The neoplasm table in the Alphabetic Index should be referenced first. If the histological term is documented, that term should be referenced first, rather than going immediately to the Neoplasm Table, in order to determine which column in the Neoplasm Table is appropriate. For example, if the documentation indicates "adenoma," refer to the term in the Alphabetic Index to review the entries under this term and the instructional note to "see also neoplasm, by site, benign." The table provides the proper code based on the type of neoplasm and the site. It is important to select the proper column in the table that corresponds to the type of neoplasm. The tabular should then be referenced to verify that the correct code has been selected from the table and that a more specific site code does not exist.

A. If the treatment is directed at the malignancy, designate the malignancy as the principal diagnosis.

B. When a patient is admitted because of a primary neoplasm with metastasis and treatment is directed toward the secondary site only, the secondary neoplasm is designated as the principal diagnosis even though the primary malignancy is still present.

C. Coding and sequencing of complications associated with the malignant neoplasm or with the therapy thereof are subject to the following guidelines:

1. When admission/encounter is for management of an anemia associated with the malignancy, and the treatment is only for anemia, the anemia is designated at the principal diagnosis and is followed by the appropriate code(s) for the malignancy.

2. When the admission/encounter is for management of an anemia associated with chemotherapy or radiotherapy and the only treatment is for the anemia, the anemia is sequenced first followed by the appropriate code(s) for the malignancy.

3. When the admission/encounter is for management of dehydration due to the malignancy or the therapy, or a combination of both, and only the dehydration is being treated (intravenous rehydration), the dehydration is sequenced first, followed by the code(s) for the malignancy.

4. When the admission/encounter is for treatment of a complication resulting from a surgical procedure performed for the treatment of an intestinal malignancy, designate the complication as the principal or first-listed diagnosis if treatment is directed at resolving the complication.

D. When a primary malignancy has been previously excised or eradicated from its site and there is no further treatment directed to that site and there is no evidence of any existing primary malignancy, a code from category V10, Personal history of malignant neoplasm, should be used to indicate the former site of the malignancy. Any mention of extension, invasion, or metastasis to another site is coded as a secondary malignant neoplasm to that site. The secondary site may be the principal or first-listed with the V10 code used as a secondary code.

E. Admissions/Encounters involving chemotherapy and radiation therapy

1. When an episode of care involves the surgical removal of a neoplasm, primary or secondary site, followed by chemotherapy or radiation treatment, the neoplasm code should be assigned as principal or first-listed diagnosis. When an episode of inpatient care involves surgical removal of a primary site or secondary site malignancy followed by adjunct chemotherapy or radiotherapy, code the malignancy as the principal or first-listed diagnosis, using codes in the 140-198 series or where appropriate in the 200-203 series.

2. If a patient admission/encounter is solely for the administration of chemotherapy or radiation therapy code V58.0, Encounter for radiation therapy, or V58.1, Encounter for chemotherapy, should be the first-listed or principal diagnosis. If a patient receives both chemotherapy and radiation therapy both codes should be listed, in either order of sequence.

3. When a patient is admitted for the purpose of radiotherapy or chemotherapy and develops complications such as uncontrolled nausea and vomiting or dehydration, the principal or first-listed diagnosis is V58.0, Encounter for radiotherapy, or V58.1, Encounter for chemotherapy.

F. When the reason for admission/encounter is to determine the extent of the malignancy, or for a procedure such as paracentesis or thoracentesis, the primary malignancy or appropriate metastatic site is designated as the principal or first-listed diagnosis, even though chemotherapy or radiotherapy is administered.

G. Symptoms, signs, and ill-defined conditions listed in Chapter 16 characteristic of, or associated with, an existing primary or secondary site malignancy cannot be used to replace the malignancy as principal or first-listed diagnosis, regardless of the number of admissions or encounters for treatment and care of the neoplasm.

C3. Endocrine, Nutritional, and Metabolic Diseases and Immunity Disorders

Reserved for future guideline expansion

C4. Diseases of Blood and Blood Forming Organs

Reserved for future guideline expansion

C5. Mental Disorders

Reserved for future guideline expansion

C6. Diseases of Nervous System and Sense Organs

Reserved for future guideline expansion

C7. Diseases of Circulatory System

A. Hypertension

The Hypertension Table, found under the main term, "Hypertension", in the Alphabetic Index, contains a complete listing of all conditions due to or associated with hypertension and classifies them according to malignant, benign, and unspecified.

1. Hypertension, Essential, or NOS Assign hypertension (arterial) (essential) (primary) (systemic) (NOS) to category code 401 with the appropriate fourth digit to indicate malignant (.0), benign (.1), or unspecified (.9). Do not use either .0 malignant or .1 benign unless medical record documentation supports such a designation.

2. Hypertension with Heart Disease

Heart conditions (425.8, 429.0-429.3, 429.8, 429.9) are assigned to a code from category 402 when a causal relationship is stated (due to hypertension) or implied (hypertensive). Use an additional code from category 428 to identify the type of heart failure in those patients with heart failure. More than one code from category 428 may be assigned if the patient has systolic or diastolic failure and congestive heart failure.

The same heart conditions (425.8, 428, 429.0-429.3, 429.8, 429.9) with hypertension, but without a stated causal relationship, are coded separately. Sequence according to the circumstances of the admission/encounter.

3. Hypertensive Renal Disease with Chronic Renal Failure

Assign codes from category 403, Hypertensive renal disease, when conditions classified to categories 585-587 are present. Unlike hypertension with heart disease, ICD-9-CM presumes a cause-and-effect relationship and classifies renal failure with hypertension as hypertensive renal disease.

4. Hypertensive Heart and Renal Disease

Assign codes from combination category 404, Hypertensive heart and renal disease, when both hypertensive renal disease and hypertensive heart disease are stated in the diagnosis. Assume a relationship between the hypertension and the renal disease, whether or not the condition is so designated. Assign an additional code from category 428, to identify the type of heart failure. More than one code from category 428 may be assigned if the patient has systolic or diastolic failure and congestive heart failure.

5. Hypertensive Cerebrovascular Disease

First assign codes from 430-438, Cerebrovascular disease, then the appropriate hypertension code from categories 401-405.

6. Hypertensive Retinopathy

Two codes are necessary to identify the condition. First assign the code from subcategory 362.11, Hypertensive retinopathy, then the appropriate code from categories 40-05 to indicate the type of hypertension.

7. Hypertension, Secondary

Two codes are required: one to identify the underlying etiology and one from category 405 to identify the hypertension. Sequencing of codes is determined by the reason for admission/encounter.

8. Hypertension, Transient

Assign code 796.2, Elevated blood pressure reading without diagnosis of hypertension, unless patient has an established diagnosis of hypertension. Assign code 642.3x for transient hypertension of pregnancy.

9. Hypertension, Controlled

Assign appropriate code from categories 401-405. This diagnostic statement usually refers to an existing state of hypertension under control by therapy.

10. Hypertension, Uncontrolled

Uncontrolled hypertension may refer to untreated hypertension or hypertension not responding to current therapeutic regimen. In either case, assign the appropriate code from categories 401-405 to designate the stage and type of hypertension. Code to the type of hypertension.

11. Elevated Blood Pressure

For a statement of elevated blood pressure without further specificity, assign code 796.2, Elevated blood pressure reading without diagnosis of hypertension, rather than a code from category 401.

B. Late Effects of Cerebrovascular Disease

Category 438 is used to indicate conditions classifiable to categories 430-437 as the causes of late effects (neurologic deficits), themselves classified elsewhere. These "late effects" include neurologic deficits that persist after initial onset of conditions classifiable to 430-437. The neurologic deficits caused by cerebrovascular disease may be present from the onset or may arise at any time after the onset of the condition classifiable to 430-437.

Codes from category 438 may be assigned on a health care record with codes from 430-437, if the patient has a current cerebrovascular accident (CVA) and deficits from an old CVA. Assign code V12.59 (and not a code from category 438) as an additional code for history of cerebrovascular disease when no neurologic deficits are present.

C8. Diseases of Respiratory System

Reserved for future guideline expansion

C9. Diseases of Digestive System

Reserved for future guideline expansion

C10. Diseases of Genitourinary System

Reserved for future guideline expansion

C11. Complications of Pregnancy, Childbirth, and the Puerperium

A. General Rules for Obstetric Cases

1. Obstetric cases require codes from chapter 11, codes in the range 630-677, Complications of Pregnancy, Childbirth, and the Puerperium. Should the physician document that the pregnancy is incidental to the encounter, then code V22.2 should be used in place of any chapter 11 codes. It is the physician's responsibility to state that the condition being treated is not affecting the pregnancy.

2. Chapter 11 codes have sequencing priority over codes from other chapters. Additional codes from other chapters may be used in conjunction with chapter 11 codes to further specify conditions. For example, sepsis and septic shock associated with abortion, ectopic pregnancy, and molar pregnancy are classified to category codes in Chapter 11 (630-639).

3. Chapter 11 codes are to be used only on the maternal record, never on the record of the newborn.

4. Categories 640-648, 651-676 have required fifth-digits, which indicate whether the encounter is antepartum, postpartum and whether a delivery has also occurred.

5. The fifth-digits, which are appropriate for each code number, are listed in brackets under each code. The fifth-digits on each code should all be consistent with each other. That is, should a delivery occur all of the fifth-digits should indicate the delivery.

6. For prenatal outpatient visits for patients with high-risk pregnancies, a code from category V23, Supervision of high-risk pregnancy, should be used as the principal or first-listed diagnosis. Secondary chapter 11 codes may be used in conjunction with these codes if appropriate. A thorough review of any pertinent excludes note is necessary to be certain that these V codes are being used properly.

7. An outcome of delivery code, V27.0-V27.9, should be included on every maternal record when a delivery has occurred. These codes are not to be used on subsequent records or on the newborn record.

8. For routine outpatient prenatal visits when no complications are present codes V22.0, Supervision of normal first pregnancy, and V22.1,

Supervision of other normal pregnancy, should be used as the first-listed diagnoses. These codes should not be used in conjunction with chapter 11 codes.

B. Selection of OB Principal or First-listed Diagnosis

1. In episodes when no delivery occurs, the principal diagnosis should correspond to the principal complication of the pregnancy, which necessitated the encounter. Should more than one complication exist, all of which are treated or monitored, any of the complications codes may be sequenced first.

2. When a delivery occurs, the principal diagnosis should correspond to the main circumstances or complication of the delivery.

    In cases of cesarean delivery, the selection of the principal diagnosis should correspond to the reason the cesarean delivery was performed unless the reason for admission/encounter was unrelated to the condition resulting in the cesarean delivery.

C. Fetal Conditions Affecting the Management of the Mother

Codes from category 655, Known or suspected fetal abnormality affecting management of the mother, and category 656, Other fetal and placental problems affecting the management of the mother, are assigned only when the fetal condition is actually responsible for modifying the management of the mother, i.e., by requiring diagnostic studies, additional observation, special care, or termination of pregnancy. The fact that the fetal condition exists does not justify assigning a code from this series to the mother's record.

D. HIV Infection in Pregnancy, Childbirth and the Puerperium

During pregnancy, childbirth or the puerperium, a patient admitted because of an HIV-related illness should receive a principal diagnosis of 647.6X, Other specified infectious and parasitic diseases in the mother classifiable elsewhere, but complicating the pregnancy, childbirth or the puerperium, followed by 042 and the code(s) for the HIV-related illness(es). This is an exception to the sequencing rule found in above.

Patients with asymptomatic HIV infection status admitted during pregnancy, childbirth, or the puerperium should receive codes of 647.6X and V08.

E. Normal Delivery, 650

1. Code 650 is for use in cases when a woman is admitted for a full-term normal delivery and delivers a single, healthy infant without any complications antepartum, during the delivery, or postpartum during the delivery episode.

2. Code 650 may be used if the patient had a complication at some point during her pregnancy but the complication is not present at the time of the admission for delivery.

3. Code 650 is always a principal diagnosis. It is not to be used if any other code from chapter 11 is needed to describe a current complication of the antenatal, delivery, or perinatal period. Additional codes from other chapters may be used with code 650 if they are not related to or are in any way complicating the pregnancy.

4. V27.0, Single liveborn, is the only outcome of delivery code appropriate for use with 650.

F. The Postpartum Period

1. The postpartum period begins immediately after delivery and continues for six weeks following delivery.

2. A postpartum complication is any complication occurring within the six-week period.

3. Chapter 11 codes may also be used to describe pregnancy-related complications after the six-week period should the physician document that a condition is pregnancy related.

4. Postpartum complications that occur during the same admission as the delivery are identified with a fifth digit of "2." Subsequent admissions/encounters for postpartum complications should identified with a fifth digit of "4."

5. When the mother delivers outside the hospital prior to admission and is admitted for routine postpartum care and no complications are noted, code V24.0, Postpartum care and examination immediately after delivery, should be assigned as the principal diagnosis.

6. A delivery diagnosis code should not be used for a woman who has delivered prior to admission to the hospital. Any postpartum procedures should be coded.

G. Code 677, Late effect of complication of pregnancy, childbirth, and the puerperium

1. Code 677, Late effect of complication of pregnancy, childbirth, and the puerperium is for use in those cases when an initial complication of a pregnancy develops a sequelae requiring care or treatment at a future date.

2. This code may be used at any time after the initial postpartum period.

3. This code, like all late effect codes, is to be sequenced following the code describing the sequelae of the complication.

H. Abortions

1. Fifth-digits are required for abortion categories 634-637. Fifth-digit 1, incomplete, indicates that all of the products of conception have not been expelled from the uterus. Fifth-digit 2, complete, indicates that all products of conception have been expelled from the uterus prior to the episode of care.

2. A code from categories 640-648 and 651-657 may be used as additional codes with an abortion code to indicate the complication leading to the abortion.

   Fifth digit 3 is assigned with codes from these categories when used with an abortion code because the other fifth digits will not apply. Codes from the 660-669 series are not to be used for complications of abortion.

3. Code 639 is to be used for all complications following abortion. Code 639 cannot be assigned with codes from categories 634-638.

4. Abortion with Liveborn Fetus.

   When an attempted termination of pregnancy results in a liveborn fetus assign code 644.21, Early onset of delivery, with an appropriate code from category V27, Outcome of Delivery. The procedure code for the attempted termination of pregnancy should also be assigned.

5. Retained Products of Conception following an abortion.

Subsequent admissions for retained products of conception following a spontaneous or legally induced abortion are assigned the appropriate code from category 634, Spontaneous abortion, or legally induced abortion, with a fifth digit of "1" (incomplete). This advice is appropriate even when the patient was discharged previously with a discharge diagnosis of complete abortion.

C12. Diseases Skin and Subcutaneous Tissue

Reserved for future guideline expansion

C13. Diseases of Musculoskeletal and Connective Tissue

Reserved for future guideline expansion

C14. Congenital Anomalies

Reserved for future guideline expansion

C15. Newborn (Perinatal) Guidelines

For coding and reporting purposes the perinatal period is defined as birth through the 28th day following birth. The following guidelines are provided for reporting purposes. Hospitals may record other diagnoses as needed for internal data use.

A. General Perinatal Rule

All clinically significant conditions noted on routine newborn examination should be coded. A condition is clinically significant if it requires:

clinical evaluation; or

therapeutic treatment; or

diagnostic procedures; or

extended length of hospital stay; or

increased nursing care and/or monitoring; or

has implications for future health care needs.

Note: The perinatal guidelines listed above are the same as the general coding guidelines for "additional diagnoses," except for the final point regarding implications for future health care needs. Whether or not a condition is clinically significant can only be determined by the physician.

B. Use of Codes V30-V39

When coding the birth of an infant, assign a code from categories V30-V39, according to the type of birth. A code from this series is assigned as a principal diagnosis, and assigned only once to a newborn at the time of birth.

C. Newborn Transfers

If the newborn is transferred to another institution, the V30 series is not used at the receiving hospital.

D. Use of Category V29

   1. Assign a code from category V29, Observation and evaluation of newborns and infants for suspected conditions not found, to identify those instances when a healthy newborn is evaluated for a suspected condition that is determined after study not to be present. Do not use a code from category V29 when the patient has identified signs or symptoms of a suspected problem; in such cases, code the sign or symptom.

   2. A V29 code is to be used as a secondary code after the V30, Outcome of delivery, code. It may also be assigned as a principal code for readmissions or encounters when the V30 code no longer applies. It is for use only for healthy newborns and infants for which no condition after study is found to be present.

E. Maternal Causes of Perinatal Morbidity

   Codes from categories 760-763, Maternal causes of perinatal morbidity and mortality, are assigned only when the maternal condition has actually affected the fetus or newborn. The fact that the mother has an associated medical condition or experiences some complication of pregnancy, labor or delivery does not justify the routine assignment of codes from these categories to the newborn record.

F. Congenital Anomalies

   Assign an appropriate code from categories 740-759, Congenital Anomalies, as an additional diagnosis when a specific abnormality is diagnosed for an infant. Congenital anomalies may also be the principal or first listed diagnosis for admissions/encounters subsequent to the newborn admission. Such abnormalities may occur as a set of symptoms or multiple malformations. A code should be assigned for each presenting manifestation of the syndrome if the syndrome is not specifically indexed in ICD-9-CM.

G. Coding of Additional Perinatal Diagnoses

   1. Assign codes for conditions that require treatment or further investigation, prolong the length of stay, or require resource utilization.

   2. Assign codes for conditions that have been specified by the physician as having implications for future health care needs.

   Note: This guideline should not be used for adult patients.

   3. Assign a code for Newborn conditions originating in the perinatal period (categories 760-779), as well as complications arising during the current episode of care classified in other chapters, only if the diagnoses have been documented by the responsible physician at the time of transfer or discharge as having affected the fetus or newborn.

H. Prematurity and Fetal Growth Retardation

   Codes from category 764 and subcategories 765.0 and 765.1 should not be assigned based solely on recorded birthweight or estimated gestational age, but on the attending physician's clinical assessment of maturity of the infant. NOTE: Since physicians may utilize different criteria in determining prematurity, do not code the diagnosis of prematurity unless the physician documents this condition.

A code from subcategory 765.2, Weeks of gestation, should be assigned as an additional code with category 764 and codes from 765.0 and 765.1 to specify weeks of gestation as documented by the physician.

C16. Signs, Symptoms and Ill-Defined Conditions

Reserved for future guideline expansion

C17. Injury and Poisoning

A. Coding of Injuries

When coding injuries, assign separate codes for each injury unless a combination code is provided, in which case the combination code is assigned. Multiple injury codes are provided in ICD-9-CM, but should not be assigned unless information for a more specific code is not available. These codes are not to be used for normal, healing surgical wounds or to identify complications of surgical wounds.

The code for the most serious injury, as determined by the physician, is sequenced first.

1. Superficial injuries such as abrasions or contusions are not coded when associated with more severe injuries of the same site.

2. When a primary injury results in minor damage to peripheral nerves or blood vessels, the primary injury is sequenced first with additional code(s) from categories 950-957, Injury to nerves and spinal cord, and/or 900-904, Injury to blood vessels. When the primary injury is to the blood vessels or nerves, that injury should be sequenced first.

B. Coding of Fractures

The principles of multiple coding of injuries should be followed in coding fractures. Fractures of specified sites are coded individually by site in accordance with both the provisions within categories 800-829 and the level of detail furnished by medical record content. Combination categories for multiple fractures are provided for use when there is insufficient detail in the medical record (such as trauma cases transferred to another hospital), when the reporting form limits the number of codes that can be used in reporting pertinent clinical data, or when there is insufficient specificity at the fourth-digit or fifth-digit level. More specific guidelines are as follows:

1. Multiple fractures of same limb classifiable to the same three-digit or four-digit category are coded to that category.

2. Multiple unilateral or bilateral fractures of same bone(s) but classified to different fourth-digit subdivisions (bone part) within the same three-digit category are coded individually by site.

3. Multiple fracture categories 819 and 828 classify bilateral fractures of both upper limbs (819) and both lower limbs (828), but without any detail at the fourth-digit level other than open and closed type of fractures.

4. Multiple fractures are sequenced in accordance with the severity of the fracture and the physician should be asked to list the fracture diagnoses in the order of severity.

C. Coding of Burns

Current burns (940-948) are classified by depth, extent and by agent (E code). Burns are classified by depth as first degree (erythema), second degree (blistering), and third degree (full-thickness involvement).

1. Sequence first the code that reflects the highest degree of burn when more than one burn is present.

2. Classify burns of the same local site (three-digit category level, (940-947) but of different degrees to the subcategory identifying the highest degree recorded in the diagnosis.

3. Non-healing burns are coded as acute burns.

   Necrosis of burned skin should be coded as a non-healed burn.

4. Assign code 958.3, Posttraumatic wound infection, not elsewhere classified, as an additional code for any documented infected burn site.

5. When coding burns, assign separate codes for each burn site. Category 946 Burns of Multiple specified sites, should only be used if the location of the burns are not documented.

   Category 949, Burn, unspecified, is extremely vague and should rarely be used.

6. Assign codes from category 948, Burns classified according to extent of body surface involved, when the site of the burn is not specified or when there is a need for additional data. It is advisable to use category 948 as additional coding when needed to provide data for evaluating burn mortality, such as that needed by burn units. It is also advisable to use category 948 as an additional code for reporting purposes when there is mention of a third-degree burn involving 20 percent or more of the body surface.

   In assigning a code from category 948:

   > Fourth-digit codes are used to identify the percentage of total body surface involved in a burn (all degree).

   > Fifth-digits are assigned to identify the percentage of body surface involved in third-degree burn.

   > Fifth-digit zero (0) is assigned when less than 10 percent or when no body surface is involved in a third-degree burn.

   Category 948 is based on the classic "rule of nines" in estimating body surface involved: head and neck are assigned nine percent, each arm nine percent, each leg 18 percent, the anterior trunk 18 percent, posterior trunk 18 percent, and genitalia one percent. Physicians may change these percentage assignments where necessary to accommodate infants and children who have proportionately larger heads than adults and patients who have large buttocks, thighs, or abdomen that involve burns.

7. Encounters for the treatment of the late effects of burns (i.e., scars or joint contractures) should be coded to the residual condition (sequelae) followed by the appropriate late effect code (906.5-906.9). A late effect E code may also be used, if desired.

8. When appropriate, both a sequelae with a late effect code, and a current burn code may be assigned on the same record.

D. Coding of Debridement of Wound, Infection, or Burn

Excisional debridement may be performed by a physician and/or other health care provider and involves an excisional, as opposed to a mechanical (brushing, scrubbing, washing) debridement.

For coding purposes, excisional debridement, 86.22.

Nonexcisional debridement is assigned to 86.28.

Modified based on *Coding Clinic*, 2nd Quarter 2000, p. 9.

E. Adverse Effects, Poisoning and Toxic Effects

The properties of certain drugs, medicinal and biological substances or combinations of such substances, may cause toxic reactions. The occurrence of drug toxicity is classified in ICD-9-CM as follows:

1. Adverse Effect

   When the drug was correctly prescribed and properly administered, code the reaction plus the appropriate code from the E930-E949 series. Codes from the E930-E949 series must be used to identify the causative substance for an adverse effect of drug, medicinal and biological substances, correctly prescribed and properly administered. The effect, such as tachycardia, delirium, gastrointestinal hemorrhaging, vomiting, hypokalemia, hepatitis, renal failure, or respiratory failure, is coded and followed by the appropriate code from the E930-E949 series.

   Adverse effects of therapeutic substances correctly prescribed and properly administered (toxicity, synergistic reaction, side effect, and idiosyncratic reaction) may be due to (1) differences among patients, such as age, sex, disease, and genetic factors, and (2) drug-related factors, such as type of drug, route of administration, duration of therapy, dosage, and bioavailability.

2. Poisoning

   a. When an error was made in drug prescription or in the administration of the drug by physician, nurse, patient, or other person, use the appropriate poisoning code from the 960-979 series.

   b. If an overdose of a drug was intentionally taken or administered and resulted in drug toxicity, it would be coded as a poisoning (960-979 series).

   c. If a nonprescribed drug or medicinal agent was taken in combination with a correctly prescribed and properly administered drug, any drug toxicity or other reaction resulting from the interaction of the two drugs would be classified as a poisoning.

   d. When coding a poisoning or reaction to the improper use of a medication (e.g., wrong dose, wrong substance, wrong route of administration) the poisoning code is sequenced first, followed by a code for the manifestation. If there is also a diagnosis of drug abuse or dependence to the substance, the abuse or dependence is coded as an additional code.

C18. Classification of Factors Influencing Health Status and Contact with Health Service

A. ICD-9-CM provides codes to deal with encounters for circumstances other than a disease or injury. The Supplementary Classification of Factors Influencing Health Status and Contact with Health Services (V01.0-V83.89) is provided to deal with occasions when circumstances other than a disease or injury (codes 001-999) are recorded as a diagnosis or problem.

There are four primary circumstances for the use of V codes:

1. When a person who is not currently sick encounters the health services for some specific reason, such as to act as an organ donor, to receive prophylactic care, such as inoculations or health screenings, or to receive counseling on health related issue.

2. When a person with a resolving disease or injury, or a chronic, long-term condition requiring continuous care, encounters the health care system for specific aftercare of that disease or injury (e.g., dialysis for renal disease; chemotherapy for malignancy; cast change). A diagnosis/symptom code should be used whenever a current, acute, diagnosis is being treated or a sign or symptom is being studied.

3. When circumstances or problems influence a person's health status but are not in themselves a current illness or injury.

4. For newborns, to indicate birth status.

B. V codes are for use in both the inpatient and outpatient setting but are generally more applicable to the outpatient setting. V codes may be used as either a first listed (principal diagnosis code in the inpatient setting) or secondary code depending on the circumstances of the encounter. Certain V codes may only be used as first listed, others only as secondary codes.

C. V Codes indicate a reason for an encounter. They are not procedure codes. A corresponding procedure code must accompany a V code to describe the procedure performed.

D. Categories of V Codes

1. Contact/Exposure

   Category V01 indicates contact with or exposure to communicable diseases. These codes are for patients who do not show any sign or symptom of a disease but have been exposed to it by close personal contact with an infected individual or are in an area where a disease is epidemic. These codes may be used as a first listed code to explain an encounter for testing, or, more commonly, as a secondary code to identify a potential risk.

2. Inoculations and vaccinations

   Categories V03-V06 are for encounters for inoculations and vaccinations. They indicate that a patient is being seen to receive a prophylactic inoculation against a disease. The injection itself must be represented by the appropriate procedure code. A code from V03-V06 may be used as a secondary code if the inoculation is given as a routine part of preventive health care, such as a well-baby visit.

3. Status

   Status codes indicate that a patient is either a carrier of a disease or has the sequelae or residual of a past disease or condition. This includes such things as the presence of prosthetic or mechanical devices resulting from past treatment. A status code is informative because the status may affect the course of treatment and its outcome. A status code is distinct from a history code. The his-tory code indicates that the patient no longer has the condition.

The status V codes/categories are:

V02   Carrier or suspected carrier of infectious diseases

> Carrier status, indicates that a person harbors the specific organisms of a disease without manifest symptoms and is capable of transmitting the infection.

V08   Asymptomatic HIV infection status

> This code indicates that a patient has tested positive for HIV but has manifested no signs or symptoms of the disease.

V09   Infection with drug-resistant microorganisms

> This category indicates that a patient has an infection which is resistant to drug treatment. Sequence the infection code first.

V21   Constitutional states in development

V22.2   Pregnant state, incidental

> This code is a secondary code only for use when the pregnancy is in no way complicating the reason for visit. Otherwise, a code from the obstetric chapter is required.

V26.5x   Sterilization status

V42   Organ or tissue replaced by transplant

V43   Organ or tissue replaced by other means

V44   Artificial opening status

V45   Other postsurgical states

V46   Other dependence on machines

V49.6   Upper limb amputation status

V49.7   Lower limb amputation status

V48.81   Postmenopausal status

V49.82   Dental sealant status

V58.6   Long-term (current) drug use

> This subcategory indicates a patient's continuous use of a prescribed drug (including such things as aspirin therapy) for the long-term treatment of a condition or for prophylactic use. It is not for use for patients who have addictions to drugs.

V83   Genetic carrier status

> Categories V42-V46, and subcategories V49.6, V49.7are for use only if there are no complications or malfunctions of the organ or tissue replaced, the amputation site or the equipment on which the patient is dependent. These are always secondary codes.

4. History (of)

There are two types of history V codes, personal and family. Personal history codes explain a patient's past medical condition that no longer exists and is not receiving any treatment but that has the potential for recurrence, and, therefore, may require continued monitoring. The exceptions to this general rule are category V14, Personal history of allergy to medicinal agents and subcategory V15.0, Allergy, other than to medicinal agents. A person who has had an allergic episode to a substance or food in the past should always be considered allergic to the substance.

Family history codes are for use when a patient has a family member(s) who has had a particular disease that causes the patient to be at higher risk of also contracting the disease.

Personal history codes may be used in conjunction with follow-up codes and family history codes may be use in conjunction with screening codes to explain the need for a test or procedure. History codes are also acceptable on any medical record regardless of the reason for visit. A history of an illness, even if no longer present, is important information that may alter the type of treatment ordered.

The history V code categories are:

V10   Personal history of malignant neoplasm

V12   Personal history of certain other diseases

V13   Personal history of other diseases

> Except: V13.4, Personal history of arthritis, and V13.6, Personal history of congenital malformations. These conditions are life-long so are not true history codes.

V14   Personal history of allergy to medicinal agents

V15   Other personal history presenting hazards to health

> Except: V15.7, Personal history of contraception.

V16   Family history of malignant neoplasm

V17   Family history of certain chronic disabling diseases

V18   Family history of certain other specific diseases

V19   Family history of other conditions

5. Screening

Screening is the testing for disease or disease precursors in seemingly well individuals so that early detection and treatment can be provided for those who test positive for the disease. Screenings that are recommended for many subgroups in a population include: routine mammograms for women over 40, a fecal occult blood test for everyone over 50, an amniocentesis to rule out a fetal anomaly for pregnant women over 35, because the incidence of breast cancer and colon cancer in these subgroups is higher than in the general population, as is the incidence of Down's syndrome in older mothers.

The testing of a person to rule out or confirm a suspected diagnosis because the patient has some sign or symptom is a diagnostic examination, not a screening. In these cases, the sign or symptom is used to explain the reason for the test.

A screening code may be a first listed code if the reason for the visit is specifically the screening exam. It may also be used as an additional code if the screening is done during an office visit for other health problems. A screening code is not necessary if the screening is inherent to a routine examination, such as a pap smear done during a routine pelvic examination.

Should a condition be discovered during the screening then the code for the condition may be assigned as an additional diagnosis.

The V code indicates that a screening exam is planned. A procedure code is required to confirm that the screening was performed.

The screening V code categories:

V28   Antenatal screening

V73-V82   Special screening examinations

6. Observation

There are two observation V code categories. They are for use in very limited circumstances when a person is being observed for a suspected condition that is ruled out. The observation codes are not for use if an injury or illness or any signs or symptoms related to the suspected condition are present. In such cases the diagnosis/symptom code is used with the corresponding E code to identify any external cause.

The observation codes are to be used as principal diagnosis only. The only exception to this is when the principal diagnosis is required to be a code from the V30, Live born infant, category. Then the V29 observation code is sequenced after the V30 code. Additional codes may be used in addition to the observation code but only if they are unrelated to the suspected condition being observed.

The observation V code categories:

V29   Observation and evaluation of newborns for suspected condition not found

> A code from category V30 should be sequenced before the V29 code.

V71   Observation and evaluation for suspected condition not found

7. Aftercare

Aftercare visit codes cover situations when the initial treatment of a disease or injury has been performed and the patient requires continued care during the healing or recovery phase, or for the long-term consequences of the disease. The aftercare V code should not be used if treatment is directed at a current, acute disease or injury, the diagnosis code is to be used in these cases. Exceptions to this rule are codes V58.0, Radiotherapy, and V58.1, Chemotherapy. These codes are to be first listed, followed by the diagnosis code when a patient's encounter is solely to receive radiation therapy or chemotherapy for the treatment of a neoplasm. Should a patient receive both chemotherapy and radiation therapy during the same encounter code V58.0 and V58.1 may be used together on a record with either one being sequenced first.

The aftercare codes are generally first listed to explain the specific reason for the encounter. An aftercare code may be used as an additional code when some type of aftercare is provided in addition to the reason for admission and no diagnosis code is applicable. An example of this would be the closure of a colostomy during an encounter for treatment of another condition.

Certain aftercare V code categories need a secondary diagnosis code to describe the resolving condition or sequelae, for others, the condition is inherent in the code title.

Additional V code aftercare category terms include, fitting and adjustment, and attention to artificial openings.

The aftercare V category/codes:

V52	Fitting and adjustment of prosthetic device and implant
V53	Fitting and adjustment of other device
V54	Other orthopedic aftercare
V55	Attention to artificial openings
V56	Encounter for dialysis and dialysis catheter care
V57	Care involving the use of rehabilitation procedures
V58.0	Radiotherapy
V58.1	Chemotherapy
V58.3	Attention to surgical dressings and sutures
V58.41	Encounter for planned post-operative wound closure
V53.42	Aftercare, surgery, neoplasm
V53.43	Aftercare, surgery, trauma
V58.49	Other specified aftercare following surgery
V53.71-V53.78	Aftercare following surgery
V58.81	Fitting and adjustment of vascular catheter
V58.82	Fitting and adjustment of non-vascular catheter
V53.83	Monitoring therapeutic drug
V58.89	Other specified aftercare

8. Follow-up

The follow-up codes are for use to explain continuing surveillance following completed treatment of a disease, condition, or injury. They infer that the condition has been fully treated and no longer exists. They should not be confused with aftercare codes which explain current treatment for a healing condition or its sequelae. Follow-up codes may be used in conjunction with history codes to provide the full picture of the healed condition and its treatment. The follow-up code is sequenced first, followed by the history code.

A follow-up code may be used to explain repeated visits. Should a condition be found to have recurred on the follow-up visit, then the diagnosis code should be used in place of the follow-up code.

The follow-up V code categories:

V24 Postpartum care and evaluation

V67 Follow-up examination

9. Donor

Category V59 is the donor codes. They are for use for living individuals who are donating blood or other body tissue. These codes are only for individuals donating for others, not for self donations. They are not for use to identify cadaveric donations.

10. Counseling

Counseling V codes are for use for when a patient or family member receives assistance in the aftermath of an illness or injury, or when support is required in coping with family or social problems. They are not necessary for use in conjunction with a diagnosis code when the counseling component of care is considered integral to standard treatment.

The counseling V categories/codes:

V25.0   General counseling and advice for contraceptive management

V26.3   Genetic counseling

V26.4   General counseling and advice for procreative management

V61   Other family circumstances

V65.1   Person consulted on behalf of another person

V65.3   Dietary surveillance and counseling

V65.4   Other counseling, not elsewhere classified

11. Obstetrics and related conditions

See the Obstetrics guidelines for further instruction on the use of these codes.

V codes for pregnancy are for use in those circumstances when none of the problems or complications included in the codes from the Obstetrics chapter exist (a routine prenatal visit or postpartum care) V22.0, Supervision of normal first pregnancy, and V22.1, Supervision of other normal pregnancy, are always first listed and are not to be used with any other code from the OB chapter.

The outcome of delivery, category V27, should be included on all maternal delivery records. It is always a secondary code.

V codes for family planning (contraceptive) or procreative management and counseling should be included on an obstetric record either during the pregnancy or the postpartum stage, if applicable.

Obstetrics and related conditions V code categories:

V22   Normal pregnancy

V23   Supervision of high-risk pregnancy

> Except: V23.2, Pregnancy with history of abortion. Code 646.3, Habitual aborter, from the OB chapter is required to indicate a history of abortion during a pregnancy.

V24   Postpartum care and evaluation

V25   Encounter for contraceptive management

> Except V25.0x (See counseling above)

V26   Procreative management

> Except V26.5x, Sterilization status, V26.3 and V26.4 (Counseling)

V27   Outcome of delivery

V28   Antenatal screening

See Screening- see section 5 of this article

12. Newborn, infant and child

See the newborn guidelines for further instruction on the use of these codes.

Newborn V code categories:

V20   Health supervision of infant or child

V29   Observation and evaluation of newborns for suspected condition not found—see Observation, section 6 of this article.

V30-V39   Liveborn infant according to type of birth

13. Routine and administrative examinations

The V codes allow for the description of encounters for routine examinations, such as, a general check-up, or, examinations for administrative purposes, such as, a pre-employment physical. The codes are for use as first listed codes only and are not to be used if the examination is for diagnosis of a suspected condition or for treatment purposes. In such cases the diagnosis code is used. During a routine exam, should a diagnosis or condition be discovered, it should be coded as an additional code. Pre-existing and chronic conditions, and history codes may also be included as additional codes as long as the examination is for administrative purposes and not focused on any particular condition.

Pre-operative examination V codes are for use only in those situations when a patient is being cleared for surgery and no treatment is given.

The V codes categories/code for routine and administrative examinations:

V20.2   Routine infant or child health check

Any injections given should have a corresponding procedure code.

V70   General medical examination

V72   Special investigations and examinations

Except V72.5 and V72.6

14. Miscellaneous V codes

The miscellaneous V codes capture a number of other health care encounters that do not fall into one of the other categories. Certain of these codes identify the reason for the encounter, others are for use as additional codes which provide useful information on circumstances which may affect a patient's care and treatment.

Miscellaneous V code categories/codes:

V07   Need for isolation and other prophylactic measures

V50   Elective surgery for purposes other than remedying health states

V58.5   Orthodontics

V60   Housing, household, and economic circumstances

V62   Other psychosocial circumstances

V63   Unavailability of other medical facilities for care

V64   Persons encountering health services for specific procedures, not carried out

V66   Convalescence and Palliative Care

V68   Encounters for administrative purposes

V69   Problems related to lifestyle

15. Nonspecific V codes

Certain V codes are so non-specific, or potentially redundant with other codes in the classification that there can be little justification for their use in the inpatient setting. Their use in the outpatient setting should be limited to those instances when there is no further documentation to permit more precise coding. Otherwise, any sign or symptom or any other reason for visit which is captured in another code should be used.

Nonspecific V code categories/codes:

V11   Personal history of mental disorder

> A code from the mental disorders chapter, with an in remission fifth-digit, should be used.

V13.4   Personal history of arthritis

V13.6   Personal history of congenital malformations

V15.7   Personal history of contraception

V23.2   Pregnancy with history of abortion

V40   Mental and behavioral problems

V41   Problems with special senses and other special functions

V47   Other problems with internal organs

V48   Problems with head, neck, and trunk

V49   Problems with limbs and other problems

> Exceptions:
>
> > V49.6   Upper limb amputation status
> >
> > V49.7   Lower limb amputation status
> >
> > V49.81   Postmenopausal status
> >
> > V49.82   Dental sealant status

V51   Aftercare involving the use of plastic surgery

V58.2   Blood transfusion, without reported diagnosis

V58.9   Unspecified aftercare

V72.5   Radiological examination, NEC

V72.6   Laboratory examination

> Codes V72.5 and V72.6 are not to be used if any sign or symptoms, or reason for a test is documented. See section K and L of the outpatient guidelines.

C19. Supplemental Classification of External Causes of Injury and Poisoning (E-codes)

Introduction: These guidelines are provided for those who are currently collecting E codes in order that there will be standardization in the process. If your institution plans to begin collect-ing E codes, these guidelines are to be applied. The use of E codes is supplemental to the application of ICD-9-CM diagnosis codes. E codes are never to be recorded as principal diagnosis (first-listed in noninpatient setting) and are not required for reporting to CMS.

External causes of injury and poisoning codes (E codes) are intended to provide data for injury research and evaluation of injury prevention strategies. E codes capture how the injury or poisoning happened (cause), the intent (unintentional or accidental; or intentional, such as suicide or assault), and the place where the event occurred. Some major categories of E codes include:

transport accidents

poisoning and adverse effects of drugs, medicinal substances and biologicals

accidental falls

accidents caused by fire and flames

accidents due to natural and environmental factors

late effects of accidents, assaults or self injury

assaults or purposely inflicted injury

suicide or self inflicted injury

These guidelines apply for the coding and collection of E codes from records in hospitals, outpatient clinics, emergency departments, other ambulatory care settings and physician offices, and nonacute care settings, except when other specific guidelines apply. (See Section III, Reporting Diagnostic Guidelines for Hospital-based Outpatient Services/Reporting Requirements for Physician Billing.)

A. General E Code Coding Guidelines

1. An E code may be used with any code in the range of 001-V83.89, which indicates an injury, poisoning, or adverse effect due to an external cause.

2. Assign the appropriate E code for all initial treatments of an injury, poisoning, or adverse effect of drugs.

3. Use a late effect E code for subsequent visits when a late effect of the initial injury or poisoning is being treated. There is no late effect E code for adverse effects of drugs.

4. Use the full range of E codes to completely describe the cause, the intent and the place of occurrence, if applicable, for all injuries, poisonings, and adverse effects of drugs.

5. Assign as many E codes as necessary to fully explain each cause. If only one E code can be recorded, assign the E code most related to the principal diagnosis.

6. The selection of the appropriate E code is guided by the Index to External Causes, which is located after the alphabetical index to diseases and by Inclusion and Exclusion notes in the Tabular List.

7. An E code can never be a principal (first listed) diagnosis.

B. Place of Occurrence Guideline

Use an additional code from category E849 to indicate the Place of Occurrence for injuries and poisonings. The Place of Occurrence describes the place where the event occurred and not the patient's activity at the time of the event.
Do not use E849.9 if the place of occurrence is not stated.

C. Adverse Effects of Drugs, Medicinal and Biological Substances Guidelines

1. Do not code directly from the Table of Drugs and Chemicals. Always refer back to the Tabular List.

2. Use as many codes as necessary to describe completely all drugs, medicinal or biological substances.

3. If the same E code would describe the causative agent for more than one adverse reaction, assign the code only once.

4. If two or more drugs, medicinal or biological substances are reported, code each individually unless the combination code is listed in the Table of Drugs and Chemicals. In that case, assign the E code for the combination.

5. When a reaction results from the interaction of a drug(s) and alcohol, use poisoning codes and E codes for both.

6. If the reporting format limits the number of E codes that can be used in reporting clinical data, code the one most related to the principal diagnosis. Include at least one from each category (cause, intent, place) if possible.
   If there are different fourth digit codes in the same three digit category, use the code for "Other specified" of that category. If there is no "Other specified" code in that category, use the appropriate "Unspecified" code in that category.
   If the codes are in different three digit categories, assign the appropriate E code for other multiple drugs and medicinal substances.

7. Codes from the E930-E949 series must be used to identify the causative substance for an adverse effect of drug, medicinal and biological substances, correctly prescribed and properly administered. The effect, such as tachycardia, delirium, gastrointestinal hemorrhaging, vomiting, hypokalemia, hepatitis, renal failure, or respiratory failure, is coded and followed by the appropriate code from the E930-E949 series.

D. Multiple Cause E Code Coding Guidelines

If two or more events cause separate injuries, an E code should be assigned for each cause. The first listed E code will be selected in the following order:

E codes for child and adult abuse take priority over all other E codes—see Child and Adult abuse guidelines.

E codes for terrorism events take priority over all other E codes except child and adult abuse.

E codes for cataclysmic events take priority over all other E codes except child and adult abuse and terrorism.

E codes for transport accidents take priority over all other E codes except cataclysmic events and child and adult abuse and terrorism.

The first-listed E code should correspond to the cause of the most serious diagnosis due to an assault, accident, or self-harm, following the order of hierarchy listed above.

E. Child and Adult Abuse Guideline

1. When the cause of an injury or neglect is intentional child or adult abuse, the first listed E code should be assigned from categories E960-E968, Homicide and injury purposely inflicted by other persons, (except category E967). An E code from category E967, Child and adult battering and other maltreatment, should be added as an additional code to identify the perpetrator, if known.

2. In cases of neglect when the intent is determined to be accidental E code E904.0, Abandonment or neglect of infant and helpless person, should be the first listed E code.

F. Unknown or Suspected Intent Guideline

1. If the intent (accident, self-harm, assault) of the cause of an injury or poisoning is unknown or unspecified, code the intent as undetermined E980-E989.

2. If the intent (accident, self-harm, assault) of the cause of an injury or poisoning is questionable, probable or suspected, code the intent as undetermined E980-E989.

G. Undetermined Cause

When the intent of an injury or poisoning is known, but the cause is unknown, use codes: E928.9, Unspecified accident, E958.9, Suicide and self-inflicted injury by unspecified means, and E968.9, Assault by unspecified means.

These E codes should rarely be used, as the documentation in the medical record, in both the inpatient outpatient and other settings, should normally provide sufficient detail to determine the cause of the injury.

H. Late Effects of External Cause Guidelines

1. Late effect E codes exist for injuries and poisonings but not for adverse effects of drugs, misadventures and surgical complications.

2. A late effect E code (E929, E959, E969, E977, E989, or E999.1) should be used with any report of a late effect or sequela resulting from a previous injury or poisoning (905-909).

3. A late effect E code should never be used with a related current nature of injury code.

I. Misadventures and Complications of Care Guidelines

1. Assign a code in the range of E870-E876 if misadventures are stated by the physician.

2. Assign a code in the range of E878-E879 if the physician attributes an abnormal reaction or later complication to a surgical or medical procedure, but does not mention misadventure at the time of the procedure as the cause of the reaction.

J. Terrorism Guidelines

1. When the cause of an injury is identified by the Federal Government (FBI) as terrorism, the first-listed E-code should be a code from category E979, Terrorism. The definition of terrorism employed by the FBI is found at the inclusion note at E979. The terrorism E-code is the only E-code that should be assigned. Additional E codes from the assault categories should not be assigned.

2. When the cause of an injury is suspected to be the result of terrorism a code from category E979 should not be assigned. Assign a code in the range of E codes based circumstances on the documentation of intent and mechanism.

3. Assign code E979.9, Terrorism, secondary effects, for conditions occurring subsequent to the terrorist event. This code should not be assigned for conditions that are due to the initial terrorist act.

4. For statistical purposes these codes will be tabulated within the category for assault, expanding the current category from E960-E969 to include E979 and E999.1.

SECTION II SELECTION OF PRINCIPAL DIAGNOSIS(ES) FOR INPATIENT, SHORT-TERM, ACUTE CARE HOSPITAL RECORDS

The circumstances of inpatient admission always govern the selection of principal diagnosis. The principal diagnosis is defined in the Uniform Hospital Discharge Data Set (UHDDS) as "that condition established after study to be chiefly responsible for occasioning the admission of the patient to the hospital for care."

The UHDDS definitions are used by acute care short-term hospitals to report inpatient data elements in a standardized manner. These data elements and their definitions can be found in the July 31, 1985, Federal Register (Vol. 50, No, 147), pp. 31038-40.

In determining principal diagnosis the coding conventions in the ICD-9-CM, Volumes I and II take precedence over these official coding guidelines. (See Section IA).

The importance of consistent, complete documentation in the medical record cannot be overemphasized. Without such documentation the application of all coding guidelines is a difficult, if not impossible, task.

A. Codes for symptoms, signs, and ill-defined conditions

Codes for symptoms, signs, and ill-defined conditions from Chapter 16 are not to be used as principal diagnosis when a related definitive diagnosis has been established.

B. Two or more interrelated conditions, each potentially meeting the definition for principal diagnosis.

When there are two or more interrelated conditions (such as diseases in the same ICD-9-CM chapter or manifestations characteristically associated with a certain disease) potentially meeting the definition of principal diagnosis, either condition may be sequenced first, unless the circumstances of the admission, the therapy provided, the Tabular List, or the Alphabetic Index indicate otherwise.

C. Two or more diagnoses that equally meet the definition for principal diagnosis.

In the unusual instance when two or more diagnoses equally meet the criteria for principal diagnosis as determined by the circumstances of admission, diagnostic workup and/or therapy provided, and the Alphabetic Index, Tabular List, or another coding guidelines does not provide sequencing direction, any one of the diagnoses may be sequenced first.

D. Two or more comparative or contrasting conditions.

In those rare instances when two or more contrasting or comparative diagnoses are documented as "either/or" (or similar terminology), they are coded as if the diagnoses were confirmed and the diagnoses are sequenced according to the circumstances of the admission. If no further determination can be made as to which diagnosis should be principal, either diagnosis may be sequenced first.

E. A symptom(s) followed by contrasting/comparative diagnoses.

When a symptom(s) is followed by contrasting/comparative diagnoses, the symptom code is sequenced first. All the contrasting/comparative diagnoses should be coded as additional diagnoses.

F. Original treatment plan not carried out.

Sequence as the principal diagnosis the condition, which after study occasioned the admission to the hospital, even though treatment may not have been carried out due to unforeseen circumstances.

G. Complications of surgery and other medical care.

When the admission is for treatment of a complication resulting from surgery or other medical care, the complication code is sequenced as the principal diagnosis. If the complication is classified to the 996-999 series, an additional code for the specific complication may be assigned.

H. Uncertain Diagnosis.

If the diagnosis documented at the time of discharge is qualified as "probable", "suspected", "likely", "questionable", "possible", or "still to be ruled out", code the condition as if it existed or was established. The bases for these guidelines are the diagnostic workup, arrangements for further workup or observation, and initial therapeutic approach that correspond most closely with the established diagnosis.

SECTION III REPORTING ADDITIONAL DIAGNOSES FOR INPATIENT, SHORT-TERM, ACUTE CARE HOSPITAL RECORDS

GENERAL RULES FOR OTHER (ADDITIONAL) DIAGNOSES

For reporting purposes the definition for "other diagnoses" is interpreted as additional conditions that affect patient care in terms of requiring:

clinical evaluation; or

therapeutic treatment; or

diagnostic procedures; or

extended length of hospital stay; or

increased nursing care and/or monitoring.

The UHDDS item #11-b defines Other Diagnoses as "all conditions that coexist at the time of admission, that develop subsequently, or that affect the treatment received and/or the length of stay. Diagnoses that relate to an earlier episode which have no bearing on the current hospital stay are to be excluded." UHDDS definitions apply to inpatients in acute care, short-term, hospital setting The UHDDS definitions are used by acute care short-term hospitals to report inpatient data elements in a standardized manner. These data elements and their definitions can be found in the July 31, 1985, Federal Register (Vol. 50, No, 147), pp. 31038-40.

The following guidelines are to be applied in designating "other diagnoses" when neither the Alphabetic Index nor the Tabular List in ICD-9-CM provide direction. The listing of the diagnoses in the patient record is the responsibility of the attending physician.

A. Previous conditions

If the physician has included a diagnosis in the final diagnostic statement, such as the discharge summary or the face sheet, it should ordinarily be coded. Some physicians include in the diagnostic statement resolved conditions or diagnoses and status-post procedures from previous admission that have no bearing on the current stay. Such conditions are not to be reported and are coded only if required by hospital policy.

However, history codes (V10-V19) may be used as secondary codes if the historical condition or family history has an impact on current care or influences treatment.

B. Abnormal findings

Abnormal findings (laboratory, x-ray, pathologic, and other diagnostic results) are not coded and reported unless the physician indicates their clinical significance. If the findings are outside the normal range and the attending physician has ordered other tests to evaluate the condition or prescribed treatment, it is appropriate to ask the physician whether the abnormal finding should be added.

Please note: This differs from the coding practices in the outpatient setting for coding encounters for diagnostic tests that have been interpreted by a physician.

C. Uncertain Diagnosis

If the diagnosis documented at the time of discharge is qualified as "probable", "suspected", "likely", "questionable", "possible", or "still to be ruled out", code the condition as if it existed or was established. The bases for these guidelines are the diagnostic workup, arrangements for further workup or observation, and initial therapeutic approach that correspond most closely with the established diagnosis.

SECTION IV DIAGNOSTIC CODING AND REPORTING GUIDELINES FOR OUTPATIENT SERVICES

These coding guidelines for outpatient diagnoses have been approved for use by hospitals/physicians in coding and reporting hospital-based outpatient services and physician office visits.

Information about the use of certain abbreviations, punctuation, symbols, and other conventions used in the ICD-9-CM Tabular List (code numbers and titles), can be found in Section IA of these guidelines, under "Conventions Used in the Tabular

List." Information about the correct sequence to use in finding a code is also described in Section I.

The terms encounter and visit are often used interchangeably in describing outpatient service contacts and, therefore, appear together in these guidelines without distinguishing one from the other.

Though the conventions and general guidelines apply to all settings, coding guidelines for outpatient and physician reporting of diagnoses will vary in a number of instances from those for inpatient diagnoses, recognizing that:

The Uniform Hospital Discharge Data Set (UHDDS) definition of princi-pal diagnosis applies only to inpatients in acute, short-term, general hospitals.

Coding guidelines for inconclusive diagnoses (probable, suspected, rule out, etc.) were developed for inpatient reporting and do not apply to outpatients.

A. Selection of first-listed condition

In the outpatient setting, the term first-listed diagnosis is used in lieu of principal diagnosis.

In determining the first-listed diagnosis the coding conventions of ICD-9-CM, as well as the general and disease specific guidelines take precedence over the outpatient guidelines.

Diagnoses often are not established at the time of the initial encounter/visit. It may take two or more visits before the diagnosis is confirmed.

The most critical rule involves beginning the search for the correct code assignment through the Alphabetic Index. Never begin searching initially in the Tabular List as this will lead to coding errors.

B. The appropriate code or codes from 001.0 through V83.89 must be used to identify diagnoses, symptoms, conditions, problems, complaints, or other reason(s) for the encounter/visit.

C. For accurate reporting of ICD-9-CM diagnosis codes, the documentation should describe the patient's condition, using terminology which includes specific diagnoses as well as symptoms, problems, or reasons for the encounter. There are ICD-9-CM codes to describe all of these.

D. The selection of codes 001.0 through 999.9 will frequently be used to describe the reason for the encounter. These codes are from the section of ICD-9-CM for the classification of diseases and injuries (e.g. infectious and parasitic diseases; neoplasms; symptoms, signs, and ill-defined conditions, etc.).

E. Codes that describe symptoms and signs, as opposed to diagnoses, are acceptable for reporting purposes when a diagnosis has not been established (confirmed) by the physician. Chapter 16 of ICD-9-CM, Symptoms, Signs, and Ill-defined conditions (codes 780.0-799.9) contain many, but not all codes for symptoms.

F. ICD-9-CM provides codes to deal with encounters for circumstances other than a disease or injury. The Supplementary Classification of factors Influencing Health Status and Contact with Health Services (V01.0-V83.89) is provided to deal with occasions when circumstances other than a disease or injury are recorded as diagnosis or problems.

G. Level of Detail in Coding

1. ICD-9-CM is composed of codes with either 3, 4, or 5 digits. Codes with three digits are included in ICD-9-CM as the heading of a category of codes that may be further subdivided by the use of fourth and/or fifth digits, which provide greater specificity.

2. A three-digit code is to be used only if it is not further sub-divided. Where fourth-digit subcategories and/or fifth-digit subclassifications are provided, they must be assigned. A code is invalid if it has not been coded to the full number of digits required for that code. See also discussion under Section I, General Coding Guidelines, Level of Detail.

H. List first the ICD-9-CM code for the diagnosis, condition, problem, or other reason for encounter/visit shown in the medical record to be chiefly responsible for the services provided. List additional codes that describe any coexisting conditions.

I. Do not code diagnoses documented as "probable", "suspected," "questionable," "rule out," or "working diagnosis". Rather, code the condition(s) to the highest degree of certainty for that encounter/visit, such as symptoms, signs, abnormal test results, or other reason for the visit.

Please note: This differs from the coding practices used by hospital medical record departments for coding the diagnosis of acute care, short-term hospital inpatients.

J. Chronic diseases treated on an ongoing basis may be coded and reported as many times as the patient receives treatment and care for the condition(s).

K. Code all documented conditions that coexist at the time of the encounter/visit, and require or affect patient care treatment or management. Do not code conditions that were previously treated and no longer exist. However, history codes (V10-V19) may be used as secondary codes if the historical condition or family history has an impact on current care or influences treatment.

L. For patients receiving diagnostic services only during an encounter/visit, sequence first the diagnosis, condition, problem, or other reason for encounter/visit shown in the medical record to be chiefly responsible for the outpatient services provided during the encounter/visit. Codes for other diagnoses (e.g., chronic conditions) may be sequenced as additional diagnoses.

For outpatient encounters for diagnostic tests that have been interpreted by a physician, and the final report is available at the time of coding, code any confirmed or definitive diagnosis(es) documented in the interpretation. Do not code related signs and symptoms as additional diagnoses.

Please note: This differs from the coding practice in the hospital inpatient setting regarding abnormal findings on test results.

M. For patients receiving therapeutic services only during an encounter/visit, sequence first the diagnosis, condition, problem, or other reason for encounter/visit shown in the medical record to be chiefly responsible for the outpatient services provided during the encounter/visit. Codes for other diagnoses (e.g., chronic conditions) may be sequenced as additional diagnoses.

The only exception to this rule is that when the primary reason for the admission/encounter is chemotherapy, radiation therapy, or rehabilitation, the appropriate V code for the service is listed first, and the diagnosis or problem for which the service is being performed listed second.

N. For patient's receiving preoperative evaluations only, sequence a code from category V72.8, Other specified examinations, to describe the pre-op consultations. Assign a code for the condition to describe the reason for the surgery as an additional diagnosis. Code also any findings related to the pre-op evaluation.

O. For ambulatory surgery, code the diagnosis for which the surgery was performed. If the postoperative diagnosis is known to be different from the preoperative diagnosis at the time the diagnosis is confirmed, select the postoperative diagnosis for coding, since it is the most definitive.

P. For routine outpatient prenatal visits when no complications are present codes V22.0, Supervision of normal first pregnancy, and V22.1, Supervision of other normal pregnancy, should be used as principal diagnoses. These codes should not be used in conjunction with chapter 11 codes.

Appendix B

Medical Terminology

ablation	removal by cutting
abortion	termination of pregnancy
actinotherapy	treatment of acne using ultraviolet rays
adenoidectomy	removal of adenoids
adipose	fatty
adrenal	glands, located at the top of the kidneys, that produce steroid hormones
albinism	water-soluble protein
allograft	homograft, same species graft
alopecia	condition in which hair falls out
amniocentesis	percutaneous aspiration of amniotic fluid
amniotic sac	sac containing the fetus and amniotic fluid
A-mode	one-dimensional ultrasonic display reflecting the time it takes a sound wave to reach a structure and reflect back; maps the structure's outline
anastomosis	surgical connection of two tubular structures, such as two pieces of the intestine
aneurysm	sac formed outside the vessel, artery, or heart
angina	sudden pain
angiography	radiography of the blood vessels
angioplasty	surgical or percutaneous procedure in a vessel to dilate the vessel opening; used in the treatment of atherosclerotic disease

anhidrosis	deficiency of sweat
anomaloscope	instrument used to test color vision
anoscopy	procedure that uses a scope to examine the anus
antepartum	before childbirth
anterior (ventral)	in front of
anterior segment	those parts of the eye in the front of and including the lens, orbit, extraocular muscles, and eyelid
anteroposterior	from front to back
antigen	a substance that produces a specific response
aortography	radiographic recording of the aorta
apexcardiography	recording of the movement of the chest wall
aphakia	absence of the lens of the eye
apicectomy	excision of a portion of the temporal bone
apnea	stop breathing
arthrocentesis	injection and/or aspiration of joint
arthrodesis	surgical fixation of joint
arthrography	radiography of joint
arthroplasty	reshaping or reconstruction of joint
arthroscopy	use of scope to view inside joint
arthrotomy	incision into joint
articular	pertains to joint
asphyxia	lack of oxygen
aspiration	use of a needle and a syringe to withdraw fluid
assignment	Medicare's payment for the service, which participating physicians agree to accept as payment in full
asthma	shortage of breath caused by contraction of bronchi
astigmatism	condition in which the refractive surfaces of the eye are unequal
atelectasis	incomplete expansion of lung
atherectomy	removal of plaque by percutaneous method
atrophy	wasting away
audiometry	hearing test
aural atresia	congenital absence of the external auditory canal
auscultation	listening to sounds, such as to lung sounds
autograft	from patient's own body
axillary nodes	lymph nodes located in the armpit
bacilli	plural of bacillus, a bacterium

barium enema	radiographic contrast medium
beneficiary	person who benefits from health or life insurance
bifocal	two focuses in eyeglasses, one usually for close work and the other for improvement of distance vision
bilateral	occurring on two sides
biliary	refers to gallbladder, bile, or bile duct
bilobectomy	surgical removal of two lobes of a lung
biofeedback	process of giving a person self-information
biometry	application of a statistical measure to a biologic fact
biopsy	removal of a small piece of living tissue for diagnostic purposes
block	frozen piece of a sample
brachytherapy	therapy using radioactive sources that are placed inside the body
bronchiole	smaller division of bronchial tree
bronchography	radiographic recording of the lungs
bronchoplasty	surgical repair of the bronchi
bronchoscopy	inspection of the bronchial tree using a bronchoscope
B-scan	two-dimensional display of tissues and organs
bulbocavernosus	muscle that constricts the vagina in a female and the urethra in a male
bulbourethral	gland rounded mass of the urethra
bundle of His	muscular cardiac fibers that provide the heart rhythm to the ventricles; blockage of this rhythm produces heart block
bundled codes	one code that represents a package of services
bunion	hallux valgus, abnormal increase in size of metatarsal head that results in displacement of the great toe
burr	drill used to create an entry into the cranium
bursa	fluid-filled sac that absorbs friction
bursitis	inflammation of bursa
bypass	to go around
calcaneal	heel bone
calculus	concretion of mineral salts, also called a stone
calycoplasty	surgical reconstruction of a recess of the renal pelvis
calyx	recess of the renal pelvis
cancellous	lattice-type structure, usually of bone
cardiopulmonary	refers to the heart and lungs
cardiopulmonary bypass	blood bypasses the heart through a heart-lung machine during open-heart surgery
cardioversion	electrical shock to the heart to restore normal rhythm

cardioverter-defibrillator	surgically placed device that directs an electrical current shock to the heart to restore rhythm
carotid body	located on each side of the common carotid artery, often a site of tumor
cartilage	connective tissue
cataract	opaque covering on or in the lens
catheter	tube placed into the body to put fluid in or take fluid out
caudal	same as inferior; away from the head, or the lower part of the body
causalgia	burning pain
cauterization	destruction of tissue by the use of cautery
cavernosa	saphenous vein shunt creation of a connection between the cavity of the penis and a vein
cavernosography	radiographic recording of a cavity, e.g., the pulmonary cavity or the main part of the penis
cavernosometry	measurement of the pressure in a cavity, e.g., the penis
central nervous system	brain and spinal cord
cervical	pertaining to the neck or to the cervix of the uterus
cervix uteri	rounded, cone-shaped neck of the uterus
cesarean	surgical opening through abdominal wall for delivery
cholangiography	radiographic recording of the bile ducts
cholangiopancreatography	ERCP, radiographic recording of the biliary system or pancreas
cholecystectomy	surgical removal of the gallbladder
cholecystoenterostomy	creation of a connection between the gallbladder and intestine
cholecystography	radiographic recording of the gallbladder
cholesteatoma	tumor that forms in middle ear
chondral	referring to the cartilage
chordee	condition resulting in the penis being bent downward
chorionic villus sampling	CVS, biopsy of the outermost part of the placenta
circumflex	a coronary artery that circles the heart
Cloquet's node	also called a gland; it is the highest of the deep groin lymph nodes
closed fracture repair	not surgically opened with/without manipulation and with/without traction
closed treatment	fracture site that is not surgically opened and visualized
coccyx	caudal extremity of vertebral column
collagen	protein substance of skin
Colles' fracture	fracture at lower end of radius that displaces the bone posteriorly
colonoscopy	fiberscopic examination of the entire colon that may include part of the terminal ileum

colostomy	artificial opening between the colon and the abdominal wall
component	part
computed axial tomography	CAT or CT, procedure by which selected planes of tissue are pinpointed through computer enhancement, and images may be reconstructed by analysis of variance in absorption of the tissue
conjunctiva	the lining of the eyelids and the covering of the sclera
contraction	drawn together
contralateral	opposite side
cordectomy	surgical removal of the vocal cord(s)
cordocentesis	procedure to obtain a fetal blood sample; also called a percutaneous umbilical blood sampling
corneosclera	cornea and sclera of the eye
corpectomy	removal of vertebrae
corpora cavernosa	the two cavities of the penis
corpus uteri	uterus
crackle	abnormal sound when breathing
craniectomy	permanent, partial removal of skull
craniotomy	opening of the skull
cranium	that part of the skeleton that encloses the brain
curettage	scraping of a cavity using a spoon-shaped instrument
curette	spoon-shaped instrument used to remove material from a cavity
cutdown	incision into a vessel for placement of a catheter
cyanosis	bluish
cystocele	herniation of the bladder into the vagina
cystography	radiographic recording of the urinary bladder
cystolithectomy	removal of a calculus (stone) from the urinary bladder
cystolithotomy	cystolithectomy
cystometrogram	CMG, measurement of the pressures and capacity of the urinary bladder
cystoplasty	surgical reconstruction of the bladder
cystorrhaphy	suture of the bladder
cystoscopy	use of a scope to view the bladder
cystostomy	surgical creation of an opening into the bladder
cystotomy	incision into the bladder
cystourethroplasty	surgical reconstruction of the bladder and urethra
cystourethroscopy	use of a scope to view the bladder and urethra
dacryocystography	radiographic recording of the lacrimal sac or tear duct sac

dacryostenosis	narrowing of the lacrimal duct
debridement	cleansing of or removal of dead tissue from a wound
deductible	amount the patient is liable for before the payer begins to pay for covered services
delayed flap	pedicle of skin with blood supply that is separated from origin over time
delivery	childbirth
dermabrasion	planing of the skin by means of sander, brushes, or sandpaper
dermatologist	physician who treats conditions of the skin
dermatoplasty	surgical repair of skin
dialysis	filtration of blood
dilation	stretching
diskectomy	removal of a vertebral disk
diskography	radiographic recording of an intervertebral joint
dislocation	placement in a location other than the original location
distal	farther from the point of attachment or origin
diverticulum	protrusion in the wall of an organ
Doppler	ultrasonic measure of blood movement
dosimetry	scientific calculation of radiation emitted from various radioactive sources
drainage	free flow or withdrawal of fluids from a wound or cavity
duodenography	radiographic recording of the duodenum or first part of the small intestine
dysphagia	difficulty swallowing
dysphonia	speech impairment
dyspnea	shortage of breath
echocardiography	radiographic recording of the heart or heart walls or surrounding tissues
echoencephalography	ultrasound of the brain
echography	ultrasound procedure in which sound waves are bounced off an internal organ and the resulting image is recorded
ectopic	pregnancy outside the uterus (i.e., in the fallopian tube)
edema	swelling due to abnormal fluid collection in the tissue spaces
elective surgery	nonemergency procedure
electrocardiogram	ECG, written record of the electrical action of the heart
electrocautery	cauterization by means of heated instrument
electrocochleography	test to measure the eighth cranial nerve (hearing test)
electrode	lead attached to a generator that carries the electrical current from the generator to the atria or ventricles

electroencephalogram	EEG, written record of the electrical action of the brain
electromyogram	EMG, written record of the electrical activity of the skeletal muscles
electronic claim submission	claims prepared and submitted via a computer
electronic signature	identification system of a computer
electro-oculogram	EOG, written record of the electrical activity of the eye
electrophysiology	the study of the electrical system of the heart, including the study of arrhythmias
embolectomy	removal of blockage (embolism) from vessels
emphysema	air accumulated in organ or tissue
encephalography	radiographic recording of the subarachnoid space and ventricles of the brain
endarterectomy	incision into an artery to remove the inner lining so as to eliminate disease or blockage
endomyocardial	pertaining to the inner and middle layers of the heart
endopyelotomy	procedure involving the bladder and ureters, including the insertion of a stent
endoscopy	inspection of body organs or cavities using a lighted scope that may be inserted through an existing opening or through a small incision
enterolysis	releasing of adhesions of intestine
enucleation	removal of an organ or organs from a body cavity
epicardial	over the heart
epidermolysis	superficial fungal infection
epididymectomy	surgical removal of the epididymis
epididymis	tube located at the top of the testes that stores sperm
epididymography	radiographic recording of the epididymis
epididymovasostomy	creation of a new connection between the vas deferens and epididymis
epiglottidectomy	excision of the covering of the larynx
episclera	connective covering of sclera
epistaxis	nose bleed
epithelium	surface covering of internal and external organs of the body
erythema	redness of skin
escharotomy	surgical incision into necrotic (dead) tissue
eventration	protrusion of the bowel through the viscera of the abdomen
evisceration	pulling the viscera outside of the body through an incision
evocative	tests that are administered to evoke a predetermined response
exenteration	removal of an organ all in one piece

exophthalmos	protrusion of the eyeball
exostosis	bony growth
exstrophy	condition in which an organ is turned inside out
extracorporeal	occurring outside of the body
false aneurysm	sac of clotted blood that has completely destroyed the vessel and is being contained by the tissue that surrounds the vessel
fasciectomy	removal of a band of fibrous tissue
Federal Register	official publication of all "Presidential Documents," "Rules and Regulations," "Proposed Rules," and "Notices"; government-instituted national changes are published in the *Federal Register*
fee schedule	services and payment allowed for each service
femoral	pertaining to the bone from the pelvis to knee
fenestration	creation of a new opening in the inner wall of the middle ear
fissure	groove
fistula	abnormal opening from one area to another area or to the outside of the body
fluoroscopy	procedure for viewing the interior of the body using x-rays and projecting the image onto a television screen
fracture	break in a bone
free full-thickness graft	graft of epidermis and dermis that is completely removed from donor area
fulguration	use of electrical current to destroy tissue
fundoplasty	repair of the bottom of an organ or muscle
furuncle	nodule in the skin caused by staphylococci entering through hair follicle
ganglion	knot
gastrointestinal	pertaining to the stomach and intestine
gastroplasty	operation on the stomach for repair or reconfiguration
gastrostomy	artificial opening between the stomach and the abdominal wall
gatekeeper	a physician who manages a patient's access to health care
glaucoma	eye diseases that are characterized by an increase of intraocular pressure
globe	eyeball
glottis	true vocal cords
gonioscopy	use of a scope to examine the angles of the eye
Group Practice Model	an organization of physicians who contract with a Health Maintenance Organization to provide services to the enrollees of the HMO
grouper	computer used to input the principal diagnosis and other critical information about a patient and then provide the correct DRG code

Health Maintenance Organization	HMO, a health care delivery system in which an enrollee is assigned a primary care physician who manages all the health care needs of the enrollee
hematoma	mass of blood that forms outside the vessel
hemodialysis	cleansing of the blood outside of the body
hemolytic	breakdown of red blood cells
hemoptysis	bloody sputum
hepatography	radiographic recording of the liver
hernia	organ or tissue protruding through the wall or cavity that usually contains it
histology	study of structure of tissue and cells
homograft	allograft, same species graft
hormone	chemical substance produced by the body
hydrocele	sac of fluid
hyperopia	farsightedness, eyeball is too short from front to back
hypogastric	lowest middle abdominal area
hyposensitization	decreased sensitivity
hypothermia	low body temperature; sometimes induced during surgical procedures
hypoxia	low level of oxygen in the blood of artery
hysterectomy	surgical removal of the uterus
hysterorrhaphy	suturing of the uterus
hysterosalpingography	radiographic recording of the uterine cavity and fallopian tubes
hysteroscopy	visualization of the canal of the uterine cervix and cavity of the uterus using a scope placed through the vagina
ichthyosis	skin disorder characterized by scaling
ileostomy	artificial opening between the ileum and the abdominal wall
ilium	portion of hip
imbrication	overlapping
immunotherapy	therapy to increase immunity
incarcerated	regarding hernias, a constricted, irreducible hernia that may cause obstruction of an intestine
incise	to cut into
Individual Practice Association	IPA, an organization of physicians who provide services for a set fee; Health Maintenance Organizations often contract with the IPA for services to their enrollees
inferior	away from the head or the lower part of the body; also known as caudalingual

inofemoral	referring to the groin and thigh
internal/external fixation	application of pins, wires, screws, and so on to immobilize a body part; they can be placed externally or internally
intracardiac	inside the heart
intramural	within the organ wall
intramuscular	into a muscle
intrauterine	inside the uterus
intravenous	into a vein
intravenous pyelography	IVP, radiographic recording of the urinary system
introitus	opening or entrance to the vagina from the uterus
intubation	insertion of a tube
invasive	entering the body, breaking skin
iontophoresis	introduction of ions into the body
ischemia	deficient blood supply due to obstruction of the circulatory system
island pedicle flap	contains a single artery and vein that remains attached to origin temporarily or permanently
isthmus	connection of two regions or structures
isthmus, thyroid	tissue connection between right and left thyroid lobes
isthmusectomy	surgical removal of the isthmus
jejunostomy	artificial opening between the jejunum and the abdominal wall
jugular nodes	lymph nodes located next to the large vein in the neck
keratomalacia	softening of the cornea associated with a deficiency of vitamin A
keratoplasty	surgical repair of the cornea
Kock pouch	surgical creation of a urinary bladder from a segment of the ileum
kyphosis	humpback
labyrinth	inner connecting cavities, such as the internal ear
labyrinthitis	middle ear inflammation
lacrimal	related to tears
lamina	flat plate
laminectomy	surgical excision of the lamina
laparoscopy	exploration of the abdomen and pelvic cavities using a scope placed through a small incision in the abdominal wall
laryngeal web	congenital abnormality of connective tissue between the vocal cords
laryngectomy	surgical removal of the larynx
laryngography	radiographic recording of the larynx
laryngoplasty	surgical repair of the larynx
laryngoscope	fiberoptic scope used to view the inside of the larynx

laryngoscopy	direct visualization and examination of the interior of larynx with a laryngoscope
laryngotomy	incision into the larynx
lateral	away from the midline of the body (to the side)
lavage	washing out
leukoderma	depigmentation of skin
leukoplakia	white patch on mucous membrane
ligament	fibrous band of tissue that connects cartilage or bones
ligation	binding or tying off, as in constricting the blood flow of a vessel or binding fallopian tubes for sterilization
lipocyte	fat cell
lipoma	fatty tumor
lithotomy	incision into an organ or a duct for the purpose of removing a stone
lithotripsy	crushing of a stone by sound waves or force
lobectomy	removal of lobe of lung
lordosis	anterior curve of spine
lumbodynia	pain in the lumbar area
lunate	one of the wrist (carpal) bones
lymph node	station along the lymphatic system
lymphadenectomy	excision of a lymph node or nodes
lymphadenitis	inflammation of a lymph node
lymphangiography	radiographic recording of the lymphatic vessels and nodes
lymphangiotomy	incision into a lymphatic vessel
lysis	releasing
magnetic resonance imaging	MRI, procedure that uses nonionizing radiation to view the body in a cross-sectional view
Major Diagnostic Categories	MDC, the division of all principal diagnoses into 25 mutually exclusive principal diagnosis areas within the DRG system
mammography	radiographic recording of the breasts
Managed Care Organization	MCO, a group that is responsible for the health care services offered to an enrolled group of persons
manipulation	movement by hand
manipulation or reduction	attempted restoration of a fracture or joint dislocation to its normal position
Maximum Actual Allowable Charge	MAAC, limitation on the total amount that can be charged by physicians who are not participants in Medicare

meatotomy	surgical enlargement of the opening of the urinary meatus
medial	toward the midline of the body
Medical Volume Performance Standards	MVPS, government's estimate of how much growth is appropriate for nationwide physician expenditures paid by the Part B Medicare program
Medicare Economic Index	MEI, government mandated index that ties increases in the Medicare prevailing charges to economic indicators
Medicare Fee Schedule	MFS, schedule that listed the allowable charges for Medicare services; was replaced by the Medicare reasonable charge payment system
Medicare Risk HMO	a Medicare-funded alternative to the standard Medicare supplemental coverage
melanin	dark pigment of skin
melanoma	tumor of epidermis
Ménière's disease	condition that causes dizziness, ringing in the ears, and deafness
M-mode	one-dimensional display of movement of structures
modality	treatment method
Mohs' surgery or Mohs' micrographic surgery	removal of skin cancer in layers by a surgeon who also acts as pathologist during surgery
monofocal	eyeglasses with one vision correction
muscle	organ of contraction for movement
muscle flap	transfer of muscle from origin to recipient site
myasthenia gravis	syndrome characterized by muscle weakness
myelography	radiographic recording of the subarachnoid space of the spine
myopia	near-sightedness, eyeball too long from front to back
myringotomy	incision into tympanic membrane
nasal button	a synthetic circular disk used to cover a hole in the nasal septum
nasopharyngoscopy	use of a scope to visualize the nose and pharynx
National provider identifier	NPI, a 10-digit number assigned to a physician by Medicare
nephrectomy, paraperitoneal	kidney transplant
nephrocutaneous fistula	a channel from the kidney to the skin
nephrolithotomy	removal of a kidney stone through an incision made into the kidney
nephrorrhaphy	suturing of the kidney
nephrostolithotomy	creation of an artificial channel to the kidney
nephrostolithotomy, percutaneous	procedure to establish an artificial channel between the skin and the kidney
nephrostomy	creation of a channel into the renal pelvis of the kidney
nephrostomy, percutaneous	creation of a channel from the skin to the renal pelvis
nephrotomy	incision into the kidney

neurovascular flap	contains artery, vein, and nerve
noninvasive	not entering the body, not breaking skin
nuclear cardiology	diagnostic specialty that uses radiologic procedures to aid in diagnosis of cardiologic conditions
nystagmus	rapid involuntary eye movements
ocular adnexa	orbit, extraocular muscles, and eyelid
olecranon	elbow bone
Omnibus Budget Reconciliation Act of 1989	OBRA, act that established new rules for Medicare reimbursement
oophorectomy	surgical removal of the ovary(ies)
opacification	area that has become opaque (milky)
open fracture repair	surgical opening over or remotely opening of a fracture site
open treatment	fracture site that is surgically opened and visualized
ophthalmodynamometry	test of the blood pressure of the eye
ophthalmology	body of knowledge regarding the eyes
ophthalmoscopy	examination of the interior of the eye by means of a scope, also known as funduscopy
optokinetic	movement of the eyes to objects moving in the visual field
orchiectomy	castration
orchiopexy	surgical procedure to release undescended testis
order	shows subordination of one to another, family, or class
orthopnea	difficulty in breathing unless in the upright position
orthoptic	corrective; in the correct place
osteoarthritis	degenerative condition of articular cartilage
osteoclast	absorption or removal of bone
osteotomy	cutting into bone
otitis media	noninfectious inflammation of the ear; serous otitis media produces liquid drainage (not purulent) and suppurative otitis media is purulent (pus) matter
otoscope	instrument used to examine the internal and external ear
oviduct	fallopian tube
papilledema	swelling of the optic disk (papilla)
paraesophageal hiatus hernia	hernia that is near the esophagus
parathyroid	produces a hormone to mobilize calcium from the bones to the blood
paronychia	infection around nail
Part A	Medicare's Hospital Insurance; covers hospital/facility care
Part B	Medicare's Supplemental Medical Insurance; covers physician services and durable medical equipment that are not paid for under Part A

participating provider program	Medicare providers who have agreed in advance to accept assignment on all Medicare claims
patella	knee cap
pedicle	tumor on a stem
Peer Review Organizations	PROs, groups established to review hospital admission and care
pelviolithotomy	pyeloplasty
penoscrotal	referring to the penis and scrotum
percussion	tapping with sharp blows as a diagnostic technique
percutaneous	through the skin
percutaneous fracture repair	repair of a fracture by means of pins and wires inserted through the fracture site
percutaneous skeletal fixation	considered neither open nor closed; the fracture is not visualized, but fixation is placed across the fracture site under x-ray imaging
pericardiocentesis	procedure in which a surgeon withdraws fluid from the pericardial space by means of a needle inserted percutaneously into the space
pericardium	membranous sac enclosing heart and ends of great vessels
perinephric cyst	cyst in the tissue around the kidney
perineum	area between the vulva and anus; also known as the pelvic floor
peripheral nerves	12 pairs of cranial nerves, 31 pairs of spinal nerves, and autonomic nervous system; connects peripheral receptors to the brain and spinal cord
perirenal	around the kidney
peritoneal	within the lining of the abdominal cavity
peritoneoscopy	visualization of the abdominal cavity using one scope placed through a small incision in the abdominal wall and another scope placed in the vagina
pharyngolaryngectomy	surgical removal of the pharynx and larynx
phlebotomy	cutting into a vein
phonocardiogram	recording of heart sounds
photochemotherapy	treatment by means of drugs that react to ultraviolet radiation or sunlight
physics	scientific study of energy
pilosebaceous	pertains to hair follicles and sebaceous glands
placenta	an organism that connects the fetus and mother during pregnancy
plethysmography	determining the changes in volume of an organ part or body
pleura	lines lungs and thoracic cavity
pleurectomy	surgical excision of the pleura
pleuritis	inflammation of the pleura

pneumonocentesis	surgical puncturing of a lung to withdraw fluid
pneumonolysis	surgical separation of the lung from the chest wall to allow the lung to collapse
pneumonostomy	surgical procedure in which the chest cavity is exposed and the lung is incised
pneumonotomy	incision of the lung
pneumoplethysmography	determining the changes in the volume of the lung
posterior (dorsal)	in back of
posterior segment	those parts of the eye behind the lens
posteroanterior	from back to front
postpartum	after childbirth
Preferred Provider Organization	PPO, a group of providers who form a network and who have agreed to provide services to enrollees at a discounted rate
priapism	painful condition in which the penis is constantly erect
primary care physician	PCP, physician who oversees a patient's care within a managed care organization
primary diagnosis	chief complaint of a patient in outpatient setting
prior approval	also known as a prior authorization, the payer's approval of care
proctosigmoidoscopy	fiberscopic examination of the sigmoid colon and rectum
Professional Standards Review Organization	PSRO, voluntary physicians' organization designed to monitor the necessity of hospital admissions, treatment costs, and medical records of hospitals
prognosis	probable outcome of an illness
prostatotomy	incision into the prostate
provider identification number	PIN, assigned to physicians by payers for use in claims submission
pyelography	radiographic recording of the kidneys, renal pelvis, ureters, and bladder
qualitative	measuring the presence or absence of
quantitative	measuring the presence or absence of and the amount of
rad	radiation-absorbed dose, the energy deposited in patient's tissues
radiation oncology	branch of medicine concerned with the application of radiation to a tumor site for treatment (destruction) of cancerous tumors
radiograph	film on which an image is produced through exposure to x-radiation
radiologist	physician who specializes in the use of radioactive materials in the diagnosis and treatment of disease and illnesses
radiology	branch of medicine concerned with the use of radioactive substances for diagnosis and therapy
rales	coarse sound on inspiration, also known as crackle

real time	two-dimensional display of both the structures and the motion of tissues and organs, with the length of time also recorded as part of the study
reduction	replace to normal position
Relative Value Unit	RVU, unit value that has been assigned for each service
Resource-Based Relative Value Scale	RBRVS, scale designed to decrease Medicare expenditures, redistribute physician payment, and ensure quality health care at reasonable rates
resource intensity	refers to the relative volume and type of diagnostic, therapeutic, and bed services used in the management of a particular illness
retrograde	moving backward or against the usual direction of flow
rhinoplasty	surgical repair of nose
rhinorrhea	nasal mucous discharge
salpingectomy	surgical removal of the uterine tube
salpingostomy	creation of a fistula into the uterine tube
scan	mapping of emissions of radioactive substances after they have been introduced into the body; the density can determine normal or abnormal conditions
sclera	outer covering of the eye
sebaceous gland	secretes sebum
seborrhea	excess sebum secretion
sebum	oily substance
section	slice of a frozen block
segmentectomy	surgical removal of a portion of a lung
septoplasty	surgical repair of the nasal septum
serum	blood from which the fibrinogen has been removed
severity of illness	refers to the levels of loss of function and mortality that may be experienced by patients with a particular disease
shunt	divert or make an artificial passage
sialography	radiographic recording of the salivary duct and branches
sialolithotomy	surgical removal of a stone of the salivary gland or duct
sinography	radiographic recording of the sinus or sinus tract
sinusotomy	surgical incision into a sinus
skeletal traction	application of pressure to the bone by means of pins and/or wires inserted into the bone
skin traction	application of pressure to the bone by means of tape applied to the skin
skull	entire skeletal framework of the head
somatic nerve	sensory or motor nerve
specimen	sample of tissue or fluid

spirometry	measurement of breathing capacity
splenectomy	excision of the spleen
splenography	radiographic recording of the spleen
splenoportography	radiographic procedure to allow visualization of the splenic and portal veins of the spleen
split-thickness graft	all epidermis and some of dermis
spondylitis	inflammation of vertebrae
Staff Model	a Health Maintenance Organization that directly employs the physicians who provide services to enrollees
steatoma	fat mass in sebaceous gland
stem cell	immature blood cell
stereotaxis	method of identifying a specific area or point in the brain
strabismus	extraocular muscle deviation resulting in unequal visual axes
stratified	layered
stratum	layer
subcutaneous	tissue below the dermis, primarily fat cells that insulate the body
subluxation	partial dislocation
subungual	beneath the nail
superior	toward the head or the upper part of the body; also known as cephalic
supination	supine position
supine	lying on the back
Swan Ganz catheter	a catheter that measures pressure in the heart
sympathetic nerve	part of the peripheral nervous system that controls automatic body function and sympathetic nerves activated under stress
symphysis	natural junction
synchondrosis	union between two bones
tachypnea	quick, shallow breathing
tarsorrhaphy	suturing together of the eyelids
Tax Equity and Fiscal Responsibility Act	TEFRA, act that contains language to reward cost-conscious health care providers
tendon	attaches a muscle to a bone
tenodesis	suturing of a tendon to a bone
tenorrhaphy	suture repair of tendon
thermogram	written record of temperature variation
third-party payer	insurance company or entity that is liable for another's health care services
thoracentesis	surgical puncture of the thoracic cavity, usually using a needle, to remove fluids

thoracic duct	collection and distribution point for lymph, and the largest lymph vessel located in the chest
thoracoplasty	surgical procedure that removes rib(s) and thereby allows the collapse of a lung
thoracoscopy	use of a lighted endoscope to view the pleural spaces and thoracic cavity or to perform surgical procedures
thoracostomy	surgical incision into the chest wall and insertion of a chest tube
thoracotomy	surgical incision into the chest wall
thromboendarterectomy	procedure to remove plaque or clot formations from a vessel by percutaneous method
thymectomy	surgical removal of the thymus
thymus	gland that produces hormones important to the immune response
thyroglossal duct	connection between the thyroid and the pharynx
thyroid	part of the endocrine system that produces hormones that regulate metabolism
thyroidectomy	surgical removal of the thyroid
tinnitus	ringing in the ears
titer	measure of a laboratory analysis
tocolysis	repression of uterine contractions
tomography	procedure that allows viewing of a single plane of the body by blurring out all but that particular level
tonography	recording of changes in intraocular pressure in response to sustained pressure on the eyeball
tonometry	measurement of pressure or tension
total pneumonectomy	surgical removal of an entire lobe of a lung
tracheostomy	creation of an opening into trachea
tracheotomy	incision into trachea
traction	application of pressure to maintain normal alignment
transcutaneous	entering by way of the skin
transesophageal echocardiogram	TEE, echocardiogram performed by placing a probe down the esophagus and sending out sound waves to obtain images of the heart and its movement
transmastoid antrostomy	called a simple mastoidectomy, it creates an opening in the mastoid for drainage
transplantation	grafting of tissue from one source to another
transseptal	through the septum
transtracheal	across the trachea
transureteroureterostomy	surgical connection of one ureter to the other ureter
transurethral resection, prostate	procedure performed through the urethra by means of a cystoscopy to remove part or all of the prostate

transvenous	across a vein
transvesical ureterolithotomy	removal of a ureter stone (calculus) through the bladder
trephination	surgical removal of a disk of bone
trocar needle	needle with a tube on the end; used to puncture and withdraw fluid from a cavity
tubercle	lesion caused by infection of tuberculosis
tumescence	state of being swollen
tunica vaginalis	covering of the testes
tympanolysis	freeing of adhesions of the tympanic membrane
tympanometry	test of the inner ear using air pressure
tympanostomy	insertion of ventilation tube into tympanum
ultrasound	technique using sound waves to determine the density of the outline of tissue
unbundling	reporting with multiple codes that which can be reported with one code
unilateral	occurring on one side
uptake	absorption of a radioactive substance by body tissues; recorded for diagnostic purposes in conditions such as thyroid disease
ureterectomy	surgical removal of a ureter, either totally or partially
ureterocolon	pertaining to the ureter and colon
ureterocutaneous fistula	the channel from the ureter to the exterior skin
ureteroenterostomy	creation of a connection between the intestine and the ureter
ureterolithotomy	removal of a stone from the ureter
ureterolysis	freeing of adhesions of the ureter
ureteroneocystostomy	surgical connection of the ureter to a new site on the bladder
ureteropyelography	ureter and bladder radiography
ureterotomy	incision into the ureter
urethrocystography	radiography of the bladder and urethra
urethromeatoplasty	surgical repair of the urethra and meatus
urethropexy	fixation of the urethra by means of surgery
urethroplasty	surgical repair of the urethra
urethrorrhaphy	suturing of the urethra
urethroscopy	use of a scope to view the urethra
urography	same as pyelography; radiographic recording of the kidneys, renal pelvis, ureters, and bladder
uveal	vascular tissue of the choroid, ciliary body, and iris
varices	varicose vein
varicocele	swelling of a scrotal vein
vas deferens	tube that carries sperm from the epididymis to the urethra

vasogram	recording of the flow in the vas deferens
vasotomy	creation of an opening in the vas deferens
vasovasorrhaphy	suturing of the vas deferens
vasovasostomy	reversal of a vasectomy
vectorcardiogram	VCG, continuous recording of electrical direction and magnitude of the heart
venography	radiographic recording of the veins and tributaries
vertigo	dizziness
vesicostomy	surgical creation of a connection of the viscera of the bladder to the skin
vesicovaginal fistula	creation of a tube between the vagina and the bladder
vesiculectomy	excision of the seminal vesicle
vesiculography	radiographic recording of the seminal vesicles
vesiculotomy	incision into the seminal vesicle
viscera	an organ in one of the large cavities of the body
volvulus	twisted section of the intestine
vomer	flat bones of the nasal septum
xanthoma	tumor composed of cells containing lipid material
xenograft	different species graft
xeroderma	dry, discolored, scaly skin
xeroradiography	photoelectric process of radiographs

Appendix C

Combining Forms

abdomin/o	abdomen
acetabul/o	hip socket
acr/o	height/extremities
adeno/ adnen/o	gland
adenoid/o	adenoids
adip/o	fat
albin/o	white
albumin/o	albumin
alveol/o	alveolus
ambly/o	dim
amni/o	amnion
an/o	anus
andr/o	male
andren/o adreno	adrenal gland
andrenal/o adrenalo	adrenal gland
angi/o	vessel
ankyl/o	bent
aort/o	aorta
aponeur/o	tendon type
appendic/o	appendix
aque/o	water

arche/o	first
arter/o	artery
arthr/o	joint
atel/o	incomplete
atri/o	atrium
audi/o	hearing
aut/o	self
axill/o	armpit
azot/o	urea
balan/o	glans penis
bi/o	life
bil/i	bile
bilirubin/o	bile pigment
blephar/o	eyelid
brachi/o	arm
bronch/o	bronchus
bronchi/o	bronchus
bronchiol/o	bronchiole
burs/o	joint fluid sac
calc/o or calci/I	calcium
calc/o, calci/o	calcium
cardi/o	heart
carp/o	carpals (wrist bones)
cauter/o	burn
cec/o	cecum
celi/o	abdomen
cephal/o	head
cerebell/o	cerebellum
cerebr/o	cerebrum
cervic/o	neck/cervix
cervic/o	cervix
chol/e	gall
cholangio/o	bile duct
cholecyst/o	gallbladder
choledoch/o	common bile duct
cholester/o	cholesterol
chondr/o	cartilage

chori/o	chorion
clavic/o, clavicul/o	clavicle (collar bone)
col/o	colon
colp/o	vagina
coni/o	dust
conjunctiv/o	conjunctiva
cor/o coreo	pupil
corne/o	cornea
coron/o	heart
cost/o	rib
crani/o	cranium (skull)
crin/o	secrete
crypt/o	hidden
culd/o	cul-de-sac
cutane/o	skin
cyan/o	blue
cyano/ cryan/o	blue
cycl/o	ciliary body
cyst/o	bladder
dacry/o	tear
dacryocyst/o-	prefix meaning pertaining to the lacrimal sac
dent/i	tooth
derm/o	skin
diaphragmat/o	diaphragm
dips/o	thirst
disk/o	intervertebral disk
diverticul/o	diverticulum
duoden/o	duodenum
dur/o	dura mater
encephal/o	brain
enter/o	small intestine
eosin/o	rosy
epididym/o	epididymis
epiglott/o	epiglottis
episi/o	vulva
erythr/o	red
esophag/o	esophagus

estr/o	female
femor/o	thighbone
fet/o	fetus
fibul/o	fibula
galact/o	milk
gangli/o	ganglion
ganglion/o	ganglion
gastr/o	stomach
gingiv/o	gum
glomerul/o	glomerulus
gloss/o	tongue
gluc/o	sugar
glyc/o	sugar
glycos/o	sugar
gonad/o	ovaries and testes
gyn/o	female
gynec/o	female
hepat/o	liver
herni/o	hernia
heter/o	different
hidr/o	sweat
home/o	same
hormon/o	hormone
humer/o	humerus (upper arm bone)
hydr/o	water
hymen/o	hymen
hyster/o	uterus
ichthy/o	dry/scaly
ile/o	ileus
ili/o	ilium (upper pelvic bone)
immun/o	immune
inguin/o	groin
sir/o	iris
irid/o	iris
isch/o	back
jaund/o	yellow
jejun/o	jejunum

kal/i	potassium
kerat/o	hard
kerat/o	cornea
kinesi/o	movement
kyph/o	hump
lacrim/o	tear
lact/o	milk
lamin/o	lamina
lapar/o	abdomen
lapar/o	abdominal wall
laryng/o	larynx
lingu/o	tongue
lip/o	fat
lith/o	stone
lob/o	lobe
lord/o	curve
lumb/o	lower back
lute/o	yellow
lymph/o	lymph
lymphaden/o	lymph gland
mamm/o	breast
mandibul/o	mandible (lower jawbone)
mast/o	breast
maxilla/o	maxilla (upper jawbone)
meat/o	meatus
melan/o	black
men/o	menstruation, month
mening/o	meninges
menisc/o	meniscus
ment/o	mind
metacarp/o	metacarpals (hand)
metatars/o	metatarsals (foot)
metr/o	uterus, measure
metri/o	uterus
mon/o	one
muc/o	mucus
my/o, myos/o	muscle

myc/o	fungus
myel/o	bone marrow
myx/o	mucus
nas/o	nose
nati/i	birth
natr/o	sodium
necr/o	death
nephr/o	kidney
neur/o	nerve
noct/i	night
ocul/o	eye
olecran/o	olecranon (elbow)
olig/o	scant
onych/o	nail
oo/o	egg
oophor/o	ovary
ophthalm/o	eye
opt/o	eye
optic/o	eye
or/o	mouth
orch/i	testicle
orch/o	testicle
orchi/o	testicle
orchid/o	testicle
orth/o	straight
oste/o	bone
ot/o	ear
ov/o	egg
ovari/o	ovary
ovul/o	egg
ox/i	oxygen
ox/o	oxygen
pachy/o	thick
palat/o	palate
palpebr/o	eyelid
pancreat/o	pancreas
patell/o	patella (kneecap)

pelv/i	pelvis (hip)
pericardi/o	pericardium
perine/o	perineum
peritone/o	peritoneum
phac/o	eye lens
phak/o	eye lens
phalang/o	phalanges (finger or toe)
pharyng/o	pharynx
phas/o	speech
phleb/o	vein
phren/o	mind
pil/o	hair
pituitar/o	pituitary gland
pleur/o	pleura
pneumat/o	air
pneumon/o	lung/air
poli/o	gray
polyp/o	polyp
pont/o	pons
proct/o	rectum
prostat/o	prostate gland
psych/o	mind
pub/o	pubis
pulmon/o	lung
pupill/o	pupil
py/o	pus
pyel/o	renal pelvis
pylor/o	pylorus
quadr/i	four
rachi/o	spine
radi/o	radius (lower arm)
radicul/o	nerve root
rect/o	rectum
ren/o	kidney
retin/o	retina
rhin/o	nose
sacr/o	sacrum

salping/o	uterine tube
scapul/o	scapula (shoulder)
scler/o	sclera
scoli/o	bent
seb/o	sebum/oil
sept/o	septum
sial/o	saliva
sigmoid/o	sigmoid colon
sinus/o	sinus
somat/o	body
son/o	sound
sperm/o	sperm
spermat/o	sperm
sphygm/o	pulse
spir/o	breath
splen/o	spleen
spondyl/o	vertebra
staped/o	middle ear
staphyl/o	clusters
steat/o	fat
ster/o or stere/o	solid, having three dimensions
stern/o	sternum (breast bone)
steth/o	chest
stomat/o	mouth
strept/o	twisted chain
synov/o	synovial membrane
tars/o	tarsal (ankle)
ten/o	tendon
tend/o	tendon (connective tissue)
tendin/o	tendon (connective tissue)
test/o	testicle
thorac/o	chest
thromb/o	clot
thym/o	thymus gland
thyr/o	thyroid gland
thyroid/o	thyroid gland
tibi/o	shin bone

toc/o	childbirth
tonsill/o	tonsil
top/o	place
tox/o	poison
toxic/o	poison
trache/o	trachea
trich/o	hair
tympan/o	ear drum
uln/o	ulna (lower arm bone)
ungu/o	nail
ur/o	urine
ureter/o	ureter
urethr/o	urethra
urin/o	urine
uter/o	uterus
uve/o	uvea
uvul/o	uvula
vagin/o	vagina
valv/o	valve
valvul/o	valve
vas/o	vessel
vascul/o	vessel
ven/o	vein
ventriculo/ventricul/o	ventricle
vertebr/o	vertebra
vesic/o	bladder
vesicul/o	seminal vesicles
vitre/o	glass
vulv/o	vulva
xanth/o	yellow
xer/o	dry

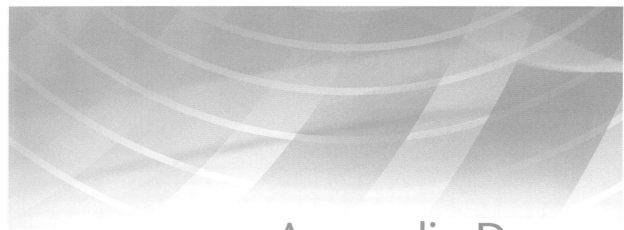

Appendix D

Prefixes

a-	not
an-	not
ante-	before
brady-	slow
de-	lack of
dys-	bad
ecto-	outside
endo-	within
epi-	on/upon
eso-	inward
eu-	good
exo-	outward
extra-	outside
hyper-	excess
hypo-	under
in-	into
inter-	between
intra-	within
multi-	many
neo-	new
nulli-	none

pan-	all
para-	beside
per-	through
peri-	surrounding
poly-	many
primi-	first
pseudo-	false
retro-	backwards
sub-	under
supra-	above
sym-	together
syn-	together
tachy-	fast
tetra-	four
tri-	three
tropin-	act on
uni-	one

Appendix E

Suffixes

-agon	assemble
-algesia	pain sensation
-algia	pain
-ar	pertaining to
-arche	beginning
-ary	pertaining to
-blast	embryonic
-capnia	carbon dioxide
-cele	hernia
-centesis	puncture to remove
-chezia	defecation
-clast, -clasia, -clasis	break
-coccus	bacterium
-cyesis	pregnancy
-desis	fusion
-dilation	widening, expanding
-drome	run
-dynia	pain
-eal	pertaining to
-ectasis	stretching
-ectomy	removal

-edema	swelling
-emia	blood
-esthesis	feeling
-gram	record
-graph	recording instrument
-graphy	recording process
-gravida	pregnancy
-ia	condition
-iatrist	physician specialist
-iatry	medical treatment
-ical	pertaining to
-in	a substance
-ine	a substance
-itis	inflammation
-listhesis	slipping
-lysis	separation
-malacia	softening
-megaly	enlargement
-meta	change
-meter	measure
-metry	measurement of
-oid	resembling
-oma	tumor
-opia	vision
-opsy	view of
-osis	condition
-oxia	oxygen
-para	woman who has given birth
-paresis	paralysis
-parous	to bear
-penia	deficient
-pexy	fixation
-phagia	eating
-phonia	sound
-phylaxis	protection
-physis	to grow
-plasty	surgical repair

-pnea	breathing
-poiesis	production
-poly	many
-porosis	spaces
-retro	behind
-rrhea	discharge
-rrhagia	bursting of blood
-rrhaphy	suture
-schisis	split
-sclerosis	hardening
-scopy	to examine
-spasm	contraction of muscle
-steat/o	fat
-stenosis	blockage
-stomy	opening
-thorax	chest
-tocia	labor
-tom/o	to cut
-tome	instrument that cuts
-tomy	incision
-tomy	cutting into
-tripsy	crush
-tropia	to turn
-tropin	act on
-uria	urine
-version	turning

Appendix F

Abbreviations

ABG	arterial blood gas
ABN	Advanced Beneficiary Notice used by CMS to notify beneficiary of payment of provider services
ACL	anterior cruciate ligament
AFB	acid-fast bacillus
AFI	amniotic fluid index
AGA	appropriate for gestational age
AGCUS	atypical glandular cells of undetermined significance
AKA	above-knee amputation
APCs	Ambulatory Patient Categories, patient classification that provides a payment system for outpatients
ARDS	adult respiratory distress syndrome
ARM	artificial rupture of membrane
ASCUS	atypical squamous cells of undetermined significance
ASCVD	arteriosclerotic cardiovascular disease
ASD	atrial septal defect
ASHD	arteriosclerotic heart disease
AV	atrioventricular
BCC	benign cellular changes
BiPAP	bi-level positive airway pressure
BKA	below-knee amputation
BPD	biparietal diameter

BPH	benign prostatic hypertrophy
BPP	biophysical profile
BV	bacterial vaginosis
bx	biopsy
C1-C7	cervical vertebrae
CABG	coronary artery bypass graft
CF	conversion factor, national-dollar amount that is applied to all services paid on the Medicare Fee Schedule basis
CHF	congestive heart failure
CHL	crown-to-heel length
CK	creatine kinase
CMS	Centers for Medicare and Medicaid Services, formerly HCFA, Health Care Financing Administration
CNM	certified nurse midwife
COB	coordination of benefits, management of payment between two or more third-party payers for a service
COPD	chronic obstructive pulmonary disease
CPAP	continuous positive airway pressure
CPD	cephalopelvic disproportion
CPK	creatine phosphokinase
CPP	chronic pelvic pain
CTS	carpal tunnel syndrome
CVI	cerebrovascular insufficiency
D&C	dilation and curettage
D&E	dilation and evacuation
derm	dermatology
DRGs	Diagnosis-Related Groups, disease classification system that relates the type of inpatients a hospital treats (case mix) to the costs incurred by the hospital
DHHS	Department of Health and Human Services
DLCO	diffuse capacity of lungs for carbon monoxide
DSE	dobutamine stress echocardiography
DUB	dysfunctional uterine bleeding
ECC	endocervical curettage
EDC	estimated date of confinement
EDI	electronic data interchange, exchange of data between multiple computer terminals
EEG	electroencephalogram
EFM	electronic fetal monitoring
EFW	estimated fetal weight

EGA	estimated gestational age
EGD	esophagogastroduodenoscopy
EGJ	esophagogastric junction
EMC	endometrial curettage
EOB	explanation of benefits, remittance advice
EPO	Exclusive Provider Organization, similar to a Health Maintenance Organization except that the providers of the services are not prepaid, but rather are paid on a fee-for-service basis
EPSDT	Early and Periodic Screening, Diagnosis, and Treatment
ERCP	endoscopic retrograde cholangiopancreatography
ERT	estrogen replacement therapy
ESRD	end-stage renal disease
FAS	fetal alcohol syndrome
FEF	forced expiratory flow
FEV_1	forced expiratory volume in one second
$FEV_1:FVC$	ratio of forced expiratory volume in one second to forced vital capacity
FHR	fetal heart rate
FI	fiscal intermediary, financial agent acting on behalf of a third-party payer
FRC	functional residual capacity
FSH	follicle-stimulating hormone
FVC	forced vital capacity
fx	fracture
GERD	gastroesophageal reflux disease
HCFA	Health Care Financing Administration, now known as Centers for Medicare and Medicaid Services (CMS)
HCVD	hypertensive cardiovascular disease
HEA	hemorrhage, exudate, aneurysm
HHN	hand-held nebulizer
HJR	hepatojugular reflux
HPV	human papillomavirus
HSG	hysterosalpingogram
HSV	herpes simplexvirus
I&D	incision and drainage
IPAP	inspiratory positive airway pressure
IVF	in vitro fertilization
L1-5	lumbar vertebrae
LBBB	left bundle branch block
LEEP	loop electrosurgical excision procedure

LGA	large for gestational age
LVH	left ventricular hypertrophy
MAT	multifocal atrial tachycardia
MDI	metered dose inhaler
MI	myocardial infarction
MRI	magnetic resonance imaging
MSLT	multiple sleep latency testing
MVV	maximum voluntary ventilation
NCPAP	nasal continuous positive airway pressure
NSR	normal sinus rhythm
OA	osteoarthritis
PAC	premature atrial contraction
PAT	paroxysmal atrial tachycardia
PAWP	pulmonary artery wedge pressure
PCWP	pulmonary capillary wedge pressure
PEAP	positive end-airway pressure
PEEP	positive end-expiratory pressure
PEG	percutaneous endoscopic gastrostomy
PERL	pupils equal and reactive to light
PERRL	pupils equal, round, and reactive to light
PERRLA	pupils equal, round, and reactive to light and accommodation
PFT	pulmonary function test
PID	pelvic inflammatory disease
PND	paroxysmal nocturnal dyspnea
PROM	premature rupture of membranes
PST	paroxysmal supraventricular tachycardia
PSVT	paroxysmal supraventricular tachycardia
PTCA	percutaneous transluminal coronary angioplasty
PVC	premature ventricular contraction
RA	remittance advice, explanation of services
RA	rheumatoid arthritis
RBBB	right bundle branch block
RDS	respiratory distress syndrome
REM	rapid eye movement
RSR	regular sinus rhythm
RV	respiratory volume
RVH	right ventricular hypertrophy

RVS	relative value studies, list of procedures with unit values assigned to each
RV:TLC	ratio of respiratory volume to total lung capacity
SHG	sonohysterogram
SROM	spontaneous rupture of membranes
subcu, subq	subcutaneous
SUI	stress urinary incontinence
SVT	supraventricular tachycardia
T1-T12	thoracic vertebrae
TAH	total abdominal hysterectomy
TEE	transesophageal echocardiography
TIA	transient ischemic attack
TLC	total lung capacity
TLV	total lung volume
TM	tympanic membrane
TMJ	temporomandibular joint
TPA	tissue plasminogen activator
TST	treadmill stress test
TURBT	transurethral resection of bladder tumor
TURP	transurethral resection of prostate
UCR	usual, customary, and reasonable, third-party payers' assessment of the reimbursement for health care services, usual that which would ordinarily be charged for the service, customary, the cost of that service in that locale, and reasonable as assessed by the payer
UPJ	ureteropelvic junction
V/Q	ventilation/perfusion scan
VBAC	vaginal birth after cesarean

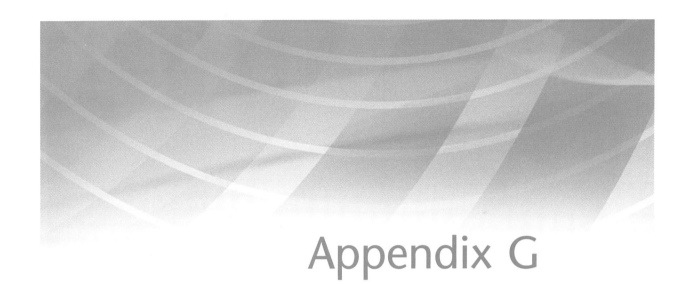

Appendix G

Further Text Resources

ANATOMY AND PHYSIOLOGY

Book Title	Author	Imprint	Publication Date	ISBN
The Anatomy and Physiology Learning System Textbook, 2nd Edition	Applegate	Saunders	2000	0-7216-8020-8
Structure and Function of the Body, 11th Edition (with CD-ROM)	Thibodeau, Patton	Mosby	2000	0-323-01081-4
Ross and Wilson—Anatomy and Physiology in Health and Illness, 9th Edition	Waugh, Grant	Churchill Livingstone	2001	0-443-06468-7

PATHOPHYSIOLOGY

Book Title	Author	Imprint	Publication Date	ISBN
Pathophysiology for the Health Related Professions, 2nd Edition	Gould	Saunders	2002	0-7216-9384-9
Essentials of Human Diseases and Conditions, 3rd Edition	Frazier, Drzymkowski, Doty	Saunders	2000	0-7216-0256-8
The Human Body in Health and Illness, 2nd Edition	Herlihy, Maebius	Saunders	2003	0-7216-9507-8
The Human Body in Health and Disease, 3rd Edition	Thibodeau, Patton	Mosby	2001	0-323-01338-4
Pathology for the Health-Related Professions, 2nd Edition	Damjanov	Saunders	2000	0-7216-8118-2

MEDICAL TERMINOLOGY

Book Title	Author	Imprint	Publication Date	ISBN
Medical Terminology: A Short Course, 2nd Edition	Chabner	Saunders	1999	0-7216-8124-7
Quick & Easy Medical Terminology, 3rd Edition	Leonard	Saunders	2000	0-7216-8271-5
Exploring Medical Language: A Student-Directed Approach, 5th Edition	LaFleur Brooks	Mosby	2001	0-323-01218-3
The Language of Medicine, 6th Edition	Chabner	Saunders	2004	0-7216-9757-7
Learning Medical Terminology, 9th Edition	Austrin, Austrin	Mosby	1998	0-323-00279-X
Medical Terminology: A Self-Learning Text, 3rd Edition	Birmingham	Mosby	1999	0-323-00406-7
Mastering Healthcare Terminology (with CD-ROM)	Shiland	Mosby	2002	0-323-01615-4
Introduction to Medical Terminology for Health Care: A Self-Teaching Package, 3rd Edition	Hutton	Churchill Livingstone	2002	0-443-07079-2
Medical Abbreviations and Eponyms, 2nd Edition	Sloane	Saunders	1997	0-7216-7088-1

INTRODUCTION TO COMPUTER

Book Title	Author	Imprint	Publication Date	ISBN
Computerized Medical Office Procedures: A Worktext	Larsen	Saunders	2002	0-7216-9213-3
Diehl & Fordney's Medical Transcribing: Techniques and Procedures, 5th Edition	Diehl Fordney	Saunders	2002	0-7216-9568-X

BASICS OF WRITING

Book Title	Author	Imprint	Publication Date	ISBN
Diehl & Fordney's Medical Transcribing: Techniques and Procedures, 5th Edition	Diehl, Fordney	Saunders	2002	0-7216-9568-X

COMPREHENSION BUILDING/STUDY SKILLS

Book Title	Author	Imprint	Publication Date	ISBN
Learning Strategies for Allied Health Students	Palau, Meltzer	Saunders	1995	0-7216-5603-X
Career Development for Health Professionals	Haroun	Saunders	2001	0-7216-8454-8
A Survivor's Guide to Study Skills and Student Assessments: For Health Care Students	Goodall	Churchill Livingstone	1997	0-443-05248-4

BASIC MATH

Book Title	Author	Imprint	Publication Date	ISBN
Basic Mathematics for the Health-Related Professions	Doucette	Saunders	2000	0-7216-7938-2
Using Maths in Health Sciences	Gunn	Churchill Livingstone	2001	0-443-07074-1

MEDICAL BILLING/INSURANCE

Book Title	Author	Imprint	Publication Date	ISBN
Insurance Handbook for the Medical Office, 8th Edition	Fordney	Saunders	2003	0-7216-0517-6
Medical Insurance Billing and Coding: An Essentials Worktext	French, Fordney	Saunders	2002	0-7216-9516-7
Medical Insurance Made Easy: A WorkText	Brown	Saunders	2001	0-7216-9187-0

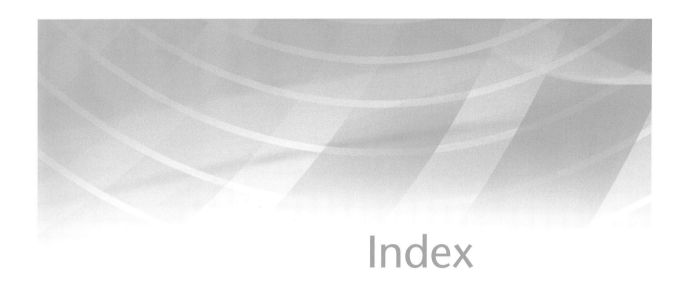

Index

5th digit. *See* Childbirth; Pregnancy; Puerperium

A

Abbreviations, 411-415
Abdomens, third-degree burn, 240-241
Abdominal aortic aneurysm, endovascular repair (34800-34832), 185
Abdominal cavity, 82
Abduction, 28
Abductor brevis, 29
ABG. *See* Arterial blood gas
Ablation, 41, 172, 375
ABN. *See* Advanced Beneficiary Notice
Abortion, 62, 337, 352-353, 375. *See also* Childbirth; Incomplete abortion; Liveborn fetus; Missed abortion; Pregnancy; Puerperium; Septic abortion; Spontaneous abortion
services (59812-59857). *See* Maternity care/delivery subsection
medical intervention, 197

Above-knee amputation (AKA), 31, 157, 411
Abuse, 132. *See also* Medicare
Accessory organs, 79, 237
Accessory sinuses, incision (31000-31090), 179
Accessory structures (10040-11646), 168-169
  benign lesions (11400-11646), 169
  biopsy (11100-11101), 169
  debridement (11000-11044), 168
  drainage (10040-10180), 168
  excision (11000-11044), 168
  incision (10040-10180), 168
  lesions, shaving (11300-11313), 169
  malignant lesions (11400-11646), 169
  paring (11055-11057), 168
  skin tag removal (11200-11201), 169
Acetabulum, 23, 35, 249, 275
Achilles tendon, 29
Acid balance, 71
Acid/base level (pH), 74
Acid-fast bacillus (AFB), 40, 411

ACL. *See* Anterior cruciate ligament
Acne, treatment, 174
ACTH. *See* Adrenocorticotropic hormone
Actinotherapy, 217, 375
Active immunization, bacteria/virus (usage), 211
Active wound care management (97601-97602). *See* Medicine section
debridement, 217
Acute care hospital records diagnoses, selection, 339-340. *See also* International Classification of Diseases (9th edition) Clinical Modification
Acute conditions, 343. *See also* Diagnosis coding
Acute cytitis, 227
Acute pancreatitis, 227
Acute renal failure (ARF), 74, 78
Acute renal insufficiency, 266, 313-314
Acute respiratory infection section, 235
Acute surgical care, 264, 309

Note: Page numbers followed by "f" refer to illustrations; page numbers followed by "t" refer to tables; page numbers followed by "b" refer to boxes.

Acute upper respiratory infection, 235

Adam's apple. *See* Trachea

Adduction, 28, 250, 276

Adenohypophysis, 99

Adenoidectomy, 41, 264, 308-309, 375

Adenoma, 346

ADH. *See* Antidiuretic hormone

Adipose, 14, 375

Admission, 155, 347
orders, 146

Adrenal cortex, 100

Adrenal gland, 100-112, 197, 250, 277, 375

Adrenal medulla, 100

Adrenocorticotropic hormone (ACTH), 99, 103

Adult abuse guidelines, 368

Adult respiratory distress syndrome (ARDS), 40, 45, 411

Adults, burns (calculation), 173f

Advanced Beneficiary Notice (ABN), 133, 411

Adverse effects, coding, 339, 357

AFB. *See* Acid-fast bacillus

AFI. *See* Amniotic fluid index

Afterbirth, 58

Aftercare, 339, 361-362

AGA. *See* Appropriate for gestational age

AGCUS. *See* Atypical glandular cells of undetermined significance

AHA, 226

AHFS. *See* American Hospital Formulary Service

AHIMA. *See* American Health Information Management Association

Airway pressure. *See* Continuous positive airway pressure; Inspiratory positive airway pressure; Nasal continuous positive airway pressure; Positive end-airway pressure

AKA. *See* Above-knee amputation

Albinism, 14, 375

Albumin, 47

Aldosterone, 100

Alimentary canal, 79

Allergen immunotherapy (95115-95199), 215-216

Allergies, 148

Allergy immunology (95004-95199), 215. *See also* Medicine section

Allergy testing (95004-95078), 215-216
coding, 215
example, 215

Allis maneuver, 260, 299

Allogenic cells, 189

Allograft, 14, 171, 252, 281, 375

Alopecia, 14, 375

Alphabetic index, 336. *See also* International Classification of Diseases (9th edition) Clinical Modification
cross references, 223
disease, etiology/manifestation, 223
eponyms, 223
neoplasm, 223
notes, 223
terms, 223

AMA. *See* American Medical Association

Ambulance modifiers. *See* Health Care Financing Administration Common Procedure Coding System

Ambulance services, 218

Ambulatory blood pressure monitoring, 187

Ambulatory Patient Categories (APCs), 136, 254, 411

American Health Information Management Association (AHIMA), 1, 226

American Hospital Formulary Service (AHFS), 225

American Medical Association (AMA), 140, 144

American Society of Anesthesiology (ASA), 257, 292

Amniocentesis, 62, 196, 375

Amniotic fluid index (AFI), 61, 411

Amniotic sac, 62, 375

A-mode ultrasound, 203, 375

Amphiarthroses, 25, 36

Amputation. *See* Above-knee amputation; Below-knee amputation

Amylase, 88

Anastomosis, 53, 84, 88, 375

Anatomic pathology (88000-88099), 206. *See also* Pathology/laboratory section
example, 210

Anatomic site arrangement, 177-178

Anatomy. *See* Final examination
quiz answers, 121-123
text resources, 417

Ancillary service, 133

Androgen, 100

And/with, usage, 222

Anesthesia, 140-142, 257-258, 261-262. *See also* Final examination; Unusual anesthesia
administering. *See* Surgeon
answers, 299-301, 320-321
formula, 160
section (00100-01999), 159-161
services, 257-258, 292-293
usage. *See* Multiple surgical procedures
uses, 149

Anesthesiologist, 159

Aneurysm, 53, 268, 375. *See also* False aneurysm; Venous reconstruction
endovascular repair. *See* Abdominal aortic aneurysm

Angina, 53, 252, 282-283, 375

Angiography, 53, 202-203, 375. *See also* Diagnostic radiology

Angioplasty, 53, 375. *See also* Venous reconstruction

Anhidrosis, 14, 376

Anomaloscope, 376

Anoscopy, 376

ANS. *See* Autonomic Nervous System

Answer sheet final. *See* Final examination

Antepartum, 62, 195, 237, 376

Antepartum care. *See* Maternity care/delivery subsection
(59990-59051), 196
delivery, inclusion, 196
episiotomies, 197
excision (59100-59160), 196
forceps, usage, 197
global routine care/delivery, physician (providing), 197
introduction (59200), 196
repair (59300-59350), 196
routine global obstetric care, 196-197

Anterior cruciate ligament (ACL), 31, 411

Anterior pituitary, 99-100

Anterior segment, 117, 376

Anterior (ventral), 376

Anteroposterior, 376

Antibodies, 47

Antidiuretic hormone (ADH), 100, 103

Antigen, 376

Antrum, 87

Aortic valve, 50, 55

Aortography, 376

APCs. *See* Ambulatory Patient Categories

Apexcardiography, 376

Block, 377
Block 21, 220
Block 24E, 220
Block 24-G, 192
Block 27, 127
    example, 141f
Blood, 47
    bank codes, 209
    cells. *See* Leukocytes
        formation, 19
    cleansing, dialysis (usage), 213
    diseases, 337. *See also*
        International Classification
        of Diseases (9th edition)
        Clinical Modification
    draw, 209
    formed part, 47
    gas. *See* Arterial blood gas
    liquid part, 47
Blood-forming organs, diseases.
    See International
    Classification of Diseases (9th
    edition) Clinical
    Modification
Blood pressure (BP), 195, 234,
    337, 349
    elevation, 235
    monitoring. *See* Ambulatory
        blood pressure monitoring
Blood urea nitrogen (BUN), 74,
    272, 328-329
Body, planes, 200-202, 201f
    component
        coding, 200
        modifiers, 201-202
    global procedures, 201
    position/projection, 200
    professional component,
        200-201
    technical component, 201
Bold type, usage, 22
Bones, 176. *See also* Ear; Flat
    bones; Irregular bones; Long
    bones; Sesamoid bones; Short
    bones
    classification, 19
    fragment, 262, 304
    grafts, 176
    marrow, 97, 168, 250, 277
    names, 28-29
    structure, 20f
    tendons, connection, 28
Botulism antitoxin, 211
BP. *See* Blood pressure
BPD. *See* Biparietal diameter
BPH. *See* Benign prostatic
    hypertrophy
BPP. *See* Biophysical profile
Braces (punctuation), usage, 222
Brachiocephalic family, 184f

Brachytherapy, 270, 323, 377. *See
    also* Intracoronary
        brachytherapy; Radiation
        oncology
Brackets
    codes. *See* Primary diagnosis
    usage, 221. *See also* Slanted
        brackets
Brain, 101, 105-107, 106f. *See also*
    Nervous system subsection
Brainstem, 105-106, 250, 278
Breasts, 58, 168
    biopsies, 259, 298
    procedures (19000-19499), 174
    structure, 58f
Bronchi, 38, 45
Bronchi (31600-31899), 180
    incision (31600-31614), 180
    introduction (31700-31730), 180
    repair (31750-31830), 180
Bronchiole, 41, 377
Bronchitis, 235
Bronchography, 377
Bronchoplasty, 41, 377
Bronchoscopy, 41, 377
B-scan ultrasound, 203-204, 377
Bulbocavernosus, 74, 377
Bulbourethral, 69, 74, 377
    gland, 65, 251, 279
BUN. *See* Blood urea nitrogen
Bundled codes, 377
Bundled procedures, 189
Bundled services, 216
Bundle of His, 50, 53-55, 187,
    250, 278, 377
Bunion, 32, 377
Burns. *See* Abdomens; Chemicals;
    Drugs; Thighs
    category 948, 240
    classification, 240
    coding, 339, 355-356
    depth, 240
    estimation. *See* Children
    example, 240-241
Burns (16000-16036), 172
    calculation. *See* Adults
    estimation. *See* Children
Burr, 109, 249, 275, 377
Bursa, 25, 377
Bursitis, 32, 377
BV. *See* Bacterial vaginosis
bx. *See* Biopsy
Bypass, 53, 377. *See also*
    Cardiopulmonary

C

C1-C7. *See* Cervical vertebrae
CAB. *See* Coronary Artery Bypass
CABG. *See* Coronary artery
    bypass graft

Calcaneal, 377
Calcaneus, 249, 275
Calculus, 74, 377
Calyces, 72, 77
Calycoplasty, 74, 377
Calyx, 74, 377
Cancellous, 377
Cannula, 179
Capillaries, 48, 55
Carbuncles, 252
Cardiac catheterization, 186, 252,
    282-283
Cardiac tissues, 27
Cardiac valves (33400-33496), 183
    Coronary Artery Bypass (CAB),
        183
Cardiogram. *See*
    Electrocardiogram;
    Phonocardiogram;
    Vectorcardiogram
Cardiography. *See*
    Apexcardiography
Cardiology. *See* Nuclear
    cardiology
    coding terminology, 181
    consultation, 255
Cardiopulmonary (CP), 53, 377
    bypass, 53, 182, 377
    resuscitation, 273, 332
Cardiovascular (CV) system, 47-
    56, 256, 289. *See also* Final
    examination
    forms, combination, 50-51
    medical abbreviations, 52-53
    medical terms, 53-54
    prefixes, 51-52
    quiz, 55-56
        answers, 121
    suffixes, 52
Cardiovascular (CV) system
    (33010-37799), 181-185
    arteries (34001-37799), 183-
        184
    cardiology coding terminology,
        181
    repairs (34501-34530), 184-
        185
    usage. *See* Medicine section;
        Radiology section; Surgery
        section
    veins (34001-37799), 183-184
    venous reconstruction (34501-
        34530), 184-185
Cardiovascular disease. *See*
    Arteriosclerotic
    cardiovascular disease
Cardioversion, 186, 377
Cardioverter-defibrillators, 53,
    378. *See also* Heart;
    Pericardium

Dual energy X-ray absorptiometry (DEXA), 284
DUB. *See* Dysfunctional uterine bleeding
Ducts, 65, 69. *See also* Bile duct; Cystic duct; Hepatic duct; Pancreatic duct; Thyroglossal duct
Duodenography, 380
Duodenum, 80, 87, 249, 275
Durable Medical Equipment (DME), 133, 135, 218
Dysfunctional uterine bleeding (DUB), 61, 412
Dysphagia, 84, 380
Dysphonia, 42, 380
Dysplasia, 264
Dyspnea, 42, 380. *See also* Paroxysmal nocturnal dyspnea
Dysuria, 74

E

Ear. *See* External ear; Inner ear; Internal ear; Middle ear
bones, 21, 35
structure, 21f
Early and Periodic Screening Diagnosis and Treatment (EPSDT), 413
ECC. *See* Endocervical curettage
ECG. *See* Electrocardiogram
Echocardiogram. *See* Transesophageal echocardiogram
Echocardiography, 204, 380. *See also* Dobutamine stress echocardiography; Transesophageal echocardiography
Echoencephalography, 380
Echography, 380
E codes, 224, 366-369. *See also* International Classification of Diseases (9th edition) Clinical Modification
guidelines, 239, 366-367
identity, 239
intent, 239
Ectopic, 62, 380
pregnancy, 267, 316
ED. *See* Emergency department
EDC. *See* Estimated date of confinement
EDD. *See* Estimated date of delivery
Edema, 53, 380
EDI. *See* Electronic Data Interchange; Electronic data interchange

EEG. *See* Electroencephalogram
EFM. *See* Electronic fetal monitoring
EFW. *See* Estimated fetal weight
EGA. *See* Estimated gestational age
EGD. *See* Esophagogastroduodenoscopy
EGJ. *See* Esophagogastric junction
EIN. *See* Employer Identification Number
Elbow, tip, 36
Elective surgery, 380
Electrical stimulation, 176
Electrocardiogram (ECG), 144, 186, 380
Electrocautery, 15, 380
Electrocochleography, 380
Electrode, 53, 380
Electroencephalogram (EEG), 109, 216, 274, 334, 381, 412
Electroencephalography, 109
Electrolysis, 174
Electrolytes, maintenance, 71
Electromyogram, 381
Electromyography, 216
Electronic analysis, 187
Electronic claim submission, 381
Electronic Data Interchange (EDI), 133
Electronic data interchange (EDI), 412
Electronic fetal monitoring (EFM), 61, 412
Electronic signature, 381
Electro-oculogram, 381
Electrophysiologic operative procedures. *See* Heart; Pericardium
Electrophysiology (EP), 53, 181, 381
system. *See* Heart
Elevated blood pressure. *See* Blood
E/M. *See* Evaluation/management
Embolectomy, 54 , 381. *See also* Arteries; Veins
Embolus, 184
Embryo, 58
EMC. *See* Endometrial curettage
Emergency department (ED) codes (99291, 99292), 156-157
services (99281-99288), 156
Emphysema, 42, 381
Employer Identification Number (EIN), 133
Encephalography, 381
Encounters, 347
form, 133
Endarterectomy, 54, 381
Endocardium, 49, 55

Endocervical curettage (ECC), 61, 412
Endocrine diseases, 348. *See also* International Classification of Diseases (9th edition) Clinical Modification
Endocrine glands, disorders, 232-233
Endocrine system, 47, 99-104, 99f
forms, combination, 101-102
medical terms, 102
prefixes, 102
quiz, 103-104
answers, 122
suffixes, 102
Endocrine system (60000-60599), 197-198
thyroid gland, excision category (60001-60281), 198
Endometrial curettage (EMC), 61, 413
Endometrium, 57, 63
repair, 58
Endomyocardial, 381
Endopyelotomy, 74, 381
Endoscopic catheterization, 270, 322-323
Endoscopic retrograde cholangiopancreatography (ERCP), 83, 88, 413
Endoscopy, 32, 381. *See also* Digestive system
(29800-29999), 177
(56820-56821), 193
(57420, 57421), 193
codes, 190
rules, 178
terminology, 189
Endosteum, 35
Endothelium, 47
Endotracheal intubation, 180
Endovascular repair, 184. *See also* Abdominal aortic aneurysm
End-stage renal disease (ESRD), 74, 78, 126, 213, 274, 333, 413
dialysis services, 214
ENT, 178
Enterolysis, 84, 381
Enucleation, 117, 381
EOBs. *See* Explanation of benefits
Eosinophils, 47
EP. *See* Electrophysiology
Epicardial, 54, 381
approach, 182
Epicardium, 49, 55
Epidermis, 237
Epidermolysis, 15, 381

Herniated disk, 269, 319-320
Herpes simplex virus (HSV), 61, 413
HHN. *See* Hand-held nebulizer
High-complexity MDM, 152
High-risk pregnancy, supervision, 363
High-risk presenting problem, 154
His, bundle. *See* Bundle of His
Histology, 383
History, 359-360. *See also* Comprehensive history; Detailed history; Family history; Past Family and Social History; Problem-focused history
  elements, 147, 150f
  levels, 148-149
History of Present Illness (HPI), 147-149
HIV. *See* Human Immunodeficiency Virus
HJR. *See* Hepatojugular reflux
HMO. *See* Health Maintenance Organization
Holter monitor, 186
Holter report, 251-252, 280
Home health care, 128
Home services (99341-99350), 157
Homograft, 15, 383
Hormone, 99-100, 102, 383
  release, 101
Hospice care, 128
Hospital
  care. *See* Initial hospital care; Subsequent hospital care
  codes, 163
  discharge services (99238, 99239), 155
  inpatient services (99221-99239), 155
  types, 155
  observation status (99217-99220; 99234-99239), 154-155
  services, 145
  setting, 155
Hospitalizations, 148
H&P, 195. *See also* Newborn
HPI. *See* History of Present Illness
HPV. *See* Human papilloma virus
HSG. *See* Hysterosalpingogram
HSV. *See* Herpes simplex virus
Human Chorionic Gonadotropin (HCG), 103
  production, 59, 101

Human Immunodeficiency Virus (HIV) (Section I, C1). *See* International Classification of Diseases (9th edition) Clinical Modification
HIV-related illness, previous diagnosis, 231, 345
  inconclusive laboratory test, 231
  infections, 344-346, 351
  pregnancy, relationship, 231
  screening, 231
  sequencing, 231
  testing, 345-346
Human papilloma virus (HPV), 61, 413
Humerus, 24, 36
Hydrocele, 74, 383
Hymen, 57
Hyoid bones, 21-22
Hyperextension, 28
Hyperopia, 117, 383
Hypertension, 258, 293, 337, 348. *See also* Controlled hypertension; Uncontrolled hypertension
  heart disease, interaction, 234
  types, 234-235
Hypertensive cardiovascular disease (HCVD), 53, 413
Hypertensive cerebrovascular disease, 234, 337, 349
Hypertensive heart disease, 234, 337, 349
Hypertensive renal disease, 337, 349
  chronic renal failure, 234, 348
Hypertensive retinopathy, 234, 349
Hypogastric, 383
Hypophysis. *See* Pituitary gland
Hyposensitization, 383
Hypothalamus, 100-101, 106, 250, 277
Hypothermia, 383
Hypoxemia, 54
Hypoxia, 54, 383
Hysterectomy, 62, 383. *See also* Total abdominal hysterectomy
Hysterorrhaphy, 62, 383
Hysterosalpingogram (HSG), 61, 413
Hysterosalpingography, 383
Hysteroscopy, 62, 383

I

ICD-9-CM. *See* International Classification of Diseases (9th edition) Clinical Modification
ICF. *See* Intermediate care facility

Ichthyosis, 15, 383
I&D. *See* Incision and drainage
Ideopathic respiratory distress syndrome (IRDS), 41
Ileostomy, 84, 383
Ileum, 80, 87, 249, 275
Iliopsoas, 29
Ilium, 23, 35, 383
Ill-defined conditions, 338, 355. *See also* International Classification of Diseases (9th edition) Clinical Modification
Illnesses, 148
  severity, 390
Imbrication, 84, 383
Immune function, 93
Immune globulins (90281-90399). *See* Medicine section
  codes, division, 211-212
  dose division, 212
  method division, 211
  type division, 211
Immunity disorders, 348. *See also* International Classification of Diseases (9th edition) Clinical Modification section, 233
Immunizations, 148, 273, 330. *See also* Active immunization; Medicine section; Passive immunization administration (90471-90474). *See* Medicine section
  methods, 212
  administration coding, 273
  report administration, 212
Immunology (86000-86849). *See* Pathology/laboratory section
Immunotherapy, 383. *See also* Allergen immunotherapy
Impending condition, 344
Incarcerated, 84, 383
Incise, 15, 383
Incision, 163, 174. *See also* Ovary; Oviduct
  (10040-10180), 168
  (30000-30020), 179
  (31000-31090), 179
  (31600-31614), 180
  (31750-31830), 181
  (56405-56441), 192
Incision and drainage (I&D), 14, 168, 413
Includes notes, usage, 222, 341
Incomplete abortion, 197
Incus, 21, 35, 114, 119
Individual Practice Association (IPA), 383
Industrial accidents. *See* Appendices

Positron Emission Tomography (PET), 219
  example, 219
  modifiers. *See* Health Care Financing Administration Common Procedure Coding System
Posterior, 389. *See also* Dorsal
  posterior
  segment, 117, 389
Posterior pituitary, 100
Posteroanterior, 389
Postoperative diagnosis, 264-265, 310-312
Postoperative management (-55), 163
Postoperative period
  operating room, return (-78), 164
  staged/related (-58), 161
  unrelated E/M services, physician usage (-24), 161
  unrelated procedure (-79), 174
Postoperative procedures, 166-167
Postpartum, 62-63, 237, 389
  care, 196
  curettage, 196
  period, 337, 352. *See also* Childbirth; Pregnancy; Puerperium
PPO. *See* Preferred Provider Organization
Practice examination, 244
Preferred Provider Organization (PPO), 132, 389
Prefixes, 405-406
Pregnancy, 57-64, 101, 363-364
  abortions, 237
  complications, 338, 350-353. *See also* International Classification of Diseases (9th edition) Clinical Modification
  general rules, 236
  late effect, 352
  fifth (5th) digit, 237
  forms, combination, 59-60
  medical abbreviations, 61-62
  medical terms, 62
  postpartum period, 237
  prefixes, 60
  primary diagnosis, selection, 236
  quiz, 63-64
    answers, 121
  relationship. *See* Human Immunodeficiency Virus; Menstruation
  repair, 196
  suffixes, 60-61
  terminology, 57-58

Premalignant tissue, 172
Premature atrial contraction (PAC), 53, 414
Premature rupture of membranes (PROM), 62
Premature ventricular contraction (PVC), 53, 414
Prematurity, 338, 354-355
Premenstruation, 58
Prenatal outpatient visits, 350
Preoperative diagnosis, 261-262, 264-265, 268
  answers, 302-305, 310-312, 318-319
Preoperative procedures, 166-167
Presenting problem. *See also* High-risk presenting problem; Low-risk presenting problem; Minimal presenting problem; Moderate-risk presenting problem; Self-limiting presenting problem
  levels, 153-154
  nature, 153
Pressure ulcers (15920-15999), 172
Presurgical discontinuance, 162
Preventive medicine services (99381-99429), 158
Priapism, 67, 389
Primary care physician (PCP), 389
Primary diagnosis, 389
  brackets, codes (section I, C17), 228
  interrelated conditions (section II, B), 228
  selection. *See* Childbirth; International Classification of Diseases (9th edition) Clinical Modification; Pregnancy; Puerperium
Primary thyroid hyperplasia, 233
Prior approval, 389
Prior authorization, 134
PRL. *See* Prolactin
PRO. *See* Peer Review Organization
Problem-focused examination, 149. *See also* Expanded problem-focused examination
Problem-focused history, 148-149. *See also* Expanded problem-focused history
Procedural service. *See* Distinct procedural service; Unusual procedural service

Procedure. *See* Bilateral procedure; Discontinued procedure; Infants; Multiple procedure; Multiple surgical procedures; Separate procedures; Tissue
  codes, 167. *See also* Unlisted procedure codes
  service. *See* Repeat procedure/service
Procreative management, 363
Proctosigmoidoscopy, 85, 189, 389
Professional component (-26), 162
Professional Standards Review Organization (PSRO), 389
Progesterone, 99, 101, 103
Progestin, 100
Prognosis, 389
Prolactin (PRL), 100
Proliferation phase, 58
Prolonged E/M service (-21), 161
Prolonged services (99354-99359), 158
PROM. *See* Premature rupture of membranes
Pronation, 28, 250, 276
Proprioceptors, 115, 119
Prostate cancer, 270, 323
Prostate gland, 65, 69, 191, 251, 279
Prostate specific antigen (PSA) tests, 253, 283
Prostate transurethral resection, 67, 392
Prostatotemy, 67, 389
Provider Identification Number (PIN), 134, 389
PSA. *See* Prostate specific antigen
PSRO. *See* Professional Standards Review Organization
PSVT. *See* Paroxysmal supraventicular tachycardia
Psychiatric treatment, 213
Psychiatry (90801-90802). *See* Medicine section
Psychoses, 233
PTCA. *See* Percutaneous transluminal coronary angioplasty
PTH. *See* Parathyroid hormone
Pubis, 23
  symphysis, 23
Puerperium, complications, 338, 350-353. *See also* International Classification of Diseases (9th edition) Clinical Modification
  abortions, 237
  fifth (5th) digit, 237
  late effect, 352
  postpartum period, 237

SUI. *See* Stress urinary incontinence
Summing up formula, 160-161
Superior, 391
Supination, 28, 33, 391
Supine, 391
Suppression testing (80400-80440), 206. *See also* Pathology/laboratory section
consultations (clinical pathology) (80500-80502), 208
Supraventicular tachycardia (SVT), 415
Surgeon. *See* Assistant surgeon; Minimum assistant surgeon
anesthesia, administering (-47), 162
usage (-64), 164
Surgery, 142. *See also* Elective surgery; Intersex surgery; Invasive surgery; Mohs' micrographic surgery; Mohs' surgery; Noninvasive surgery
codes, 181
complications, 370
decision (-57), 163
Surgery section (10021-69990), 165-199
codes, 164
format, 165
notes/guidelines, 165-166
subsection (10021-10022), 168
Surgery section (10021-69990), CV usage, 181-183
cardiac valves (33400-33496), 183
heart (33010-33999), 182
pericardium (33010-33496), 182
procedures, codes, 181
Surgical arthroscopy, 177
Surgical care (-54), 163
Surgical packages, guidelines, 166-168
Surgical pathology (88300-88399), 206. *See also* Pathology/laboratory section
codes, inclusion, 211
examples, 210-211
levels, 210-211
terminology, 210
Surgical team (-66), 164
Surgical tray, 168
SVT. *See* Supraventicular tachycardia
Swan Ganz catheter, 54, 273, 332, 391
Sweat glands, 237

Sympathetic nerve, 109, 391
Sympathetic system, 107. *See also* Parasympathetic system
Symphysis, 391
Synarthroses, 24, 36
Synchondrosis, 33, 391
Synovial fluid, sacs, 25
Systole, 50, 55

T

T. *See* Time
T1-T12. *See* Thoracic vertebrae
Tabular list, 336. *See also* International Classification of Diseases (9th edition) Clinical Modification
diseases/injuries, classification, 225
divisions, 225
divisions, 224
Tachycardia. *See* Multifocal atrial tachycardia; Paroxysmal atrial tachycardia; Paroxysmal supraventicular tachycardia; Supraventicular tachycardia
history, 256, 289
Tachypnea, 42, 391
TAH. *See* Total abdominal hysterectomy
Tarsal, 24, 36. *See also* Metatarsal
dislocation, 260
Tarsorrhaphy, 118, 391
Taste, 115
Tax Equity and Fiscal Responsibility Act (TEFRA), 391
TEE. *See* Transesophageal echocardiography
Teeth, 79
TEFRA. *See* Tax Equity and Fiscal Responsibility Act
Temporal, 21, 28
Temporomandibular joint (TMJ), 32, 415
Tendons, 33, 391
connection. *See* Bones
Tenodesis, 33, 391
Tenorrhaphy, 33, 391
TENS. *See* Transcutaneous electrical nerve stimulator
Tenue, 249, 275
Terminology, quiz answers, 121-123
Terrorism guidelines, 369
Testes (gonads), 65, 69, 101, 191, 197-198
Testosterone, 65, 99, 101
Thalamus, 100, 106

Therapeutic drug assays (80150-80299), 206. *See also* Pathology/laboratory section example, 207
Therapeutic infusions (90780-90781). *See* Medicine section
Therapeutic services, 373. *See also* Medicine section
Therapeutic sinus tract injection procedures, 176
Thermograms, 187, 391
Thermoreceptors, 115, 119
Thighs, 29
second-degree burn, 240-241
Third-degree burn. *See* Abdomens
Third-party payer, 133, 134, 202, 391
confirmatory consultations, 144, 156
services/providers, 140
Thoracentesis, 43, 181, 391
Thoracic cage, 24f
Thoracic cavity, 89, 91
Thoracic duct, 95, 392
Thoracic vertebrae (T1-T12), 22, 32, 415
Thoracoplasty, 43, 392
Thoracostomy, 43, 54, 392
Thoracotomy, 43, 181, 392
Thorascopy, 43, 392
Thorax, bones, 22-23
Threatened condition, 344
Three-digit categories. *See* Appendices
Throat. *See* Pharynx
Thrombectomy. *See* Arteries; Percutaneous thrombectomy; Veins
Thromboendarterectomy, 54, 392
Thrombolysis, 186
Thrombus, 184
Thymectomy, 102, 392
Thymosin, 93, 100, 103
Thymus, 93, 97, 100-103, 197, 250, 277, 392
Thyroglossal duct, 102, 392
Thyroidectomy, 102, 268, 317, 392
Thyroid gland, 100, 102, 197, 392. *See also* Parathyroid gland
Thyroid isthmus, 102, 384
Thyroid-stimulating hormone (TSH), 100, 272, 327
Thyroxine (T4), 100
TIA. *See* Transient ischemic attack
Tibia, 24
Tibialis anterior, 29
Time-based code, usage, 163

Ureteroenterostomy, 75, 393
Ureterolithotomy, 75, 393. *See* Transvesical ureterolithotomy
Ureterolysis, 75, 393
Ureteroneocystostomy, 75, 393
Ureteropelvic junction (UPJ), 74, 415
Ureteropyelography, 75, 393
Ureterotomy, 75, 393
Ureters, 71-72
  subheading. *See* Kidneys
Urethra, 71, 77
Urethrocystography, 75, 393
Urethromeatoplasty, 75, 393
Urethropexy, 75, 393
Urethroplasty, 75, 393
Urethrorrhaphy, 75, 393
Urethroscopy, 75, 393
URI. *See* Upper respiratory infection
Urinalysis (81000-81099), 206. *See also* Pathology/laboratory section
  chemistry (82000-84999), 208-209
  equipment, usage, 208
  tests (number), performing, 208
Urinalysis (UA), 74, 271, 327
Urinary bladder, 71-73, 77
Urinary meatus, 73
Urinary system, 71-78, 71f
  forms, combination, 73
  medical abbreviations, 74
  medical terms, 74-75
  organs, 71-73
  prefixes, 73
  quiz, 77-78
    answers, 122
  suffixes, 73
Urinary system (50010-53899), 190-191
  anatomic division, 190
  kidney, subheading (50010-50590), 190-191
Urinary tract infection (UTI), 74
Urine, tests, 208
Urodynamics. *See* Kidneys
Urography, 393
URQ. *See* Upper right quadrant
Use additional code, usage, 222
Usual customary and reasonable (UCR), 134, 415
Uterine bleeding. *See* Dysfunctional uterine bleeding
Uterine serosa, 57
Uterine wall, 59
Uterus (womb), 57
UTI. *See* Urinary tract infection

Uveal, 118, 393
Uvula, 87

V

Vaccinations, 252, 282, 330, 358. *See also* Routine vaccinations
Vaccines. *See* Medicine section; Pneumococcal vaccine; Substance vaccine
  examples, 212
  reporting rule, 213
Vagina, 57, 63
Vagina (57000-57421), 193
  endoscopy (57420, 57421), 193
  introduction (57150-57180), 193
  manipulation (57400-57415), 193
  repair (57200-57335), 193
Vaginal birth after cesarean (VBAC), 62, 197, 415
Vaginalis. *See* Tunica vaginalis
Vaginosis. *See* Bacterial vaginosis
Value
  scale. *See* Resource-based relative value scale
  unit. *See* Relative value
Valves, 50
Varices, 85, 393
Varicocele, 67, 393
Vascular diagnostic studies. *See* Medicine section
Vascular families, 184f. *See also* Arteries; Veins
Vascular injection procedures. *See* Venous reconstruction
Vascular studies, 204. *See also* Medicine section
Vas deferens, 65, 67, 191, 393
Vasogram, 67, 394
Vasotomy, 67, 394
Vasovasorrhaphy, 67, 394
Vasovasostomy, 67, 394
VBAC. *See* Vaginal birth after cesarean
V codes, 224, 339, 358-366. *See also* International Classification of Diseases (9th edition) Clinical Modification
  categories, 358-359
  example, 228
  history, 359-360, 372
  neoplasms, relationship, 232
  usage, 358
  V30-V39, usage, 338, 353
Vectorcardiogram, 394
Veins, 48, 55. *See also* Circulatory system; Saphenous vein

Veins (34001-37799), 183-184
  embolectomy (34001-34490), 184
  thrombectomy (34001-34490), 184
  vascular families, 184
Venography, 394
Venous grafting. *See* Coronary Artery Bypass
Venous reconstruction. *See* Cardiovascular system
  aneurysm, 184-185
  angioplasty, 185
  arteriovenous fistula, repair (35180-35190), 185
  atherectomy, 185
  noncoronary bypass grafts (35500-35671), 185
  repair, types, 184
  vascular injection procedures (36000-36015), 185
Ventilation/perfusion scan (V/Q), 41, 415
Ventral. *See* Anterior
Ventricles, 56, 107
Ventricular fibrillation, 251, 280
Ventricular tachycardia, 251, 280
Venules, 48
Vertebrae, 107. *See also* Cervical vertebrae; Lumbar vertebrae; Thoracic vertebrae
Vertebral column, anterior view, 23f
Vertebrectomy, 109
Vertigo, 118, 255, 287, 394
Vesicostomy, 75, 394
Vesicovaginal fistula, 62, 394
Vesiculectomy, 67, 394
Vesiculography, 394
Vesiculotomy, 67, 394
Vessels, 47-48, 184f
  damage. *See* Chemicals; Drugs
  function, 47
  ligation, 170
  types, 47-48
Vestibule, 114, 119, 250, 278
Virus. *See* Herpes simplex virus; Human papilloma virus
  usage. *See* Active immunization
Viscera, 394
Visceral pericardium, 50
Visceral tissues, 28
Vitreous humor, 114, 119
Vocal cords, 38
Voice box. *See* Larynx
Volvulus, 85, 394
Vomer, 21, 394
V/Q. *See* Ventilation/perfusion scan
Vulva, 57

Vulva (56405-56821). *See* Female
  genital system
  destruction (56501-56515), 192
  endoscopy (56820-56821), 193
  excision (56605-56704), 192
    biopsy, 192
  incision (56405-56441), 192
  marsupialization, 192
  repair (56800-56810), 193
  vulvectomy, 192-193
Vulvectomy. *See* Introitus;
  Perineum; Vulva

W

WBCs. *See* White blood cells
Wedge pressure. *See* Pulmonary
  artery wedge pressure;
  Pulmonary capillary wedge
  pressure

White blood cells (WBCs), 209,
  271, 326. *See also* Leukocytes
Windpipe. *See* Trachea
Witzel technique, 265
Womb. *See* Uterus
Workers' Compensation, 162
Wound care management. *See*
  Medicine section
Wound exploration, 170
  (20100-20103), 175
Wound repair
  codes, inclusion, 170
  grouping, 170
    restrictions, 170
  repair factors, 170
  types, 170
Writing (basics), text resources,
  418

X

Xanthoma, 16, 394
Xenograft, 16, 171, 394
Xeroderma, 16, 394
Xeroradiography, 394

Z

Zygoma, 35
Zygomatic process, 21
Zygomaticus, 28